Nursing the Feline Patient

Nursing the Feline Patient

Editors

Linda E. Schmeltzer, RVT

Gary D. Norsworthy, DVM, DABVP (Feline)

WILEY-BLACKWELL

A John Wiley & Sons, Ltd., Publication

This edition first published 2012 © 2012 by John Wiley & Sons, Inc

Wiley-Blackwell is an imprint of John Wiley & Sons, formed by the merger of Wiley's global Scientific, Technical and Medical business with Blackwell Publishing.

Registered Office
John Wiley & Sons, Ltd, The Atrium, Southern Gate, Chichester, West Sussex, PO19 8SQ, UK

Editorial Offices
2121 State Avenue, Ames, Iowa 50014-8300, USA
The Atrium, Southern Gate, Chichester, West Sussex, PO19 8SQ, UK
9600 Garsington Road, Oxford, OX4 2DQ, UK

For details of our global editorial offices, for customer services and for information about how to apply for permission to reuse the copyright material in this book please see our website at www.wiley.com/wiley-blackwell.

Library of Congress Cataloging-in-Publication Data

Nursing the feline patient / editors, Linda E. Schmeltzer, Gary D. Norsworthy.
    p. ; cm.
  Includes bibliographical references and index.
  ISBN 978-0-470-95901-5 (pbk. : alk. paper)
I. Schmeltzer, Linda E. II. Norsworthy, Gary D.
[DNLM: 1. Cat Diseases–nursing. 2. Animal Technicians. SF 985]
  636.8′0896–dc23
                            2011036439

A catalogue record for this book is available from the British Library.

Wiley also publishes its books in a variety of electronic formats. Some content that appears in print may not be available in electronic books.

Set in 8/10pt Palatino by SPi Publisher Services, Pondicherry, India
Printed and bound in Malaysia by Vivar Printing Sdn Bhd

1 2012

Dedications

Linda E. Schmeltzer

I would like to dedicate this book to all veterinary technicians, formally trained or trained on the job, who are always interested in furthering their education and knowledge of the patients in their care.

To my husband, Eric, thank you for believing in me. To my sweet Katlyn, thank you for reminding me to take time out to be silly. To my mom and sister, you helped me more than you will ever know.

I am blessed to work with an awesome team of people everyday. Thank you for your dedication and for making work fun.

Dr. Norsworthy, my boss and coeditor, thank you for trusting me to lead your technician team. I've learned so much from you and have truly enjoyed sharing this project with you. Thank you for giving me this opportunity.

Gary D. Norsworthy

I would like to dedicate this book to the technicians who have made the rigors of private practice efficient and enjoyable for me and my colleagues. I would like to specifically mention Linda Schmeltzer, my head technician for over 10 years and my coeditor, and Emily Boulet, my personal technician for the last 2 years. Both of you have allowed me to concentrate on patient care at the veterinarian's level knowing that the details of patient care would be handled by you. I hope that my colleagues have technicians who are as efficient, competent, and fun to work with as these two special ladies.

Contents

Clinical cases, Q&As for downloading, and images from the book in PowerPoint are available for download at www.wiley.com/go/schmeltzernorsworthy.

Editors

Linda E. Schmeltzer, RVT
Head Technician
Alamo Feline Health Center
San Antonio, Texas

Gary D. Norsworthy, DVM, DABVP (Feline)
Chief of Staff
Alamo Feline Health Center
San Antonio, Texas
Adjunct Professor
College of Veterinary Medicine
Mississippi State University

Contributors

Barbara Bockstahler, PhD, DVM, CCRP
Head of Physical Therapy
University of Veterinary Medicine
Clinic for Surgery and Ophthalmology
Vienna, Austria

Susan Bryant, CVT, VTS (Anesthesia)
Veterinary Technician Manager
Tufts Cummings School of Veterinary Medicine
North Grafton, Massachusetts

Rick L. Cowell, DVM, MS, MRCVS, DACVP
IDEXX Laboratories
Stillwater, Oklahoma

Keith DeJong, DVM, Dipl. ACVP
Clinical Pathologist
Professional Services Veterinarian, Northwest Area
Abaxis North American Animal Health
Union City, California

J. Scot Estep, DVM, DACVP
Chief of Comparative Pathology
US ARMY Institute of Surgical Research
Spring Branch, Texas

Diana Eubanks, DVM, MS, DABVP, FAVD
Associate Clinical Professor
Mississippi State University College of Veterinary Medicine
Mississippi State, Mississippi

Sharon Fooshee Grace, MAgric, MS, DVM, DABVP (Canine-Feline), DACVIM (Small Animal)
Clinical Professor
Program Leader for Student Affairs
Mississippi State University College of Veterinary Medicine Department of Clinical Sciences
Mississippi State, Mississippi

Merrilee Holland, DVM, DACVR
Associate Professor
Radiology
Auburn University College of Veterinary Medicine
Auburn, Alabama

Judith Hudson, DVM, PhD, DACVR
Professor
Auburn University College of Veterinary Medicine
Auburn, Alabama

Nicole Atkens Humphreys, MBA, RVT
Critical Care Specialist and Sales
The Pet Blood Bank, Inc.
Lago Vista, Texas

Laura V. Lane, DVM, DACVP
Resident (Clinical Pathology)
Department of Veterinary Pathobiology
Oklahoma State University
Stillwater, Oklahoma

David Levine, PT, PhD, DPT, OCS, CCRP
Walter M. Cline Chair of Excellence in Physical Therapy
Professor
Department of Physical Therapy
The University of Tennessee at Chattanooga
Chattanooga, Tennessee

Karen M. Lovelace DVM
Veterinarian
Ventura, California

Ludovic Pelligand, DVM, MRCVS, Dipl. ECVAA
North Hymms, Hatfield
Royal Veterinary College
Hertfordshire, United Kingdom (England)

Eric Schmeltzer, DVM
Veterinarian
Boerne, Texas

Craig M. Tockman, DVM
Director of Professional Services
Abaxis North American Animal Health
Wildwood, Missouri

Teija Kaarina Viita-aho, DVM
Helsinki, Finland

Preface

According to the 2011–2012 American Pet Products Association survey, there are 86.4 million cats owned in the United States and 78.2 million dogs. Veterinary technicians should be well educated in the unique qualities of the feline patient. The goal of this book is to address all aspects of feline nursing from the examination room to the surgical suite. I hope it proves to be an excellent resource for any practicing veterinary technician as well as a useful reference for technician students.

Linda Schmeltzer, RVT

SECTION

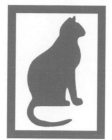

1

Patient Management

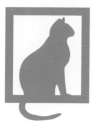

CHAPTER 1

Patient History and Physical Examination

Nicole Atkens Humphreys

Introduction

One of the most important parts of a medical record is the patient history. Without an accurate and detailed history, the most experienced veterinarian may not be able to define the problems of a particular patient. A thorough history may be time consuming, but in a busy practice, a technician can begin the history-taking process thus allowing the veterinarian to ask the client other pertinent questions. The key to history taking is asking the right questions to obtain the most important information. History-taking questions are important details that alert the veterinarian or veterinary technician to problems or symptoms that may be contributing factors to the patient's ailment. Questions will vary among species being evaluated, but in general they should remain unbiased so as not to lead the client toward a specific answer.

Because cats cannot speak, the owner is relied upon during the patient history-taking process. Asking a question in an unbiased fashion may require the owner to reflect on a change in the pet's behavior and overall health and draw conclusions whether this change has been a positive or negative one. More often than not, a question may have to be asked more than once but phrased in a slightly different way to make sure the owner understands the question and is consistent with answers. When asking specific questions be mindful of the owner's ability or inability to observe the cat. Questions such as "Does your cat have diarrhea?" may not be as suitable as "Have you noticed a change in your cat's stool?"

The medical record is comprised of pertinent facts about the patient's life and health history. It can be used to describe past and present illnesses as well as treatments that were ordered by the clinician. The history provided by the animal's owner, the veterinarians' observations, and results of any laboratory tests that were performed help determine a diagnosis or course of treatment for a particular patient.

It is important to create a complete patient history. Begin with owner's name, address, and telephone numbers (home, work, cell, pager, fax, etc.). The cat should be assigned an identification number or a case number. The cat's name and signalment (age, gender, breed, and species) should also be entered into the chart so the correct history is linked to the patient.

Use of a standard history form ensures that all of the pertinent questions are asked (Table 1-1).

Signalment

The signalment of an animal is the age, gender, breed, and species; these are crucial pieces of data for developing the history and ruling out specific problems. Certain disease processes and ailments are inherited or are more common in certain breeds. Age is relevant in obtaining a history for many reasons. Older patients may show similar symptoms but for different reasons than younger ones. For example, a young energetic and curious cat may vomit due to a foreign body. An older more geriatric cat may vomit due to chronic pancreatitis, renal disease, or small bowel disease. Knowing the age of the patient may alert the technician or veterinarian to ask age-appropriate questions regarding the issues. Knowing the breed of an animal is especially helpful when trying to rule out

genetic diseases. Maine Coon cats commonly develop hypertrophic cardiomyopathy (HCM). When a Maine Coon cat has cardiac signs, the veterinarian will consider HCM and perform relevant tests. Knowing reproductive status helps when considering disorders related to gender.

Chief Complaint and History of Illness

It is important to determine the primary reason for the visit. This is known as the chief complaint. It is crucial that that the owner is given time to elaborate on the reason the cat was brought in. Because this process can be prolonged if the conversation is not controlled, specific questions will quickly lead to a definitive reason for the visit. Not focusing on the primary complaint can lead to improper tests or misdiagnoses.

Understanding the chief complaint will lead to questions regarding severity and duration. This information will determine how aggressive the diagnostic workup should be and how quickly therapy must be instituted.

Past Illness and Surgical History

Past medical illness and surgical history can lead to a more rapid diagnosis and greatly affect the outcome of certain cases. For example, a cat brought in for increased urination can have its presenting sign as a result of current furosemide administration for cardiac disease instead of renal failure or diabetes. Not knowing the cat was given a drug that can cause increased urination may result in unnecessary tests.

Dietary and Environmental History

Knowing the type of food and the daily quantity consumed will provide helpful insights when dealing with weight change (increased or decreased), obesity, and other problems such as vomiting or diarrhea. Diet is especially important when obtaining a history for feline patients because cats are frequently picky eaters only consuming highly palatable foods. The timing of a food consumption change can be helpful in understanding the duration of a problem. An understanding of a cat's dietary preferences can be helpful in establishing quality dietary intake in the hospital setting.

A cat's habitat is also important in assessing the patient. It is important to know if a cat is an indoor cat, an indoor-outdoor cat, a supervised outdoor cat, or a free-roaming outdoor cat. Environmental situations pose a wide variety of potential toxins and hazards that can contribute to problems and illnesses. Outdoor cats are more prone to ethylene glycol poisoning, retroviral conditions (feline immunodeficiency virus [FIV] feline leukemia virus [FeLV]), infections, and trauma. It is also important to understand the number of pets and species in the household because households with ten cats or more are more prone to gastrointestinal and respiratory diseases and behavior problems.

Complete Physical Examination

The physical examination is one of the most important parts of a diagnostic workup. Despite the number of blood, urine, and imaging tests available, all of those must be interpreted in light of physical

Nursing the Feline Patient, First Edition. Edited by Linda E. Schmeltzer and Gary D. Norsworthy.
© 2012 John Wiley & Sons, Inc. Published 2012 by John Wiley & Sons, Inc.

TABLE 1-1: History and Examination Record

History and Examination Record

Doctor: _____   Technician: _____

Species: _____   Sex: M Mn F Fs   Age: _____   Last visit: _____

Vaccines: ☐ Never Current Not current

Last time(s) given _____

Weight: _____   Last Weight & Date: _____   Temp: _____

Chief Complaint:

_____

Appetite: ☐ Anorexia ☐ Greatly reduced ☐ Slightly reduced Normal ☐ Slightly increased ☐ Greatly increased Duration from normal: _____

Diet: List foods, canned vs. dry, and % of each _____

Meds taken including HW and flea control products: _____

Vomiting: ☐ Never ☐ < 1/mo ☐ 1/mo ☐ 2-3/mo ☐ 1/w ☐ > 1/w

Stool: ☐ Hard ☐ Normal ☐ Watery ☐ Pancake Batter ☐ Soft Serve Ice Cream

Color: _____

Urine: ☐ Less than normal amt ☐ Normal amount ☐ More than normal amt

Blood present: _____

Activity level: ☐ Very lethargic ☐ Reduced ☐ Normal ☐ Increased ☐ Sleeps less

Exam Notes: _____

_____

_____

Plan: _____

_____

Follow-up: _____

TABLE 1-2: Sample History Questions for Body Systems

System	Sample Questions
General Attitude	Is your cat playful? Is it interested in its surroundings?
Integument	Is your cat scratching, licking, or biting more than usual? Do you notice changes in your cat's skin or hair coat?
Respiratory	Does your cat have nasal discharge? Have you noticed your cat sneezing, coughing, or wheezing?
Cardiovascular	Have you noticed a change in your cat's activity level? Is respiration rapid or labored?
Gastrointestinal	Has your cat vomited? If so, how often? Have you noticed a change in stool?
Urogenital	Is your cat intact? Have you noticed changes in your cat's urinary habits? Does your cat drink more or less than usual?
Nervous	Does your cat seem alert and aware of its surroundings? Have there been any seizures?
Musculoskeletal	Have you noticed lameness, weakness, or reluctance to move or jump?

examination findings. It is important to develop a systematic approach so no aspect of the examination is inadvertently omitted. Some choose an approach based on major body systems as described. Others prefer a "geographic" approach beginning with the head and progressing caudally. Regardless of the approach, it should be used consistently.

The physical examination process begins when the patient arrives in the examination room. The first impression of how the cat looks and acts is essential, although one must realize that some cats are unusually withdrawn or aggressive in a clinical setting. It is important to recognize the "Three A's of Examination:" Appearance, Attitude, and Awareness are significant segments of an initial examination. It is important to remember that cats like to explore. Many times when a cat is taken out of its carrier in an examination room, it wants to smell and explore its new surroundings. Take note if a cat seems uninterested or unable to respond to the new stimuli of the examination room. Is the cat trying to hide? Does the cat seem angry? These subtle observations can also determine how the cat will act during examination. It is important that every observation is documented in the patient record, and each entry be initialed by the observer. This eliminates any confusion when trying to document entries regarding history and examinations.

Another component of the physical examination is the assessment. Simply stated, each system or body region is examined for abnormalities

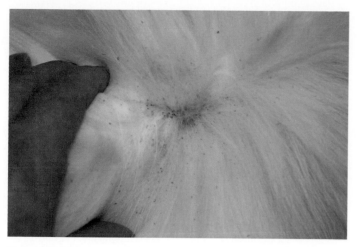

Figure 1-1 There was some evidence of flea dirt on this cat's hair coat; however, when the hair was brushed backward copious amounts of flea dirt were seen. Brushing the hair coat backward often reveals abnormalities that can easily be missed.

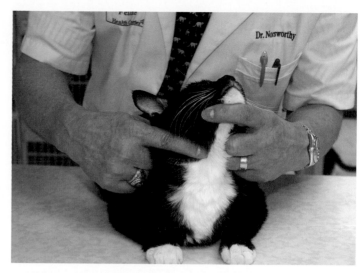

Figure 1-3 Sensitive thyroid palpation is performed on one side at a time with the tip of one's index finger placed in the groove between the trachea and the sternohyoideus muscle. It is important that the chin be lifted 45 degrees and turned 45 degrees away from the side to be palpated.

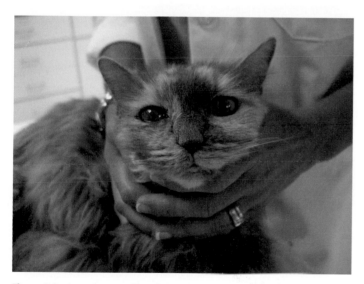

Figure 1-2 Inconsistent pupillary size, anisocoria, is an important finding that can be missed with a casual glance of the cat's eyes.

and issues. Although there is no particular order for examining body systems a usual routine pattern should be established. Most practitioners will start with the head and progress to the tail. This ensures that no system is overlooked. The veterinarian may also ask certain questions while examining each part to get a better understanding of each system (Table 1-2).

Skin, Eyes, and Ears

The integument, or skin, can be examined while examining other body systems or as an overall system itself. It is crucial to remember to examine all areas, such as the skin on the extremities as well as the underside of the cat. Many times brushing the hair coat in the opposite direction of growth will expose skin and many abnormalities that may be present (Fig. 1-1). Skin discoloration, hair loss, ulcerative or proliferative lesions, and pustules all should be marked in the record with their locations. Also note whether the hair coat is matted, oily, dry, or normal.

Following general skin appearance, the ears and eyes should be examined. An ocular examination includes examination of the external and internal ocular structures. Observe for ocular discharge and the nature of the discharge (serous or purulent), scratches on the cornea, inflammation of the conjunctiva, and cloudiness of the lenses. It is also important to note pupil size, consistency between pupil size (Fig. 1-2), and pupillary response to light.

Examining the ears involves visual as well as palpation of the external ear. Note if the pinnae exhibit hair loss, crusting, or dermatitis or if there are masses present. When examining the external ear canal, it should be clear of hair, mucus, and debris. If mucus or discharge is present, record color, smell, and consistency of the exudate. Use an otoscope to examine the ear canal for discharge, redness, ear mites, and foreign objects; evaluate the tympanic membrane for color and to determine intactness.

Respiratory System

Examining the respiratory system should begin by observing the cat's respiration rate and depth. The normal respiratory rate for feline patients is 16–30 breaths per minute. Observe for nasal discharge, abnormal sounds, such as coughing or wheezing, and any other indications of difficulty breathing. Lung sounds are heard with a stethoscope. The lung sounds of a normal cat are often heard during inspiration only. Normal air passage through the airways is usually barely audible so when feline patients present with easily heard lung sounds it is usually significant. The lack of respiratory sounds can also be significant, often signaling fluid accumulation in the pleural space (pleural effusion). Crackling or popping noises indicate abnormalities in the respiratory system and should be recorded.

Cardiovascular System

Examining the cardiovascular system begins by visualizing the cat's respiratory rate and depth. Next, the mucus membrane color and capillary refill time should be determined; they are a preliminary measure of cardiac output. Look at the color of the membranes and then blanch the color of the membranes by pressing your finger on the gums; count by seconds how long it takes to recover the color. Normal capillary refill time is 1–2 seconds. Times greater than 2 seconds can indicate poor cardiac output, which can be due to cardiac disease, dehydration, or other ailments. Palpation of the jugular and the femoral pulses is performed to monitor for adequate blood flow. Heart rate and pulse quality should also be recorded. Femoral pulses should be palpated while listening to the heart with a stethoscope to ensure there is a pulse for every beat of the heart. Cardiac auscultation should progress to listening for rate, rhythm, and the presence of a murmur. Murmurs are assessed by five indicators: intensity, grade, quality, timing, and location, which are factors in determining the need for further tests. See Chapter 20.

Gastrointestinal System

Although the gastrointestinal (GI) system is considered abdominal in location, it actually begins in the oral cavity. Examining the mouth could reveal clues to GI disease, including gastritis and GI foreign bodies. A foul odor coming from the patient's mouth may be more than just "vomit breath." Malodorous smells coming from the pharyngeal area can indicate impactions further down the gastrointestinal tract. Palpate the neck gently with one hand on both sides to feel for any masses or objects. Abdominal auscultation is used to detect gut sounds. The next step is abdominal palpation. A one-handed palpation technique may be easier to use in feline patients because of their small size. With the thumb on one side of the abdomen and four fingers on the other, the internal structures can be examined. The perineal area should be examined for masses, evidence of bowel movement problems, and inflammation.

Urogenital System

The feline kidneys can be palpated in most cats. They are about 4 cm longitudinally in the young adult cats and have a smooth surface. The full to half full urinary bladder should be palpable and is normally spherical in shape. The presence of uroliths or severe inflammation may evoke a pain response. Although the uterus and ovaries of an intact female are not palpable in the nonpregnant queen, it is crucial to examine the mammary chains for masses and the testicles of intact male cats.

Nervous System and Musculoskeletal System

The nervous and musculoskeletal systems can be harder to examine than the others. Neurological examinations are performed when a patient has central nervous system (CNS) or peripheral nerve symptoms. Examining the musculoskeletal system includes palpating joints, muscles, and bony structures. The spine is examined for pain responses and reflexes.

Miscellaneous

Several feline diseases result in enlargement of the peripheral lymph nodes. The most commonly enlarged ones are the mandibular, prescapular, and popliteal. Those lymph nodes should be palpated in a normal cat so enlargement can be appreciated.

Hyperthyroidism is common in geriatric cats. If the thyroid lobes are normal they are not palpable (Fig. 1-3). However, enlargement that is palpable justifies performance of blood tests (usually a total T4) to evaluate thyroid function.

Suggested Readings

Ettinger SJ, Feldman EC. 2000. *Textbook of Veterinary Internal Medicine*, 5th ed. Philadelphia: WB Saunders.
McCurnin DM, Bassert, JM. 2005. *Clinical Textbook for Veterinary Technicians*, 5th ed. Philadelphia: Elsevier Health Sciences.
Norsworthy GD. 2010. *The Feline Patient*, 4th ed. Ames: Wiley-Blackwell.
Poffenbarger EM, McCurnin DM. 2001. *Small Animal Physical Diagnosis and Clinical Procedures*, 2nd ed. Philadelphia: Elsevier Health Sciences.

Restraint

Linda E. Schmeltzer

One of the main reasons clients seek cat-only practices is the practice environment, which includes how cats are handled. The ability to safely and humanely restrain a cat is a vital task for every veterinary technician. The general rule of less is more is a good approach to most restraint situations. This means assessing the attitude and stress level of each patient and using the least amount of restraint required to accomplish the task. Proper restraint allows a procedure to be successfully accomplished without harm to the patient, client, or staff members involved. There is not a universal restraint technique that works for every cat that comes into a veterinary office. Loud noises outside the room, overhandling, or pain can cause the most easygoing, cooperative patient to become defensive or aggressive during a physical examination. The more methods of restraint a technician can learn, the better equipped that technician will be to handle these situations.

Restraint for Examinations

The following restraint techniques are effective for most cats during physical examination. Refer to Chapter 8 for discussion of restraint during sample collection. At the discretion of a veterinarian, chemical restraint may need to be used for aggressive patients. Technicians should never place themselves in a restraint situation with which they are not comfortable. If such a situation occurs communicate with the other staff members involved to formulate a plan to exit the situation in the safest way possible.

Restraint for Examination of the Head

During examination of the head, it is important for the restrainer to keep the cat from using its front feet to push the examiner's hands away. This is best accomplished by placing the cat on a countertop, head facing the examiner. The restrainer stands opposite the examiner, at the cat's tail. For docile cats, restrainers cradle the cat's body between their forearms and hold the cat's front legs at the elbows (Fig. 2-1). This prevents the cat from rolling to the side and pushing the examiner's hands away or scratching. Timid cats may feel more secure with a towel placed over them before the restrainer cradles them as previously described (Fig. 2-2). Using a thick bath towel to cover an aggressive cat can offer protection for restrainers and allow the examination to be accomplished successfully.

Some cats will tuck their heads down between their front legs making it difficult for the examiner to look into the eyes or mouth. Restrainers can help lift the head up by gently sliding index fingers under the cat's chin and pushing upward. If possible, place the little fingers in front of the elbows to help keep the cat's front legs down (Fig. 2-3). If using a towel for a timid or aggressive cat then be sure to keep the towel between the restraining hands and the cat.

Nursing the Feline Patient, First Edition. Edited by Linda E. Schmeltzer and Gary D. Norsworthy.

Restraint for Auscultation and Abdominal Palpation

During thoracic auscultation and abdominal palpation the restrainer should be positioned at the cat's head and the examiner at the cat's tail. The objectives of restraint during this portion of the examination are to keep the cat from leaving the examination area and to restrain the cat's head to prevent the cat from turning and biting the examiner. With docile cats this may be as easy as standing in front of the cat and petting its neck. Petting the neck distracts the patient from the examination and also puts the restrainer's hand in a position to scruff the neck should it be necessary (Fig. 2-4). Timid cats are often more cooperative when they are given a towel to hide under. If the cat is not aggressive, the restrainer should reach under the towel and scruff the neck (Fig. 2-5). For aggressive cats, it is best for the restrainer to stand to the cat's side and face toward the cat's head. Place a heavy bath towel over the cat's head and front legs. The restrainer can then apply gentle pressure over the cat's shoulders to prevent the cat from leaving the examination area (Fig. 2-6). The thick towel will act as a barrier to prevent the cat biting the restrainer or examiner. The cat may bite the towel during this part of the examination. Some aggressive or frightened cats do not tolerate this method of restraint and will become even less cooperative when covered with a towel. If this occurs do not apply stronger pressure to the shoulders because doing so can result in injury to the patient or acceleration of aggression.

A second restrainer may be needed to hold the cat's rear feet during this part of the examination if the cat uses its back feet to push the examiner's hands away during thoracic auscultation or abdominal palpation. The second restrainer stands at the cat's hindquarters and places his or her hands at the bend in the tarsus to hold the leg down (Fig. 2-7).

Restraint for Examination of Extremities

Examination of extremities works best if the cat is in lateral recumbency. This allows the examiner access to the legs and the bottom of the feet. With the cat in lateral recumbency the restrainer scruffs the cat's neck with one hand and holds the back feet with the other hand. Bracing the cat's shoulders and back against the arm that is holding the scruff may prevent the cat from wiggling (Fig. 2-8). Timid cats may feel more secure and be more cooperative if they are covered with a towel so they feel they are hiding (Fig. 2-9). For aggressive cats, place a towel between the cat's forelimbs and head as a barrier between the cat's mouth and the examiner's hands (Fig. 2-10). Some cats do not have enough loose skin to scruff or they may resist being scruffed. For these cats, the restrainer holds the cat's head by hooking thumb and index finger of his or her hand under the right and left zygomatic arches. A second restrainer or a towel may be needed to keep the cat from using its front feet to push the primary restrainer's hands away (Fig. 2-11).

Restraint for Pilling

It is often the technician's job to teach owners how to successfully pill their cats. There are several versions of a joke circulating the internet about how to give a cat a pill. Most of them involve injury to the human

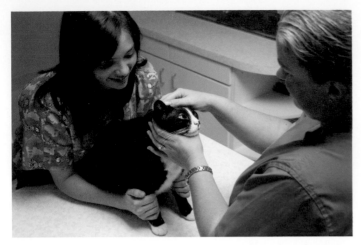

Figure 2-1 Hold the cat's front legs at the elbows and cradle the cat's body between forearms during examination of the head.

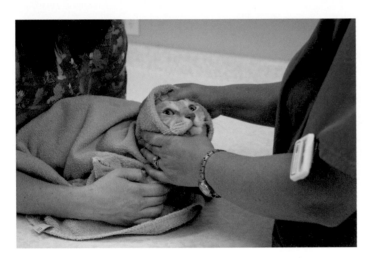

Figure 2-2 Timid cats may feel more secure with a towel placed over them.

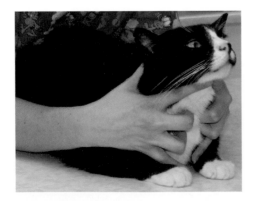

Figure 2-3 Lift the head up by gently sliding the index fingers under the cat's chin and push upward when cats tuck their heads down between their front legs during examination.

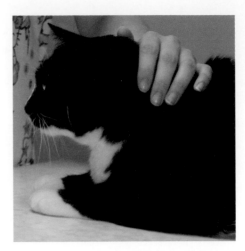

Figure 2-4 Petting the neck of docile cats distracts them during the examination and also puts the restrainer's hand in a position to scruff the neck should it become necessary.

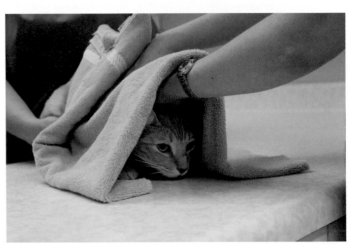

Figure 2-5 Timid cats are often more cooperative for examination when they are given a towel to hide under. If the cat is not aggressive, reach under the towel and scruff the neck.

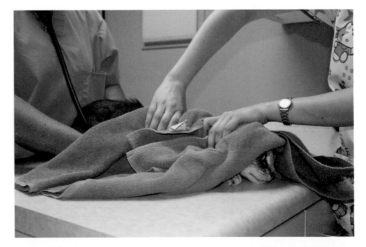

Figure 2-6 Place a heavy bath towel over an aggressive cat's head and front legs. Then apply gentle pressure over the cat's shoulders to prevent the cat from leaving the examination area.

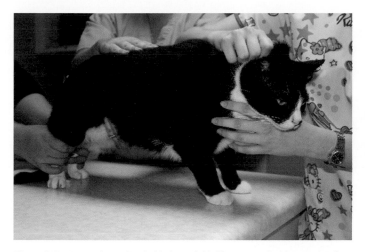

Figure 2-7 A second restrainer holds the cat's hind legs preventing the examiner from being scratched while palpating the cat's abdomen.

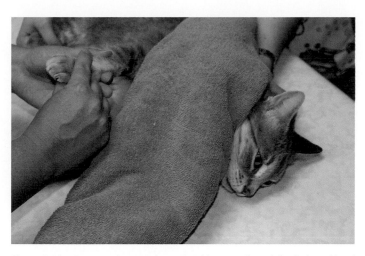

Figure 2-10 For aggressive cats, place a towel between the cat's forelimbs and head as a barrier between the cat's mouth and the examiner's hands.

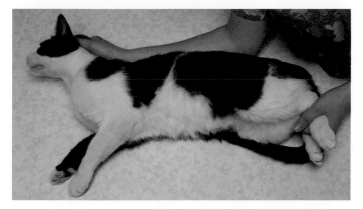

Figure 2-8 Bracing the cat's shoulders and back while restraining it in lateral recumbency may prevent the cat from wiggling.

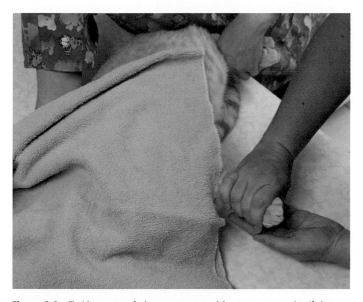

Figure 2-9 Timid cats may feel more secure and be more cooperative if they are covered with a towel so they feel they are hiding.

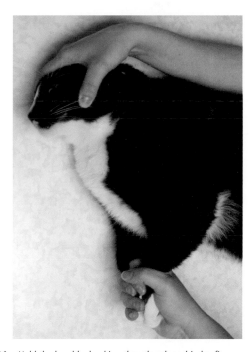

Figure 2-11 Hold the head by hooking thee thumb and index finger under the right and left zygomatic arches for cats that do not have enough loose skin to scruff or resist being scruffed. A second restrainer keeps the cat from using its front feet to push the primary restrainer's hands away.

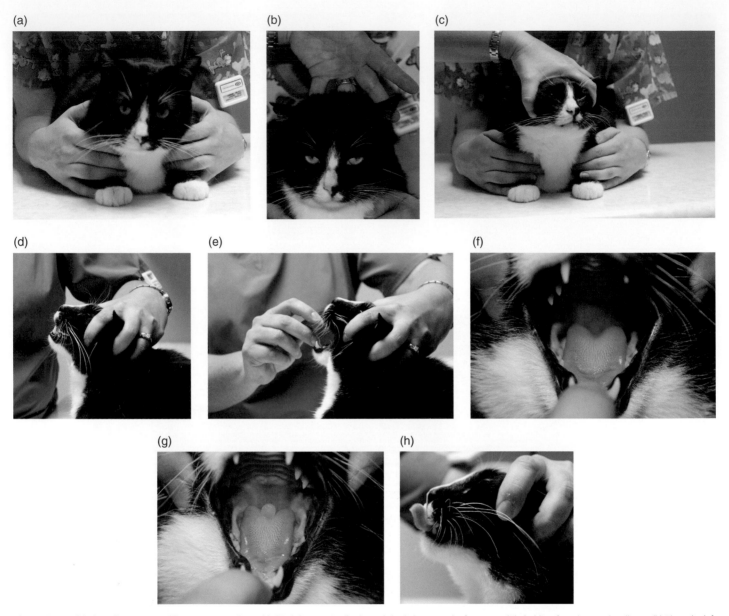

Figure 2-12 (a) Place the cat on a table or counter and stand behind the cat. Cradle the cat's body between the forearms while holding front legs at the elbows. (b) Place the left ring finger and little finger on each side of the neck at the base of the skull behind the cat's ears. (c) Hook the left index finger and thumb below the right and left zygomatic arches. (d) Tip the cat's head upward so the nose is at a 45-degree angle to the table. The cat's mouth should begin to open. (e) Hold the pill between the thumb and index finger and use the middle or ring finger to push down on the cat's lower jaw. (f) The caudal aspect of the tongue forms a groove. This is the pill slot. (g) Drop the pill into the middle of the pill slot. (h) Continue holding the chin up and wait for to the cat to stick its tongue out.

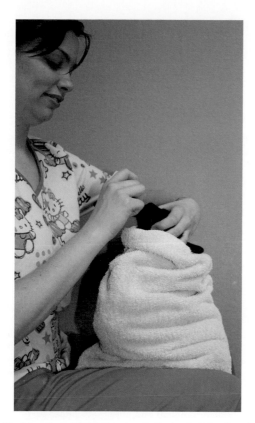

Figure 2-13 Wrap the cat tightly in a towel allowing both hands to be free when pilling a cat without an assistant.

involved, destruction of the house, and a cat that has successfully avoided taking a pill. Realistically there are few cats that cannot be pilled. Some medications must be given on an empty stomach, so wrapping them in a treat may not be possible. With proper instruction an owner can safely and successfully administer a pill to a cat without personal harm, harm to the cat, or damage to the house. Before demonstrating any technique to an owner, a technician should feel comfortable and confident using it. This allows for easier troubleshooting if problems occur for the owner.

How to Give a Cat a Pill

This technique is initially described using two people: a restrainer and a pill-giver. An alternate technique for a single person pilling a cat will be described subsequently.

Place the cat on a table or counter. The restrainer will stand behind the cat and cradle the cat's body between his or her forearms while holding the cat's front legs at the elbows (Fig. 2-12a). The pill-giver, using the nondominant hand (left in this description), places the left ring finger and little finger on each side of the neck at the base of the skull behind the cat's ears (Fig. 2-12b) and hooks the left index finger and thumb below the right and left zygomatic arches (Fig. 2-12c). This will allow for good control of the head, which is essential for success. The pill-giver then tips the cat's head upward so the nose is at a 45-degree angle to the table (Fig. 2-12d). The cat's mouth should begin to open. Hold the pill between the thumb and index finger of the dominant hand and use the middle or ring finger to push down on the cat's lower jaw, opening the mouth wider (Fig. 2-12e). Note the way the caudal aspect of the tongue forms a groove (Fig. 2-12f). This is the *pill slot*. Drop the pill into the middle of the groove (Fig. 2-12g). If it drops to one side, the cat will be able to spit it out. Do not let the cat's head drop down until the pill is swallowed. Continue holding the chin up and wait for to the cat to stick its tongue out, signaling that swallowing has occurred (Fig. 2-12h). The most common reason this method is unsuccessful is letting the head drop before the cat swallows, allowing the cat to spit the pill out.

If only one person is available for pilling, wrap the cat tightly in a towel or pillow case, allowing both hands to be free (Fig. 2-13).

Suggested Readings

French DD, Tully TN. 2006. Restraint and Handling of Animals. In DM McCurnin, JM Bassert, eds., *Clinical Textbook for Veterinary Technicians*, 6th ed., pp. 65–68. St. Louis: Elsevier Saunders.

Norsworthy GD. 2011. Restraint Techniques and Devices. In GD Norsworthy, ed., *The Feline Patient*, 4th ed., pp. 920–23. Ames: Wiley-Blackwell.

Pattengale P. 2009. Animal Restraint. In P Pattengale, ed., *Tasks for the Veterinary Technician*, 2nd ed., pp. 131–33. Ames: Wiley-Blackwell.

Rodan I, Sundahl E, Carney H, et al. 2011. AAFP and ISFM Feline-Friendly Handling Guidelines. *J Fel Med Surg*. 13(5):364–75.

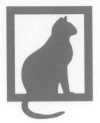

CHAPTER 3

Environmental Enrichment in the Hospital

Gary D. Norsworthy and Linda E. Schmeltzer

Overview

A hospital visit can be a terrifying event, whether as an outpatient or inpatient and regardless of species, including humans. However, when a cat visits a typical small animal practice the experience can be especially unpleasant. Many indoor cats have had no exposure to dogs and are terrified at the first and subsequent encounters, and many dogs, even those that live with a cat, find unknown cats to be objects of prey. Both of these situations are likely in a waiting room filled with canines and felines.

Veterinarians, technicians, kennel personnel, and receptionists who are not particularly fond of cats only add to the cat's anxiety. Unfortunately, some of these people are often found in the typical small animal practice. Procedures that are necessary, beginning with the rectal thermometer, further add to the cat's response of self-preservation and aggression and often result in a threatening situation for those who restrain and treat the cat.

This chapter will chronicle how the authors have tried to minimize the unpleasantries of a hospital visit. The goals of hospital environment enrichment are to make the visit as pleasant as possible for the cat and for those who treat the cat so that minimal restraint is needed and that quality health care can be provided.

Environmental enrichment in the hospital is two pronged. First, it seeks to reduce anxiety on the cat. Second, it seeks to reduce anxiety on the owner. In the process of treating the cat, a practioner must not forget that owners ultimately decide whether the cat receives the treatment that the veterinarian recommends or if the hospitals services are sought in the future.

The following ideas are based on the experience of the authors. A virtual tour of their hospital can be taken at www.alamofeline.com.

The Feline-Exclusive Practice

The first feline-exclusive practice was established in the United States in the 1960s. Although many considered it a strange concept, it had an appeal to many serious cat owners. Over the past 40 years, cats have gone from being a casual, almost disposable pet to an integral part of many families. A proliferation of feline-exclusive practices, now numbering over 300 in the United States, has accompanied the increase in feline popularity as a valued family member.

The feline-exclusive concept is based largely on three premises that cat owners find appealing. First, a veterinarian who concentrates his or her professional life on one species should become more proficient. Second, the feline practice offers a dog-free environment, which automatically produces an atmosphere that is less threatening to feline patients. Third, the feline practice is staffed with receptionists, technicians, and veterinarians who truly like cats and like working with cats.

The authors practice in a feline-exclusive practice, and the following procedures are utilized in that practice. However, most of them can also be used in a canine-feline practice either as described or with some creativity.

Nursing the Feline Patient, First Edition. Edited by Linda E. Schmeltzer and Gary D. Norsworthy.
© 2012 John Wiley & Sons, Inc. Published 2012 by John Wiley & Sons, Inc.

Reception Area

The reception area makes the first impression. It should convey the message that cats are valued as patients, and it should project cleanliness. These messages are given in the following ways:

- The dæcor should be cat themed. The decorations in small animal practice need to have equal emphasis on cats as on the other species treated. Reception areas that have a 90% canine theme send a strong negative message to the cat owner (Fig. 3-1).
- The furnishings in a feline-exclusive reception area can be living-room quality. Most cats travel in carriers. They do not have chain leashes that are raked across the furniture. They do not paw at the furniture with claws. A nicely decorated reception area will motivate your clients to rise to that level.
- Odor control is vital. The smell of cat urine often pervades the reception area. Even though it may originate in other areas of the hospital, its presence in the reception area is not acceptable. Urine must be cleaned up immediately. An effective odor-neutralizing product, such as Zero Odor Pet® (www.ZeroOdorStore.com) should be used immediately when urine is not contained within cat litter. Tom cat urine odor is especially pungent and pervasive. Either do not keep intact male cats overnight (our policy), or if they must stay, keep them in an isolation ward with a good exhaust system and use Zero Odor Pet® frequently. Their litter boxes must be cleaned immediately after urination occurs, and the wet litter should be taken to an outdoor trash receptacle.

Examination Rooms

Examination rooms are the first "medical" area. They must be efficient for patient care, and they must have appeal to clients.

- The dæcor is important. In our feline practice the six examination rooms each have a different theme based on a famous cat (Fig. 3-2). If the examination room is used for other species than just cats, its decorations should include some feline recognition. In a small animal practice, ideally one or more examination rooms should be dedicated to cats. The feline rooms do not need to be as large as those used for dogs. Their dedicated use eliminates the odors of dogs. During construction, sound board should be put in the walls to reduce or eliminate the sounds of dogs.
- If one or more examination rooms in a small animal practice are designated for feline patients, ideally they should be located out of dog traffic paths. The sound of dogs walking past and sniffing at the bottom of the door will add to a cat's level of anxiety.
- Cleanliness is paramount. Every countertop, table top, and sink should be spotlessly clean when the client enters the room. There should be no cat hair on the countertops or floor.
- Odor control is of equal importance to cleanliness. A cleaner that also deodorizes should be used. Zero Odor Pet® should be used for any residual odor. Odoriferous materials (e.g., urine, stool, and anal sac material) should be removed from the room, not just put in a trash can in the room.
- The room needs to be "cat proof." There should be no small, tight places where a cat can hide, thereby giving them the freedom to roam around the room. This is a stress reducer.

(a)

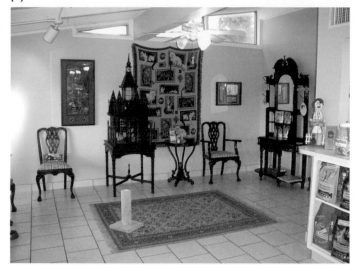

(b)

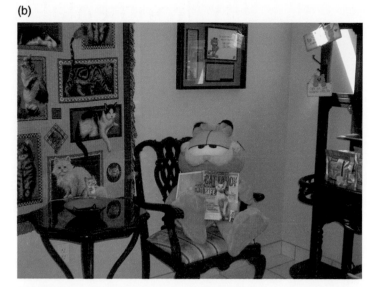

Figure 3-1 The décor of the reception room should include a feline theme proportional to the percentage of feline patients there are in the practice. Living-room quality furniture is feasible in a feline-exclusive practice.

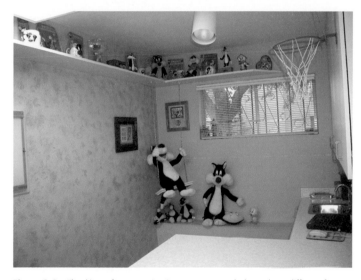

Figure 3-2 The décor of our examination rooms are each themed to a different famous cat. The examination tables are L-shaped, and a computer is located in each using a paperless system (www.avimark.com).

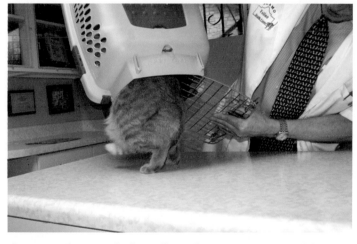

Figure 3-3 The cat can be "poured" out of its carrier. As the rear of the carrier approaches vertical, the cat will be forced to put one or more feet on the examination table. When either two front or two rear feet are on the table, the carrier can be lifted upward so the cat walks out.

- However, designated hiding places can be stress relievers. Some cats like to curl up in a sink. Others prefer a plastic pan (dish pan) or a designated cabinet. These need to be cleaned after each use.
- There should be a place for cat carriers other than on the examination table.
- Feliway® (www.feliway.com) can be helpful for calming nervous or aggressive cats. It can be sprayed on the examination table prior to use.

Examination Room Equipment and Procedures

- The first step in the examination is to remove the cat from the carrier. In many cases, the owner has done so or the cat comes out voluntarily. However, if the cat is resistant to leaving the security of its carrier

several approaches can be used. In some cases, the owner is proactive in coaxing the cat out; if not, the technician or veterinarian can remove the cat as long as the cat is reasonably willing. If not, other tactics can be employed with the goal of not inciting the cat into a defensive (or offensive) posture. The top of many plastic carriers can be removed; doing so removes the cat's need to defend its territory. If that is not feasible, the carrier door can be opened and the cat "poured" out. This should be done by tipping the rear of the carrier upward slowly while the front of the carrier rests on the examination table. The cat will slide down to the door but still try to remain in the carrier. As the rear of the carrier approaches vertical, the cat will be forced to put one or more feet on the examination table. When either two front or two rear feet are on the table, the carrier can be lifted upward so the cat walks out (Fig. 3-3). It is important that this be done slowly so the cat is not antagonized. It is also important that you not lift the carrier away if

(a)

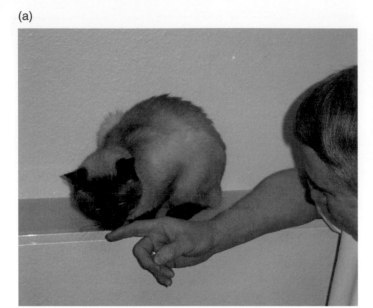

(b)

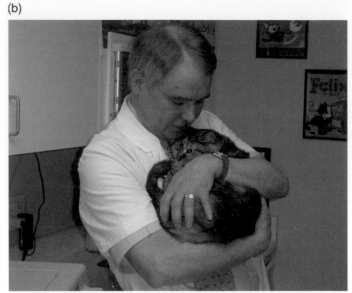

Figure 3-4 When first approaching your patient, allow it to assess you by smelling of your index finger ("the cat scan"). After that, scratch it behind the ear, stroke it a few times down the back, and, if the cat is willing, hold it a few seconds. Going through this sequence usually makes the cat less apprehensive and more cooperative during the physical examination.

(a)

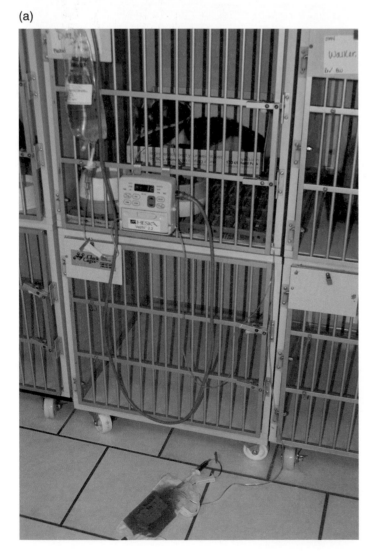

(b)

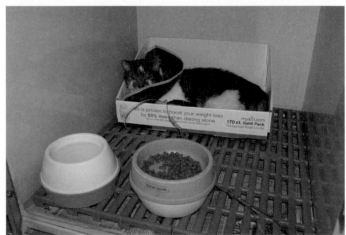

Figure 3-5 These images show several important ways to increase patient comfort even when a major illness is present. (a) The cages are fiberglass laminate; an intravenous (IV) pump hangs on the front of the cage. This cat is recovering from a urethral obstruction. His urinary collection bag is below the cage with its line entering the cage at the same point as the IV line. (b) The cat is more comfortable in a box. A soft Elizabethan collar is used to protect the IV line and urinary catheters. The bowls are elevated by taping them to a similar bowl so he can get food and water while wearing the Elizabethan collar. A slotted rack is used for flooring because a litter box is not being used for this patient.

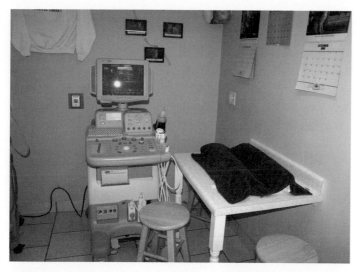

Figure 3-6 The dedicated ultrasound room has an appropriately sized table attached to the wall, a cushioned trough for the cat to lie in for an abdominal study, a spotlight that shines on the patient but not on the ultrasound screen, light switches near the table, and an oxygen outlet for use by an anesthetic machine.

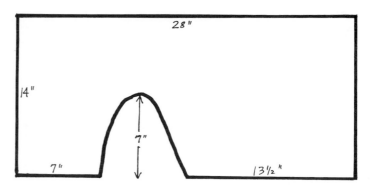

Figure 3-7 The dimensions of the echocardiogram table area shown in this drawing. It is padded, covered with vinyl, and placed on 6-inch legs. It is placed on the ultrasound table.

there is one front and one rear foot on the table. If that happens, set the carrier back down on the table and begin again.

- The next step in the examination (after greeting the client) is to assess the cat's personality. Cats tend to fall into three groups: (1) friendly, (2) apprehensive/scared, and (3) aggressive/fractious. Cats in the first two categories should be greeted with an outstretched, nonthreatening hand. If you let the cat smell your index finger (Fig. 3-4a) it will usually become less apprehensive. After it has done this, slide your finger behind the cat's ear and give it a few strokes. Follow that with a few strokes down the back. If it shows interest in your advances, stroke it a few more times or pick it up and cradle it in your arms like a baby (Fig. 3-4b). Some cats will let you do this and others will not. These proactive movements on your part will set the cat at ease and make it less likely to become aggressive during the examination. It will also send the two most important messages to the client: (1) you love cats, and (2) you love this cat.
- Aggressive or fractious cats must be handled with caution. Cat bites can create serious infections. Sedation is sometimes needed to proceed safely.
- Each of our six examination rooms is set up the same. Each is similarly equipped, and the equipment is located in the corresponding cabinets or draws. This permits efficiency when more than one doctor uses the examination rooms. It also reduces staff stress. Stressed doctors and technicians are likely to transmit anxiety to their patients.
- Our main restraint device is a heavy bath towel. Drawers in the examination tables contain three towels per examination room; they are located so they can be retrieved quickly by the veterinarian or the technician. Designate towels specifically for examination rooms making sure they are free of stains, holes, and frayed areas.
- Every cat should be weighed on every visit. We use a digital package scale (www.pelouze.com; model 4010) and place a plastic dish pan on it for the cat to stand or lie in. There is one in each examination room. It is stored in a drawer on the client's side of the examination table; when the drawer is pulled out, the scale can be used without removing it from the drawer. A strongly made drawer with heavy duty hardware is vital for long-term use.
- Veterinary otoscope cones are too large for the feline external ear canal. We use an otoscope and cones made for humans.

- Successful feline cardiac auscultation is best accomplished using a stethoscope with a 12-mm (½-inch) or 2-cm (¾-inch) bell. Feline murmurs are usually located very near the sternum.
- The cat has a strong anal reflex. A rectal thermometer should be lubricated but not forced into the rectum. Gentle pressure will result in sphincter relaxation and less resistance from the cat. For apprehensive/scared cats, take the temperature after the physical examination is complete because this procedure can result in an aggressive response.
- Blood pressure should be measured in a quiet examination room with the owner present and touching (or holding) the cat. Ideally, this should be the first event of the examination because other events will affect blood pressure causing unreliable readings.
- Blood collection can be a challenge. Most of our blood profiles are performed using a chemistry machine that requires less than 0.5 ml of blood (www.abaxis.com; VetScan VS2). Blood is taken from a medial saphenous vein. If a large quantity of blood is needed, a jugular collection procedure is used. If you are consistently proficient in drawing blood, it will impress the client; do so in the examination room. Another benefit is that this location allows you to avoid the areas of the hospital that contain dogs.

The Hospital Area

- Cleanliness and odor control are also important in this setting. Odors may be carried from the hospital to the examination rooms and reception area along hallways or through air conditioning or heating systems.
- Hospital cages are more cat friendly if they are not made of stainless steel. Laminates are quieter, warmer, and sufficiently durable for cats. Our cages (www.clarkcages.com) have been in use for 10 years and show almost no signs of wear.
- Cage size is usually a compromise between comfort, expense, and available space. Most cats are comfortable for a few days in a 24" × 24" × 24" (width, height, depth) cage. Large cats and cats that are hospitalized longer do well in 30" × 24" × 24" cages.
- Food and water bowls should be as large on the bottom as on the top so they do not turn over easily.
- We use two types of litter boxes. Small plastic ones are more appealing to cats but can consume more cage space and litter. They must be washed and disinfected between cats. Cardboard litter trays (www.chinet.com; 7" × 9" flat trays) are well accepted by most cats. They consume less litter and are disposable so disease transmission is not an issue.
- Cats on intravenous (IV) fluids, with severe diarrhea or those that are just messy do well on racks that fit into the cages (www.clarkcages.com). They allow fluids to go through while being reasonably comfortable to the cats.

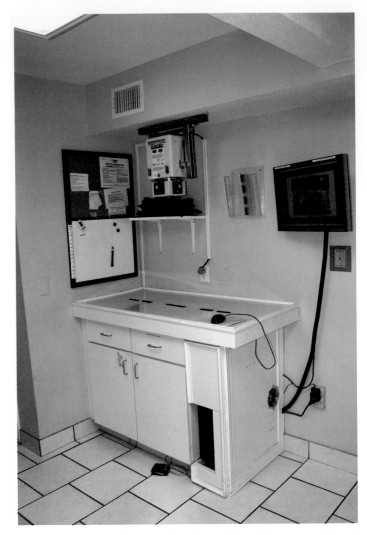

Figure 3-8 The x-ray table is made from a base cabinet with a custom made top to accommodate the digital receiving plate. It is placed in a corner of the room to help with restraint between exposures. The monitor for the digital x-ray system (www.soundeklin.com) is mounted on the back wall; the computer CPU and other x-ray system equipment are housed in a cabinet built on to the end of the base cabinet. The keyboard for the computer is located in one of the drawers in the table.

- Elizabethan collars are necessary in select situations. Use a soft collar when it is acceptable. Hard plastic collars are needed for some situations (www.kvpusa.com).
- IV catheters can be placed in several peripheral veins. Short catheters perform well in the cephalic veins for 2–3 days. Long (central venous) catheters can remain in place for up to 7 days, and blood samples can be collected through them. They can be placed in the jugular vein or in the medial saphenous vein.
- Frequently cats feel more secure when some form of seclusion is provided. Cardboard boxes can be used; they should be discarded after each use to prevent disease transmission (Fig. 3-5). Feliway can be sprayed on the boxes for added stress control.
- A deep sink is an acceptable place for bathing cats. Cats usually need less restraint and are less aggressive compared to being in a bathtub.
- Ultrasound studies are performed in a dedicated room. This room is themed like the examination rooms because owners are frequently invited to observe these studies. A spot light is attached to the ceiling and shines on the patient from behind the ultrasound screen. The spotlight is on a rheostat so the intensity can be adjusted as needed.

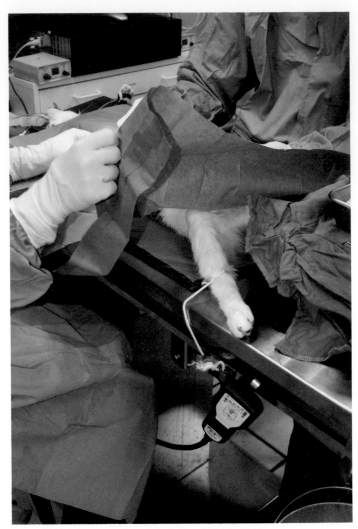

Figure 3-9 Body temperature is maintained with a controlled heat source under the cat (www.thermogear.com).

Switches for the spotlight and the room lights are located next to the ultrasound table. A sink is available for rinsing ultrasound gel off of the moist towel used for cleaning the patient. Nearby drawers contain syringes, needles, microscope slides, and other equipment used during the ultrasound procedures. An oxygen outlet is available when gas anesthesia is needed (Fig. 3-6).
- Our ultrasound table measures 25″ × 32″ and is 32 inches high. An echocardiography table is placed on it. See Figure 3-7 for size and shape; it is on 6-inch legs. Abdominal procedures are performed in a foam rubber tray that has a trough cut to fit the cat when the cat is in dorsal recumbency. It measures 18″ × 24″. A plastic bag is taped in place over it to keep body fluids from getting into the foam rubber. The tray is covered with a bath towel when in use.
- Our x-ray table is constructed from a base cabinet. A custom made top, measuring 24″ × 51″, was built to accommodate the digital x-ray sensor. It is located in a corner of the room. Although it does not permit access to both ends of the table, the enclosed corner is advantageous between exposures because cats can be released but not allowed to get off of the table (Fig. 3-8).
- Our surgery tables are stainless steel; the top measures 18.75″ × 46″. Body temperature is preserved during surgery using a warming blanket (ChillBuster® Vet Surgical Warming System by ThermoGear) placed on the surgery table (Fig. 3-9).

- Surgical monitoring is performed with a multiparameter monitor (www.vmedtech.com; PC-VetGard+) that transmits data wirelessly from the surgery table to a computer at the front of the surgery room. The data is displayed on large monitors near the ends of each surgery table.
- Declawing is performed exclusively with a carbon dioxide surgical laser (www.aesculight.com). We are convinced that cats have less pain and bleeding. This is especially evident when adult cats are declawed.
- Finally, and perhaps as important as any other suggestion, everyone on the staff should open cage doors and give some personal tender loving care to the patients. Knowing they are being cared for by caring cat lovers is reassuring to feline patients.

Boarding Facilities

- Boarding wards are separate from the hospital wards.
- The same cages as previously described are used; however, multiple sizes are available depending on the size of the cat, the number of cats the owner wants together, and the comfort level the owner desires.

- Our luxury boarding area has cages with glass backs. They are placed on an outside wall with large windows so the cats can look outdoors.
- Cats are allowed out of their kennels daily, one at a time, to roam the boarding area. Climbing trees and scratching posts are provided during the cat's exercise time.
- Toys are provided unless the owner brings cat toys. The ones we provide must be washable.

Conclusion

The goal of each item listed is to reduce patient stress and increase comfort level, even when medical procedures are performed. Thoughtfulness and planning, hopefully prior to construction, are the keys to increasing patient and owner appeal, both of which add to practice growth and income.

Suggested Readings

Norsworthy GD, Schmeltzer, L. 2010. Environmental Enrichment in the Hospital. In GD Norsworthy, ed., *The Feline Patient*, 4th ed., pp. 571–76. Ames: Wiley-Blackwell.

CHAPTER 4

Preventive Health Programs

Linda E. Schmeltzer

The Annual Visit

Many pet owners see the annual trip to the veterinarian as simply an exercise to update vaccines. In actuality it is the veterinarian's best chance to practice preventive medicine. Cats age at an average equivalent of 5 human years with the passing of one calendar year. In other words, a cat's annual examination or yearly examination is the equivalent of a person having a physical examination every 5 years.

The annual visit at Alamo Feline Health Center in San Antonio, Texas, consists of six steps:

1. Owners are asked to fill out a questionnaire that asks specific questions related to known feline diseases and aging changes (Table 4-1).
2. A single-lead electrocardiogram (ECG) is performed to identify early signs of heart disease. Hypertrophic cardiomyopathy occurs in cats as young as 1 year of age. Several early indicators occur on the ECG before the onset of congestive heart failure. See Chapter 20.
3. A thorough examination is performed beginning at the nose and ending with the tail. See Chapter 1.
4. Written recommendations regarding the health needs of each patient are provided to the client. These recommendations may include flea and heartworm prevention, diet change, dental prophylaxis, or further screening for possible disease processes.
5. After completing an individual patient risk assessment, needed vaccines are administered.
6. At checkout, clients receive a printed document listing eight things owners can do to keep their cats healthy and 18 early signs of disease of which owners should be aware (Table 4-2).

An annual wellness examination gives the veterinarian an opportunity to look for disease in its early and hopefully, treatable stages. Dental disease, thyroid disease, tumors on or under the skin, and heart disease are just a few examples of diseases that are more easily treated if diagnosed early. Consequently, this examination should be viewed seriously. The annual visit is a practitioner's annual opportunity to be proactive for the health of patients.

As cats age into the category of a senior (11–14 years) or geriatric (15 years and beyond) patient some veterinarians recommend biannual wellness visits. Twice-a-year examinations allow for even closer monitoring of patients' health. Early detection and prompt treatment of disease is especially important in the older cats so that a good quality of life can be maintained for as long as possible. As cats become older additional grooming, such as regular nail trims or brushing, may be needed. This examination allows for an additional opportunity to educate pet owners about aging changes in their cats.

Vaccination Guidelines

There is much discussion in the veterinary community regarding what constitutes the safest and most effective vaccination program.

Nursing the Feline Patient, First Edition. Edited by Linda E. Schmeltzer and Gary D. Norsworthy.
© 2012 John Wiley & Sons, Inc. Published 2012 by John Wiley & Sons, Inc.

Veterinarian recommendations vary between practices. Therefore, technicians should educate themselves with regard to the benefits and risks of the vaccination program recommended in their practice. It is important for technicians to feel comfortable with their practice recommendations so they may properly educate owners and be in agreement with the practice owners. The following vaccination guidelines are currently recommended by the American Association of Feline Practitioners.

Core Vaccinations

Core vaccinations are those recommended for all cats. Vaccines for panleukopenia virus (FPV), feline herpesvirus-1 (FHV-1), feline calicivirus (FCV), and rabies virus are in the core vaccine category.

Kittens can begin their primary series as early as 6 weeks old. They can receive a vaccination for FPV, FHV-1, and FCV every 3–4 weeks until they are 16 weeks old. A single dose of rabies virus vaccine should be administered as directed on the manufacturer's product label or by state or local regulations between the ages of 8 and 12 weeks. If rabies vaccine is given before 12 weeks of age, a booster given 2–4 weeks later is required. A second dose of rabies virus vaccine should be given 1 year after the initial dose.

Unvaccinated adult or adolescent cats (cats older than 16 weeks old) will have an amended primary series. Vaccination for FPV, FHV-1, and FCV will be administered in two doses spaced 3–4 weeks apart. A single dose of rabies virus vaccine will also be administered. A second dose of rabies virus vaccine should be given 1 year after the initial dose.

Booster vaccines for all cats are recommended. American Association of Feline Practitioners (AAFP) guidelines recommend that FPV, FHV-1, and FCV be given 1 year following the last dose in the primary series then no more frequently than every 3 years. Rabies vaccine should be given annually or as directed by local or state ordinance.

Noncore Vaccinations

Noncore vaccinations are administered to cats in specific risk categories. Vaccines for feline leukemia virus (FeLV), feline immunodeficiency virus (FIV), *Bordetella bronchiseptica*, and *Chlamydophila felis* are included in this category.

Feline Leukemia Virus Vaccine

It is highly recommended that all kittens receive FeLV vaccine. Ideally the primary series should be administered at 8 and 12 weeks old. Transdermal and injectable vaccines are available. Some products require a second dose; follow the manufacturer's recommended guidelines. A single dose should be repeated 1 year after the last dose of the initial series. Annual booster vaccines are recommended only for cats considered to be at risk of exposure.

Feline Immunodeficiency Virus Vaccine

FIV vaccine is recommended only for cats at high risk of infection. See Chapter 24. Cats should test FIV-antibody negative immediately prior to

TABLE 4-1: History Form

Give Us Some Important Information About Your Cat

Cat _____ Owner _____ Date _____

Habitat: ☐ Indoor only ☐ Mostly indoor ☐ Outdoor only ☐ Mostly outdoor ☐ In and out freely

Appetite: ☐ Very good ☐ Good ☐ Erratic ☐ Picky ☐ Poor ☐ Very poor

Change in appetite: ☐ Up ☐ Down Food(s): _____

Diet: ☐ Eats specific meals ☐ Fed free choice % table food _____ % treats_____ % dog food _____

Water Consumption: ☐ Does not drink excessively ☐ Drinks very excessively ☐ Amount up ☐ Amount down

Activity level: ☐ Very active ☐ Normal ☐ Very inactive ☐ More active ☐ Less active

YES NO

☐ ☐ Do you board your cat?

☐ ☐ Does your cat go to **cat shows**?

☐ ☐ **Lameness:** Which leg(s) _____ ☐ Constant ☐ Intermittent Duration: _____

☐ ☐ **Behavior:** Any notable change? _____

☐ ☐ **Vomiting:** If yes, how often? _____

What is vomited? _____

Is there a relationship to eating? ☐ No ☐ Yes How? _____

☐ ☐ **Diarrhea:** ☐ Occasionally ☐ Frequently Frequency:_____

If diarrhea is present: Number of bowel movements per day: _____

Straining to defecate: ☐ Yes ☐ No

☐ ☐ **Coughing:** ☐ Occasionally ☐ Frequently

☐ ☐ **Sneezing:** ☐ Occasionally ☐ Frequently

☐ ☐ **Nasal discharge:** ☐ Pus ☐ Watery ☐ Bloody Duration: _____

☐ ☐ **Itching:** ☐ Seasonal ☐ Year-round ☐ Location(s) on the cat's body: _____

☐ ☐ History of **fight wounds**: How many in the last 2 years: _____

☐ ☐ Has **tested positive** for: ☐ Feline Leukemia Virus ☐ Feline AIDS Virus If yes, how long ago? _____

☐ ☐ **Fleas or ticks** noted recently

☐ ☐ On **heartworm preventative**? ☐ Irregularly ☐ Regularly Number of months per year: _____

☐ ☐ On **flea preventative**? ☐ Irregularly ☐ Regularly Number of months per year: _____

Medications regularly taken: _____

Summary of your concerns: _____

Has your address or phone number changed since last year?

New information: _____

Our fax number: (XXX) XXX-XXX

vaccination. The initial vaccination series is three doses administered at 2- to 3-week intervals. The first dose of the primary series may be administered as early as 8 weeks old. A single dose is given 1 year following the last dose of the initial series and then annually as long as there is a risk of exposure.

Bordetella Bronchiseptica

Vaccination is recommended when cats are likely to be at risk of *B. bronchiseptica* infection. A single intranasal dose may be administered as early as 8 weeks old. Annual booster is recommended as long as the exposure risk remains.

Chlamydophila Felis

C. felis vaccine should be used only as part of a program to control disease in multicat environments where infections associated with the disease have been confirmed. The primary series is administered in two doses 3–4 weeks apart. This vaccine may be used in kittens as young as 9 weeks old. If the risk of exposure continues, an annual booster is recommended.

TABLE 4-2: Early Signs of Disease

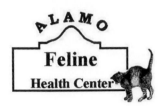

Recommendations for Cat Owners

Pet ownership carries with it the responsibility of being proactive in health care. There are certain steps that you should take to prevent health problems. We recommend the following:

1. An annual examination is essential. . . . remember, 1 year to us is an average of 5 years to your cat. That's a long time to go without a thorough physical examination.
2. Keep vaccinations current. A vaccination program should be individualized to meet the needs of your cat.
3. Brush frequently to keep hair coat from matting. Many cats do not groom themselves well.
4. Clip toenails as needed to prevent overgrowth. (Most cats younger than 10 years need no nail care.)
5. Keep plenty of fresh water available and monitor its consumption.
6. Monitor urine output by measuring the amount of wet litter in the litter box.
7. Keep other pets from preventing this one from free access to food and water.
8. Keep indoors all the time if possible but at least at night.
9. Eliminate parasites, including fleas, ticks, intestinal worms, and heartworms on a regular basis.
10. Weigh your cat on the same scale and record results at least every 60 days. Both weight loss and weight gain are noteworthy. Obesity is a serious condition that is becoming more and more common in the feline population.
11. Clean teeth are essential to continued good health. Yearly or every other year teeth cleanings are often necessary.
12. Different life stages and health conditions often require special diets. We can help you pick a diet that is appropriate for your cat's needs.

Early Signs of Disease

The following are early signs of disease. Some of these are so minor that they may not seem significant. However, our goal is to diagnose and treat diseases in their early stages when the success rate is much higher. Present your cat for an examination for any of the following:

1. Sustained, significant increase in water consumption. (Abnormal is intake greater than 50 ml/#/day or approximately 1.5 cups (8 oz cups)/day or 12 oz total for 9 pound cat.)
2. Sustained, significant increase in urination or amount of wet litter.
3. Weight loss.
4. Significant decrease in appetite or failure to eat for more than two consecutive days.
5. Significant increase in appetite.
6. Repeated vomiting.
7. Diarrhea that lasts more than 3 days.
8. Difficulty in passing stool or urine or prolonged sitting or laying in the litter box.
9. Change in litter box habits, especially if urination or defecation occurs out of the litter box.
10. Lameness that lasts more than 5 days or lameness in more than one leg.
11. Noticeable decrease in vision, especially if sudden in onset or pupils that do not constrict in bright light.
12. Masses, ulcerations (open sores), or multiple scabs on the skin that persist more than 1 week.
13. Foul mouth odor or drooling that lasts more than 2 days.
14. Increasing size of the abdomen.
15. Increasing inactivity or amount of time spent sleeping.
16. Hair loss, especially if accompanied by scratching or if in specific areas (as opposed to generalized).
17. Breathing heavily or rapid at rest.
18. Inability to chew or eat dry food.

Other Vaccines

There are other feline vaccines available. Due to lack of sufficient research or data they are not generally recommended.

Richards J, Elston T, Ford R, et al. 2006. The 2006 American Association of Feline Practitioners Feline Vaccine Advisory Panel Report. *J Amer Veter Med Assoc.* 229(9):1405–41.

Suggested Readings

Hoskins JD, Eades SC, Gill MS. 2006. Preventive Health Programs. In McCurnin DM, JM Bassert, eds., *Clinical Textbook for Veterinary Technicians*, 6th ed., pp. 337–41. St. Louis: Elsevier Saunders.

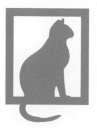

CHAPTER 5

Gestation, Parturition, and Neonatal Care

Linda E. Schmeltzer

Overview

The female cat (queen) reaches puberty by 4–12 months of age. Oriental breeds tend to reach puberty much earlier than other breeds. Long-haired breeds and British Shorthairs may not reach puberty until 1 year of age. Queens are seasonally polyestrous, meaning they come into heat (estrus) only during part of the year, typically spring.

Estrus lasts about 2–3 weeks. Queens are induced ovulators, meaning that copulation (breeding) causes a hormone release that induces ovulation. Ovulation usually occurs 24–48 hours after copulation. A single copulation may not be sufficient to induce ovulation; therefore, queens may require three or four breedings within a 24-hour period. Once ovulation has occurred, the queen will go out of heat within a day or two. If the queen is not bred, she will return to heat in 1–2 weeks. This pattern will continue for several heat cycles or until she is bred. The period of time that a queen is out of heat will vary depending on geographic and environmental factors, such as temperature and the number of daylight hours.

Gestation

The term *gestation* means the period of time when the fetuses are developing in the uterus. Gestation (pregnancy) ranges from 63 to 66 days. Increased litter size is associated with a shorter gestation period.

The only way to accurately determine the days of pregnancy is to count days from the time of breeding. Abdominal palpation to diagnose pregnancy is easiest when performed 3–4 weeks after successful breeding. Embryonic sacs are visible on ultrasound by days 11 to 17; a heartbeat can be visualized from 20 to 24 days onward. Radiography usually shows uterine enlargement about day 25 to 30. The fetal skeleton is mineralized enough to be visible by about 36 to 35 days.

Nutritional needs for Pregnancy and Lactation

A pregnant queen will have increased nutrient needs to maintain her daily energy needs and support the additional energy required for fetal development. A 4- to 5-kg (~10 pound) queen supporting four fetuses will require around 600 kilocalories per day, to include 41 grams of crude protein and 12 grams of total fat. A kitten formulation of a premium brand food should meet these needs. These diets are typically high in calories and protein and will provide all of the vitamins and minerals a queen needs.

During pregnancy, the queen's daily food consumption will often reach 1.5 times her nonpregnant level. Her body weight should increase by 40% to 50% by the end of her pregnancy. Do not withhold food; increasing the number of feedings per day is helpful in allowing her to eat enough for her needs and those of the fetuses. By the end of the nursing period, daily food consumption may exceed two times the prepregnancy amount. Weight loss during nursing is normal no matter how much the queen eats.

Nursing the Feline Patient, First Edition. Edited by Linda E. Schmeltzer and Gary D. Norsworthy.

Complications during Pregnancy

Infection, abortion, and uterine torsion are potential complications that may occur during pregnancy. It is important for clients to understand that vaginal discharge is never normal during pregnancy. Should the queen become suddenly ill and painful or have vaginal discharge, immediate veterinary examination is advised.

Parturition

During the final week of pregnancy the queen will begin to search for the most suitable place to deliver her kittens. Depending on the temperament of the queen, she will choose either a dark enclosed space away from people and noise or seek comfort from the owner and choose a location near their presence. Some queens will accept a "queening box" as a suitable place for delivery. The box should be large enough for the queen to move around freely but have low enough sides so that she can see out. The bottom of the box should be lined with several layers of newspaper or other disposable absorbent material. The upper soiled layers should be able to be removed with minimal interruption to the queen and her newborn kittens.

The process of labor and delivery is known as parturition. The signs of impending labor generally include nervousness and panting. The queen may quit eating 24 hours before labor begins. She may also have a drop in rectal temperature below 37.8°C (100°F). The temperature drop may occur intermittently for several days prior to delivery, but it will usually be constant for the last 24 hours.

Phase I of parturition is from the first observed contraction until the birth of the first kitten. The average duration is 30 to 60 minutes and typically takes less than 2 hours.

Phase II is the time between the birth of the first and last kitten. Delivery times will vary greatly. Shorthair breeds and breeds having slim heads, such as Orientals, may complete delivery in 1–2 hours. Domestic body type breeds (having large, round heads) generally require longer delivery times. Persian and other domestic body type kittens tend to be very large and have sizable heads that make delivery more difficult (Fig. 5-1). It is not unusual for Persians to rest an hour or more between each kitten. Rarely, a queen may deliver one or two kittens, then have labor stop for as long as 24 hours before the remainder of the litter is born. However, if labor does not resume within a few hours after the delivery of the first kittens, examination by a veterinarian is advised. If labor is interrupted for 24 hours or more, veterinary assistance should definitely be obtained.

Most queens experience delivery without complications; however, first-time mothers should be attended until at least one or two kittens are born. If these are born quickly and without assistance, further attendance may not be necessary, although it is desirable.

Kittens are usually born head first; however, breech presentations, in which the kitten is delivered tail-end first, occur about 40% of the time and are also considered normal. Each kitten is enclosed in a sac that is part of the placenta. The placenta is usually delivered with each kitten. However, any that do not pass will disintegrate and pass within 24 to 48 hours after delivery. If the delivery proceeds normally, a few contractions will discharge the kitten; it should exit the birth canal within 10 minutes of being visible. Once the delivery is completed, any soiled bedding should be removed with as little interruption to the queen as possible. The queen should accept the kittens readily and recline for nursing.

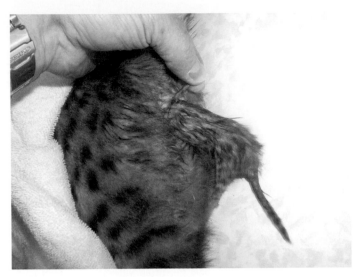

Figure 5-1 Dystocia occurs in several ways. Brachycephalic cats have proportionally larger heads that may have difficulty passing through the birth canal and result in "head lock."

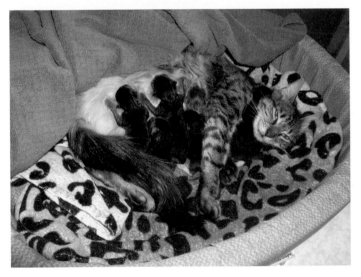

Figure 5-2 Newborn kittens have difficulty maintaining normal body temperature. They huddle together and stay with their mother to do so.

The queen and her litter should be examined by a veterinarian within 24 hours after the delivery is completed. This visit is to check the queen for complete delivery and to check the health of the newborn kittens. The mother may need to receive an injection to contract the uterus and stimulate milk production.

It is normal for the queen to have a bloody vaginal discharge for 3 to 7 days following delivery. If it continues for longer than a week, she should be examined by a veterinarian.

Problems during Delivery

Although most queens deliver without need for assistance, problems do arise that require the attention of a veterinarian. Professional assistance should be sought if any of the following occur:

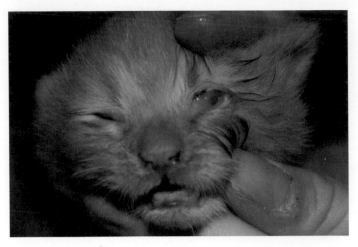

Figure 5-3 Drainage from the eye of a kitten before the eyes have fully opened can indicate infection.

Signs of problems

- No kitten is delivered after 20 minutes of intense labor.
- A kitten or a fluid-filled bubble is visible in the birth canal after 10 minutes of intense labor.
- The mother experiences acute (sudden) depression or marked lethargy.
- The mother's rectal temperature exceeds 39.4°C (103°F).
- Fresh blood discharges from the vagina for more than 10 minutes.

Difficulty delivering (dystocia) may be managed with or without surgery. The condition of the mother, size of the litter, and size of the kittens are factors used in making that decision.

Stillborn Kittens

It is not uncommon for one or two kittens in a litter to be stillborn. Although there is always a cause for this occurrence, it is often not easily determined without a necropsy that includes cultures and the submission of tissues to a pathologist. This is only recommended in special circumstances.

Newborn Kittens

The mother will spend most of her time with the kittens during the next few days. The kittens need to be kept warm and nurse frequently. They should be checked every few hours to make certain they are warm and well fed. The mother should be checked to make certain she is producing adequate milk.

Eclampsia

Eclampsia, commonly known as milk fever, is a depletion of calcium from the queen due to heavy milk production. It generally occurs to mothers with large litters, during the peak of lactation (when the kittens are 3–5 weeks old) but may occur during parturition. Clinical signs vary but may include muscle spasms resulting in rigid legs, spastic movements, and heavy panting. This can be fatal in 30 to 60 minutes, so a veterinarian should be consulted immediately. Treatment with intravenous calcium is usually successful. Heart rate should be monitored carefully during treatment and stopped if bradycardia (slow heart rate) develops.

Troubleshooting Newborn Kittens

If the mother does not stay with the kittens, their temperature must be monitored. Kittens are not capable of body temperature regulation until around their sixth day of life; therefore, supplemental heating should be provided. During the first week of life, the newborns' rectal temperature should be maintained between 35° and 36.1°C (95°–97°F). Providing a warm environment between 29.4° and 32.2°C (85°–90°F) should be sufficient. The temperature may not need to be kept as high for larger litters. As kittens huddle together, their body heat provides additional warmth (Fig. 5-2). The room temperature may gradually be decreased to 26.7°C (80°F) around the seventh to tenth day and to 22.2°C (72°F) by the end of the fourth week.

Kittens should eat or sleep 90% of the time during their first two weeks of life. Crying during or after eating can be a sign they are becoming ill or are not getting adequate milk. A newborn kitten is highly susceptible to infections. If excessive crying occurs, the queen and the entire litter should be examined by a veterinarian promptly.

When the queen's milk supply is inadequate, supplemental feeding one to three times per day is recommended and should be performed on any litter with five or more kittens. There are several milk replacement formulas available that are made to supply the needs of kittens. Some require no preparation other than warming. Milk replacement formula should be warmed to between 35° and 37.8°C (95°–100°F) before feeding. The formula temperature can be tested on one's forearm and should be about the same temperature as the skin. The commercial products have directions concerning feeding amounts. If the kittens are still nursing from their mother, the amounts recommended will be excessive. Generally, one-third to one-half of the listed amount should be the daily goal. Supplemental feeding may be continued until the kittens are old enough to eat kitten food.

If the mother does not produce milk or her milk becomes infected, the kittens will require supplemental feeding. Adopting the kittens to another nursing mother would be the most ideal. If replacement feeding is the only option, the amounts of milk listed on the product should be fed. Kittens less than 2 weeks of age should be fed every 3 to 4 hours. Kittens 2–4 weeks of age usually do well with feedings every 6 to 8 hours. Weaning, as described, should begin around 4 weeks of age.

The First Few Weeks of Life

Kittens are born with their eyes and ears closed. Their eyes will open in 7 to 14 days. Their ears usually open 24 hours after their eyes. If swelling or bulging is noted under the eyelids they should be opened gently to check for infection (Fig. 5-3). A cotton ball dampened with warm water may be used to assist opening the lids. If the swelling is due to infection, pus will drain from the opened eyelids and should be treated as prescribed by a veterinarian.

Kittens should be observed for their rate of growth, especially if they are being fed a milk replacement. Within 1 week a kitten should double its birth weight. At 2 weeks of age kittens should be alert and trying to stand. At 3 weeks they generally begin exploring their environment outside their bed or box. At 4 weeks all of the kittens should be able to walk, run, and play.

Kittens should begin eating solid food about 3½ to 4½ weeks of age. Initially, one of the milk replacers can be diluted 50:50 with water. This should be placed in a flat saucer. Once the kittens are comfortably lapping milk from the saucer, canned kitten food should be mixed into the milk until it is soggy. The amount of milk should be decreased daily until they are eating the canned food with little or no moisture added. This should occur by 4 to 6 weeks of age.

Dietary Requirements of the Growing Kitten

Proper nutrition is extremely important for a growing kitten. A kitten weighing 2 to 3 kg (~5 pounds) will need an average of 200 kilocalories per day. Kittens will eat small amounts as often as 12 times during the day. There are many commercial foods specially formulated for kittens. These foods meet the kitten's unique nutritional requirements and should be fed until 12 months of age.

Suggested Readings

Colville T. 2008. The Reproductive System. In T Colville, JM Bassert, eds., *Clinical Anatomy and Physiology for Veterinary Technicians*, 2nd ed., pp. 403–4. St. Louis: Mosby Inc.

Hoskins JD, Bolt DM, McCurnin DM, et al. 2006. Neonatal Care of the Puppy, Kitten, and Foal. In DM McCurnin, JM Bassert, eds., *Clinical Textbook for Veterinary Technicians*, 6th ed., pp. 382–88. St. Louis: Elsevier Saunders.

National Research Council of the National Academies. 2006. *Nutrient Requirements of Dogs and Cats*, pp. 39–45; 103–104; 364, 366, 368. Washington: The National Academies Press.

Norsworthy GD. 2011. Dystocia. In GD Norsworthy, ed., *The Feline Patient*, 4th ed., pp. 138–39. Ames: Wiley-Blackwell.

Tefend M, Berryhill SA, McCurnin DM, et al. 2006. Companion Animal Clinical Nutrition. In DM McCurnin, JM Bassert, eds., *Clinical Textbook for Veterinary Technicians*, 6th ed., pp. 464–65. St. Louis: Elsevier Saunders.

Viita-aho TK. 2011. Pregnancy, Parturition and Lactation. In GD Norsworthy, ed., *The Feline Patient*, 4th ed., pp. 979–81. Ames: Wiley-Blackwell.

CHAPTER 6

Geriatric Care

Karen M. Lovelace

Overview

As the field of veterinary medicine advances so does the recognition that cats need and benefit greatly from lifelong routine health care. More cats are being seen for routine wellness visits and preventative care every 6 months or less, depending on special needs. In turn, more of the cats presented for examination are older cats, and many of their owners have questions about how to increase longevity and quality of life for their feline companions. Veterinary teams must, therefore, become familiar with the special considerations and needs that an aged feline may present.

In response to this growing need, the American Animal Hospital Association (AAHA) and the American Association of Feline Practitioners (AAFP) have developed Feline Life Stage Guidelines (AAFP and AAHA) and Senior Care Guidelines (AAFP). More emphasis has been placed on recognizing the needs of cats based on life stage, especially the aging cat. The AAFP and AAHA guidelines classify cats ages 7–10 as mature, 11–14 as senior, and 15 years and older as geriatric. This chapter will highlight the considerations that deserve unique attention in these older feline groups, especially the geriatric group, in regard to semi-annual physical examination, aging changes, routine diagnostic/laboratory needs, and specific nutritional considerations.

Semi-Annual Wellness Examination

Examination findings of an older cat, when compared to examination of a younger cat, will likely center more on weight and body condition changes, dental disease, behavior related to cognitive or physical changes, osteoarthritis, grooming changes, increased incidence of hypertension, renal disease, neoplasia, endocrinopathy, pain, and quality of life assessment. General knowledge of approximate age and the special considerations pertinent to older feline life stages should be supplemented with a thorough history that includes age-directed questions. In addition to developing clues about a cat's health and quality of life that may otherwise be missed on a routine diagnostic screen or even the examination itself, this will help guide the veterinary team in making appropriate recommendations to clients about older feline patients.

If the client brought the cat in for a specific concern, questions may be posed related to this topic first, but a thorough history should still include questions relating to the whole cat and its environment, and ideally, should not be limited to questions surrounding the presenting complaint alone.

History Taking for Older Cats

History for a wellness examination may start by inquiring about specific dietary habits including brand, whether food offered is wet and/or dry, frequency and location of feeding, portions, number of animals in the home, whether animals are fed in groups or individually, any treats, nutraceuticals, herbal remedies, and/or supplements, any changes or concerns regarding eating behavior, and the cat's preferences or aversions.

Inquire as to current medications, including parasiticides, name of medication, dose, frequency, and route of administration. Ask the owner if there have been any changes in medication or administration or any concerns surrounding the cat's medication routine.

Ask for an appetite assessment such as "How would you characterize his or her appetite," and regardless of coat length, ask about frequency of vomiting, especially related to hairballs and grass.

Note if the cat has had any coughing, sneezing, or breathing changes since the last visit.

Ask about any change in social interactions with other animals or people in the home.

The client should be questioned about litter box routine and frequency and character of the cat's bowel movements and urinations. Specifically ask if the cat is consistently using the litter box, and if not, request information such as how many litter boxes are in the home, location, size, and height of box sides, litter substrate, and if the box is shared with any other cats. When probing for polyuria, ask if there has been an increase in wet litter in the litter box.

Ask about water intake and availability and if any change in thirst has been noted.

Ask questions about the availability of other resources such as scratching posts, toys, beds, hiding places, and perches or "look out" areas (i.e. vertical surfaces).

Inquire as to any changes noted in vocalization or sleeping patterns or changes in the cat's behavior from day as opposed to night.

Open-ended questions are especially helpful. For example, "What changes have you noticed?", "What concerns do you have?", "What else?", and "How is that going?" are more productive than "yes" or "no" questions or questions that lead the client or result in limited choices as answers. You may also want to use the history-taking session as an opportunity to open a dialogue about specific areas previously noted in the medical record, such as grooming or at-home dental care. Using this time to converse with clients also gives the cat a chance to acclimate to the examination room setting and may reduce the overall stress of the veterinary visit.

Physical Examination

When history taking is completed, the cat should be weighed and its temperature, pulse, and respiratory rate recorded. This is a good time to conduct a visual examination of the cat and make any notes that might be appropriate as to overall body condition, coat quality, vision, hearing, gait, ease of movement, and attitude. It is also a good time to review visual aids with the client such as body condition score charts or computer-generated graphs showing trends or changes in weight (Fig. 6-1).

If time permits and the cat is cooperative, veterinary technicians are encouraged to physically examine the patient prior to the veterinarian's examination and report these findings to the veterinarian. Involvement of multiple tiers of the veterinary team may allow the client to express a specific concern not already addressed during the history-taking session and build trust in the veterinary team. Although the veterinary technician should not make a diagnosis, sharing observations (such as showing a client dental calculus [tartar] prior to the veterinarian's examination) will likely help increase client compliance with the veterinarian's recommendations. Preliminary examination may also help to catch problems the veterinarian or client may overlook.

Nursing the Feline Patient, First Edition. Edited by Linda E. Schmeltzer and Gary D. Norsworthy.
© 2012 John Wiley & Sons, Inc. Published 2012 by John Wiley & Sons, Inc.

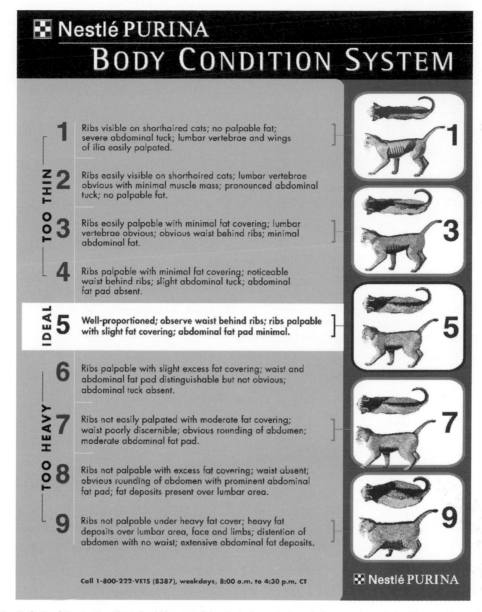

Figure 6-1 Use of the Purina Body Condition Scoring Chart should be part of the physical examination of all cats and especially older cats. The cat's conformation is judged on a 1- to 9-scale with 5 being ideal.
Used courtesy of Nestle Purina Company, St. Louis.

The next step is the physical examination itself. The veterinarian should assess each body system and should share with the client his or her findings verbally and by pointing out specific findings as they are discovered. The veterinarian should examine the cat in a systematic and repeatable fashion, such as from head to tail.

Specifics of the Physical Examination

- Quality of hair coat and skin is noted.
- The head and face are noted for symmetry.
- The eyes and vision are assessed, including fundic examination (examination of the retinas) with an ophthalmoscope.
- The eyes may be gently retropulsed (pushed back into the eye sockets) to check for masses behind the eyes.

- The ears are checked; the otoscope should be used to visualize the eardrums and check for debris. A rough assessment of hearing can be made by clapping your hands behind the cat's head, where it cannot see, and checking for response, such as movement of the pinnae.
- Airway and breath or any discharge from the nose is noted.
- The lips, teeth, and oral cavity are checked including the back of the throat and under the tongue. Examination under the tongue is most easily achieved by gently pressing a thumb or forefinger in an upward direction between the mandible (Fig. 6-2). This can be an important location to look for masses or foreign objects, such as string.
- Any abnormalities in the breath or gingiva and the presence of dental tartar are specifically noted.
- Lymph nodes at the base of the jaw (mandibular lymph nodes) are palpated, and then both sides of the neck are gently palpated to check for any thyroid gland enlargement.

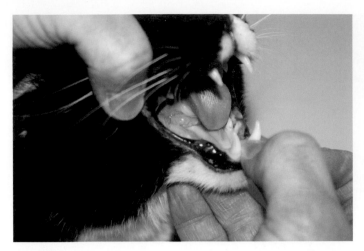

Figure 6-2 A mass is seen ventral to the tongue by pressing upward with a finger between the mandible.
Photo courtesy Dr. Gary D. Norsworthy.

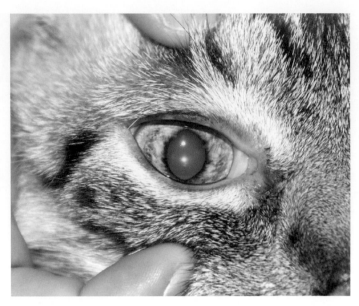

Figure 6-4 Iris atrophy results in discoloration of the iris as seen in this 16-year-old cat.
Photo courtesy Dr. Gary D. Norsworthy.

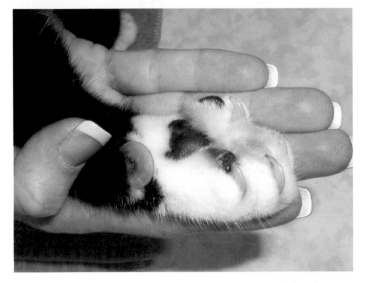

Figure 6-3 Geriatric cats often have overgrown and thickened nails. They often grow into the pads.
Photo courtesy Dr. Gary D. Norsworthy.

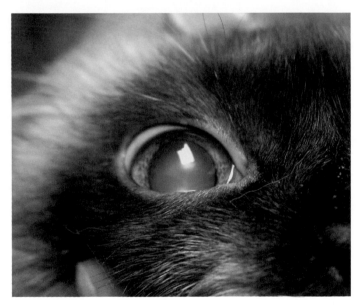

Figure 6-5 Nuclear sclerosis is not the same as a cataract, but it results in lenticular cloudiness and reduces vision.
Photo courtesy Dr. Gary D. Norsworthy.

- A stethoscope is used to assess heart rate and rhythm and to listen for murmurs and lung sounds. The cat's pulse (usually of femoral artery) may be palpated during cardiac auscultation to assess for synchronicity or pulse deficits.
- The abdomen is palpated. Size, symmetry, and shape are noted for the liver, kidneys, stomach, spleen (if enlarged), and urinary bladder, and for any thickening of the small and large bowel or mesenteric lymph nodes. A stethoscope may be used to assess motility via gut sounds, called borborygmi.
- Response to palpation including any perceived pain is noted.
- Joints are assessed for thickening, crepitus, pain, and range of motion.
- The mammary glands should be palpated in female cats to detect masses.
- The veterinarian may also do a final once over with the hands by petting the cat's entire body to check for symmetry or any lumps or areas of pain.

Any significant findings should be reported to the client and a discussion opened about diagnostic and therapeutic recommendations. Use the findings developed through the history, examination, and any diagnostic results to educate clients about the unique needs of their older feline patients and to tailor diagnostic and therapeutic advice, including dietary recommendations.

Aging Changes

Over the first year of life a cat may rapidly age up to 18 years in human terms, but then maturation slows to approximately 3 to 5 cat years for each calendar year thereafter. At age 15, a geriatric cat is comparable to

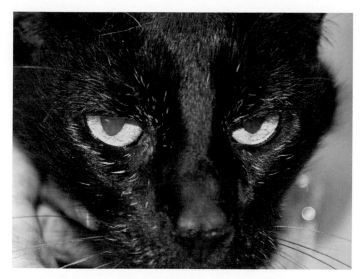

Figure 6-6 Leukotrichia (graying of the hair) is common in cats more than 15 years of age.
Photo courtesy Dr. Gary D. Norsworthy.

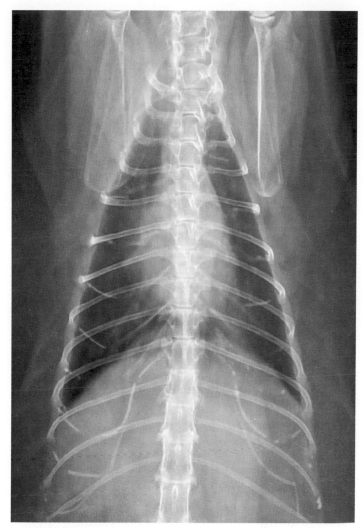

Figure 6-8 Ossification (calcification) of the rib cartilages is seen on this radiograph. It signifies aging, but it causes no functional problems.
Photo courtesy Dr. Gary D. Norsworthy.

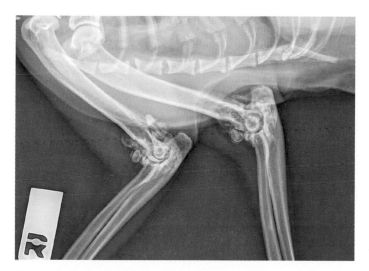

Figure 6-7 Osteoarthritis, as seen in these elbows, also commonly affects the shoulders, hips, and knees of geriatric cats.
Photo courtesy Dr. Gary D. Norsworthy.

older cats may result in more treatment options, better prognosis, and improvement in quality of life.

Diagnostic Screening

As cats mature, the incidence of specific diseases increases and cats may develop concurrent diseases that are not uncommonly chronic or complex in nature. Therefore, diagnostic screening is more important in older cats. Most notably, there is an increased incidence in hypertension, renal disease, and hyperthyroidism, but an increase in neoplasia, other endocrine disease, weight loss/decreased body condition score, dental disease, behavior problems related to cognitive or physical changes, osteoarthritis, pain, and grooming changes may also become apparent. A physical examination and a "senior panel" including blood pressure measurement, complete blood count, chemistry panel, thyroid level, and urinalysis with or without culture are recommended at 6-month intervals.

This minimum data base is recommended every 6 months as early as the mature life stage (7–10 years), but it is particularly important for cats in the senior and geriatric life stages (i.e. older than age 10). Total T4 should be used as a minimum parameter to screen the thyroid, but often

a 60- to 88-year-old human, and at age 21 it is comparable to a person that is 78–118 years old. At these advanced ages, some predictable physical and behavioral changes are commonly noted.

Physically, skin elasticity decreases, nails may become thickened and overgrown (Fig. 6-3) or brittle; eyes may show iris atrophy (Fig. 6-4) or pigment changes; and lenses may become cloudy (lenticular sclerosis, not to be confused with cataracts [Fig. 6-5]). The hair coat may show loss of pigment (grey hair also known as achromotrichia or leukotrichia [Fig. 6-6]); joints may degenerate (osteoarthritis [Fig. 6-7]); ribs may mineralize (Fig. 6-8); and sensory perception, such as hearing and olfaction, may decrease. These are some of the more predictable findings one can expect in an older cat, but every animal ages at a slightly different rate based on metabolism, genetics, and environment. Therefore, an examination and diagnostic screen every 6 months is particularly important in older cats that are aging at an accelerated rate compared to their younger counterparts. Old age is not a disease, but early detection of changes in

27

additional thyroid screening, such as free T4, may be indicated. Renal function and degeneration should be carefully monitored using a complete blood count to evaluate hematocrit; chemistry panel to monitor creatinine, blood urea nitrogen, phosphorus, calcium, and potassium; and urinalysis to assess urine specific gravity and urine protein. The urine protein-to-creatinine ratio (UPC) may be indicated as dipstick protein measurements are often inaccurate. A UPC more than 0.4 warrants further testing. Urine culture is indicated if there is active urine sediment, concurrent renal or thyroid disease, hypertension, or diabetes mellitus, or if urine specific gravity is very dilute or repeatedly below 1.035. These screening aids can help to detect otherwise occult (hidden) disease at an early, more treatable stage in a clinically normal aging cat. Hypertension and urinary tract infection are common comorbid occult diseases in cats with renal disease, thyroid disease, and diabetes mellitus; therefore, blood pressure measurement and urine culture are indicated in each of these cases.

Every attempt to keep cats comfortable and decrease stress should be made when blood pressure is measured. The cat should be placed on a soft, warm surface, such as a towel, in a quiet, dimly lit room away from loud noises and barking dogs, ideally with the owner present. It is advisable to allow the cat to acclimate to the new surroundings for up to 10 minutes with the owner present to help reduce anxiety associated with a new environment. In a clinical setting, a consultation room or a room situated away from the hospital treatment area or lobby may be best suited for this purpose. Undue anxiety can lead to false elevations in routine blood pressure measurements. An average of three, but no more than five, measurements should be taken. Beyond this many readings, the vessel or pulse quality may begin to fatigue and falsely lower the measured readings. Data collected from serum creatinine concentration, UPC ratio, and blood pressure measurements are further used to stage feline renal status to aid in the management of chronic kidney disease as based on the International Renal Interest Society (IRIS) guidelines. When examination and age-directed considerations have yielded appropriately indicated diagnostic results, these compiled findings can be used to make the best dietary recommendations for specific older felines.

Special Nutritional Considerations

Nutritional recommendations for the aged feline should be based on physical examination and diagnostic screen findings, as well as history, number of cats in the household, and any concurrent disease or painful condition. Every physical examination should involve the owner in assessment of body condition score (see Fig. 6-1). Many senior cats will have reduced body condition scores owing to decreased digestive absorption of B-vitamins (most notably cobalamin, or B_{12}) and fat, whether due to normal aging or to concurrent metabolic or inflammatory diseases; therefore, a highly digestible diet is recommended. In some instances, such as progressive weight loss, cobalamin levels and survey diagnostic imaging will be indicated. Smaller but more frequent meals with an ample fresh water supply are vital to keeping older cats hydrated and aiding in assimilating nutrition. Because some wet foods are significantly lower in complex carbohydrates and still contain adequate protein and more water, lower carbohydrate wet food is generally recommended. For cats that are obese or diabetic, wet foods are also recommended due to decreased caloric levels as related to carbohydrates. For cats with specific renal, hyperthyroid, hypertensive, or cardiac conditions, renal specific diets, which are reduced in phosphorus, salt, and carefully balanced in protein, are indicated to increase survival times and result in better control of disease and quality of life. Calculation of daily energy requirements should also take into consideration age as it pertains to activity and lifestyle. Daily energy requirement (DER) is calculated using this formula: DER = Kg × 30 + 70 times a factor for life stage, disease, or activity level, which would be less than one for desired weight loss and greater than one for conditions that necessitate increasing energy demands such as neoplasia.

Conclusion

Although age itself is not a disease, the aging process does induce complex and interrelated metabolic changes that complicate health care. Management decisions should not be based solely on the age of the patient because many conditions that affect older cats can be controlled if not cured. With the help of veterinary technicians, veterinarians treating senior cats should be adept at recognizing, managing, and monitoring chronic disease, and when possible, preventing disease progression while ensuring a good quality of life. With prevention, early detection, and treatment of health care problems, the human-animal-veterinarian bond is strengthened and the quality of life for cats improved.

As cats live longer and more cats receive more frequent veterinary care, increased attention must be paid by the entire veterinary staff to the special needs of older felines, especially regarding routine semi-annual physical examination, aging changes, routine diagnostic/laboratory needs, and specific nutritional considerations. Both veterinarians and veterinary team members alike must be trained in recognizing age-specific changes to facilitate preventative health care, improved quality of life, and a better relationship between the veterinary practice, feline patients, and their owners. This increased emphasis and training will enable the veterinary team to successfully respond to the growing trend of seeing more and older cats and will facilitate the veterinary team and clients alike in addressing health problems that an aging feline population may face and enabling cats to lead happier, healthier lives.

Suggested Readings

Bond BR. 2005. Fine Tuning the History and Physical Examination: Correlations with Miscellaneous Techniques. *Clin Tech Small Anim Pract.* 20(3):203–10. New York: Animal Medical Center Publishing Co.

Boyd LM, Langston C, Thompson K, et al. 2008. Survival in Cats with Naturally Occurring Chronic Kidney Disease. *J Vet Intern Med.* 22(5):1111–17.

Lovelace KM. 2010. Age Approximation. In GD Norsworthy, ed., *The Feline Patient*, 4th ed., pp. 933–36. Ames: Wiley-Blackwell.

Norsworthy GD. 2010. Jugular Blood Collection. In GD Norsworthy, ed., *The Feline Patient*, 4th ed., pp. 902–903. Ames: Wiley-Blackwell.

Vogt AH, Rodan I, Brown M, et al. 2010. AAFP-AAHA: Feline Life Stage Guidelines. *J Fel Med Surg.* 12(1):43–54. Philadelphia: Elsevier, www.catvets.com.

Vogt AH, Rodan I, Brown M, et al. 2010. AAFP-AAHA: Feline Life Stage Guidelines. *J Am Anim Hosp Assoc.* 46(1):70–85. Philadelphia: Elsevier, www.aahanet.org.

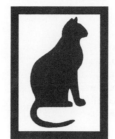

Diagnostics

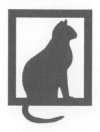

CHAPTER 7

Diagnostic Imaging of the Feline Patient

Judith Hudson and Merrilee Holland

Overview

Radiography has a multifaceted role in patient management. It is one of many possible diagnostic aids, sometimes permitting precise diagnosis, but more commonly, it aids expansion or reduction of a list of diagnoses. It can also enable better evaluation of the course of a disease whether or not therapy has been administered. Even when ultrasonography is available, abdominal radiography can help provide a complete picture of the abdomen to prevent abnormalities from being missed. Gas can obscure visualization of abdominal organs by ultrasound.

Radiation Safety

X-rays are a form of ionizing radiation. Film badges should be used to monitor radiation exposure to personnel to reduce exposure to a level that is "as low as reasonably achievable" (ALARA principle). Pregnant radiation workers should notify their superior in writing so that additional precautions can be taken to avoid radiation or keep it at a legal level.

In some instances, the patient can be sedated or anesthetized so that positioning can be achieved using tape, gauze, Velcro straps, or sandbags. If the patient must be physically restrained by hospital personnel, people holding the cat should wear protective clothing that minimally includes lead gloves, lead-lined aprons, and a thyroid collar. Protective eye glasses are also available. Remember that primary radiation can penetrate through the lead protective clothing. Hands should never be in the primary beam even when gloves are worn.

The inverse square law states that the amount of radiation exposure is inversely related to the square of the distance to the source of radiation.

New Exposure/Old Exposure = Old Distance²/New Distance²

More simply, this means that if you double the distance between you and the x-ray tube, you reduce your exposure to one-fourth of the original exposure. If you are holding a patient, extending your arms and stepping back away from the table will also reduce your level of exposure. Collimators are present on the tube assembly to restrict the primary beam to the area of the patient to be radiographed. Correct collimation can help reduce the radiation field protecting the radiographer as well as the patient from unnecessary radiation.

Technical Factors

The main technical factors include kilovoltage (kVp), milliamperage (mA), time (s), and distance (d). The process of producing x-rays begins when electrons are "boiled" off the cathode of the x-ray tube and accelerated toward the anode. X-rays are emitted when the electrons interact with the anode. kVp can be considered as controlling the quality of the x-ray beam. Increasing the kVp increases the speed of the electrons striking the anode so that the resulting x-rays are more energetic and thus, have more ability to penetrate. Reducing kVp increases the contrast of a film (fewer shades of gray). mA and time are considered together; increasing the mA or time results in the emission of more electrons from

the cathode. More electrons strike the anode producing more x-rays. Increasing mA increases exposure or the number of x-rays.

If the distance between the patient and the x-ray tube is changed, exposure to the patient will be altered according to the inverse square law. For example, halving the distance causes exposure to increase four times. Because mA can be considered as affecting the number of x-rays, mA can be changed to compensate for a change in distance. In the example in which the distance is halved, it might be desirable to keep the blackness of the film unchanged. Because halving the distance causes the effective exposure to be increased four times, mA can be decreased to one-fourth of the original value to maintain the film density.

Doubling or halving mA is roughly equivalent to increasing or decreasing kVp by approximately 15%. It should be noted, however, that a minimum kVp is necessary to penetrate the abdomen. If the kVp used is too low to penetrate the abdomen, increasing mA will not result in a diagnostic film.

Technique Chart

A technique chart for each body part should be used for consistency in determining the correct mA and kVp to use for different thicknesses (Table 7-1). An individual technique chart must be developed for each machine and film/screen system. Grid factor depends on the grid being used.

In creating a fixed mA/variable kVp chart, choose a high mA so that time can be reduced. An initial kVp is chosen using the following relationship (based on Sante's rule):

kVp = (2 × tissue thickness) + focus film distance + grid factor

TABLE 7-1: Example of a portion of a fixed milliamperage/variable kilovoltage technique chart. A technique chart should be set up for each x-ray machine. What works for one machine is not likely to work for another. Using this chart for a 12-cm abdomen, one would select 250 mA, 20 milliseconds, and 64 kVp.

TECHNIQUE CHART FOR GRID								
SELECT LARGE FOCAL SPOT AND BUCKY								
THORAX 250 mA TIME 1/120 seconds								
CM								
9	10	11	12	13	14	14	15	16
KV								
58	60	62	64	66	68	70	72	74

ABDOMEN 250 mA TIME 1/60 seconds								
CM								
9	10	11	12	13	14	14	15	16
KV								
58	60	62	64	66	68	70	72	74

PELVIS/HUMERUS/SHOULDER/FEMUR/STIFLE 300 mA TIME 1/30 seconds								
CM								
9	10	11	12	13	14	14	15	16
KV								
52	54	56	58	60	62	64	66	68

kvp, kilovoltage; ma, milliamperage.

Nursing the Feline Patient, First Edition. Edited by Linda E. Schmeltzer and Gary D. Norsworthy.

The focus film distance is normally set at 40 inches. The grid factor varies with the type of grid that is being used. A grid is unnecessary if the body part measures less than 9–11 cm.

For each body part, the chosen mA and calculated kVp are used to expose an initial film of an average-sized cat. If the film is too black, reduce kVp by increments of 15% until the exposed film is optimal. If the film is too light, increase kVp by increments of 15% until the goal is met.

The chart can now be created by starting with the exposure factors for the initial film. The mA will be fixed at the value you selected. Write the thickness of the cat and the optimal kVp on the chart. Values of kVp for other thicknesses are calculated by adding (or subtracting) 2 kVp for each 1-cm increase (or decrease) in thickness. Above 80 kVp, the amount to increase or decrease should be changed to 3 kVp. More than 100 kVp, 4 kVp should be used.

Digital Radiography

For digital radiographs, incorrect exposure does not result in the image being too black or too light. Underexposure causes an image to appear too noisy or too grainy. A certain amount of graininess is acceptable and exposure should not be increased simply to eliminate noise. Overexposure can cause some parts of the image to be lost.

Examining the Radiograph

A lateral radiograph should be placed on the view box or viewing screen with the head of the patient on the left side of the view box or screen. A ventrodorsal radiograph is positioned so that the right side of the patient is on the viewer's left. This tradition is borrowed from radiography of humans; the radiologist views the film as though he or she was about to shake hands with the patient.

The quality of a radiograph should be assessed by evaluating positioning (below) and technical factors and by checking for the presence of any artifacts (Fig. 7-1). If mA, kVp, or time is too low, the film will be underexposed appearing too light (Fig. 7-2). If kVp is too low, the body part being radiographed will be underpenetrated and borders of structures will not be visible. If mA, kVp, or time is too high, the film will be overexposed, appearing excessively black.

(a)

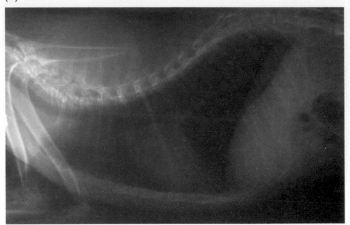

(b)

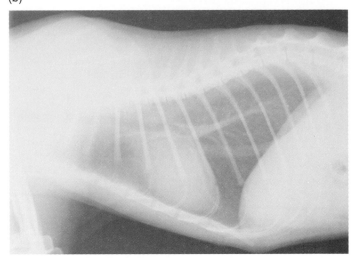

Figure 7-2 (a) The film shown is overexposed, requiring a reduction in mA or kVp. Distance should also be checked. If distance was too short, the exposure could be corrected by increasing the distance. (b) The film shown is underexposed, requiring an increase in mA or kVp. If distance was too great, the exposure could be corrected by decreasing the distance. Note that if kVp is insufficient to penetrate the patient, increasing mA will not correct the problem.

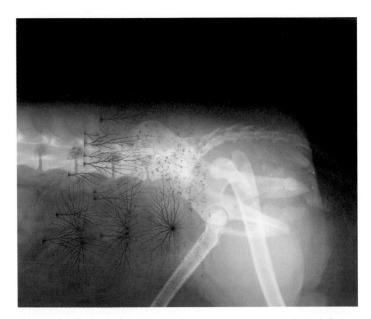

Figure 7-1 Static electricity can produce tree-like designs on your radiograph that are interesting but can hide diagnostic information.

Film processing can also affect the quality of the film. Underdevelopment can occur if chemicals are weak, their temperature is too low, or the film is left in the developer for too short a time. Overdevelopment occurs if chemicals are too strong, the temperature of development is too high, or if the film is left in the developer too long. An underdeveloped film will appear "washed out" and will appear too light. An overdeveloped film will be too black. Examination of the film label can help determine whether improper development or improper exposure has caused a film to be too light or too dark. If the blackness of the film label is correct, the problem is due to the exposure of the film and not the processing. If both the image on the radiograph and the film label are affected, the problem is due to development.

The film should be examined for any artifacts, particularly those that can interfere with interpretation of the film. If visible artifacts are likely to affect the interpretation of the film, radiography should be repeated. Common artifacts include static electricity and those caused by foreign material in the cassette or on the table or positioning sponges.

Thorax

Radiography

The typical radiographic examination of the thorax includes lateral, ventro-dorsal (VD), or dorsoventral (DV) views taken at maximum inspiration. In patients with suspected metastatic lung disease or pneumonia, both lateral views and a VD or DV view can be beneficial for complete evaluation of the thorax. In less cooperative patients, a DV view of the thorax may be impossible. A VD view using a positioning foam trough or v-shaped pad may provide some assistance with keeping the patient in position. The most common technical errors are as a result of position and motion artifacts.

Special considerations prior to taking thoracic radiographs are highlighted here.

Respiratory Status

The most important consideration before taking thoracic radiographs is to determine whether the patient's respiratory effort is normal (Fig. 7-3) or abnormal. Obese patients may require an increase in technique because of their size (Fig. 7-4). If the patient shows increased respiratory effort either by increased rate, abdominal breathing, or open mouth breathing, provide oxygen before proceeding. If fluid is suspected in the pleural space (Fig. 7-5), the radiographic technique should be increased by 5–10 kVp. When fluid is suspected, a DV view of the thorax can be obtained with minimal restraint. Remember the position of the head will determine the position of the thorax. The trick is to gently encourage the patient to face forward; the body will remain in a more symmetrical position for radiographic interpretation. This can be accomplished by placing your gloved hands outside of the front legs without pulling them forward. After evaluation of this image, a lateral view can be obtained when only minimal compression of the lungs is present from the pleural fluid. A similar approach should be done in patients with suspected heart failure (Fig. 7-6) or severe lung disease (Fig. 7-7); a DV image should be obtained prior to the lateral. Now the fluid will be within the lung parenchyma and the radiographic techniques may need to be increased by 5–10 kVp.

Positioning

The lateral view is best obtained by pulling the front legs forward with the center beam along the caudal border of the scapula. For the VD view, center the beam along the caudal border of the scapula with the front limbs pulled cranially. For the DV view, the center of the beam should be caudal to the scapula. The DV view is usually preferable to the VD view when respiratory compromise is significant.

Assessment

The front limbs should be extended forward and the radiograph should include from the caudal cervical spine/thoracic inlet to the cranial abdomen.

Extra Views

Horizontal beam views can only be done when the tube housing can be rotated horizontal to the patient. Indications for these views include distinguishing between "walled off" fluid and soft-tissue masses.

Ultrasound

After obtaining thoracic radiographs, ultrasonography can assist with distinguishing fluid from tissue. Fluid with low cellularity will appear anechoic (black) whereas tissue will typically be more hyperechoic (whiter). Pleural effusion (Fig. 7-8) or mediastinal cyst (Fig. 7-9) can be distinguished from a mediastinal mass (Fig. 7-10) or pleural mass (Fig. 7-11) within the thorax by use of ultrasound. Ultrasound can assist with localization and aspiration of fluid pockets, pleural or mediastinal

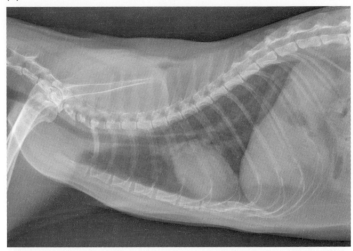
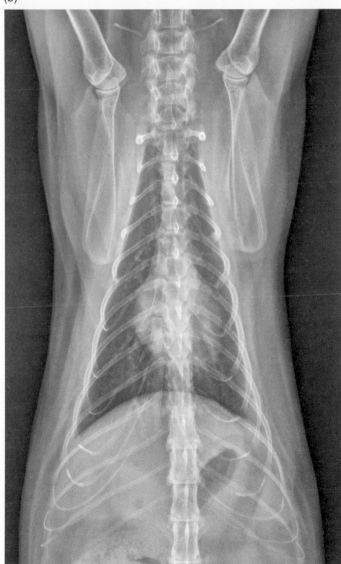

Figure 7-3 (a) Lateral and (b) ventrodorsal radiographs of a normal thorax.

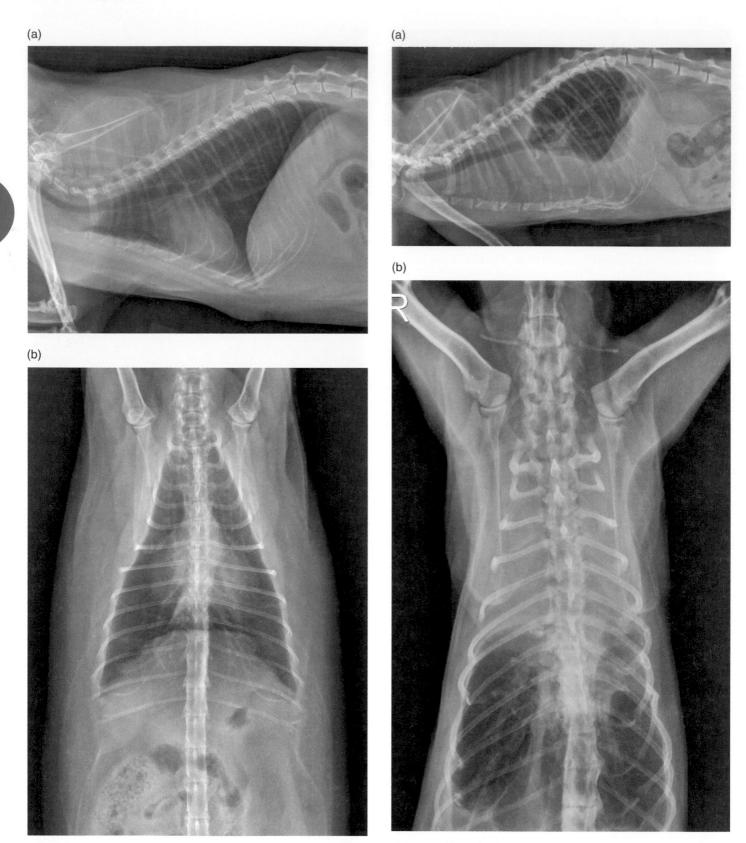

(a)

(b)

(a)

(b)

Figure 7-4 (a) Lateral and (b) ventrodorsal radiographs of a normal overweight feline patient.

Figure 7-5 (a) Lateral and (b) dorsoventral radiographs of a patient with pleural effusion.

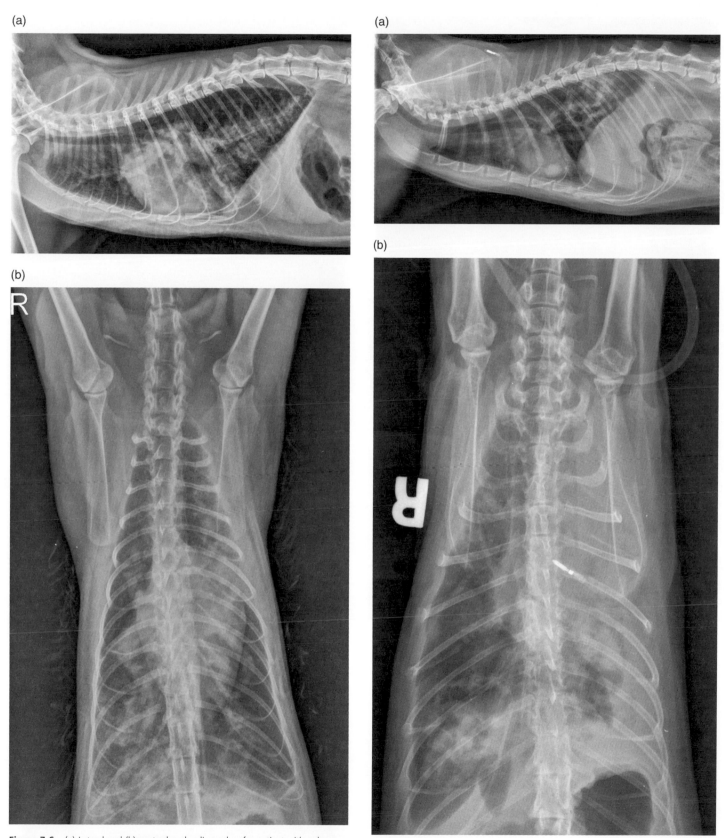

(a)

(b)

(a)

(b)

R

R

Figure 7-6 (a) Lateral and (b) ventrodorsal radiographs of a patient with pulmonary edema due to a congenital ventricular septal defect.

Figure 7-7 (a) Lateral and (b) dorsoventral radiographs of a patient with pleural effusion and lung disease.

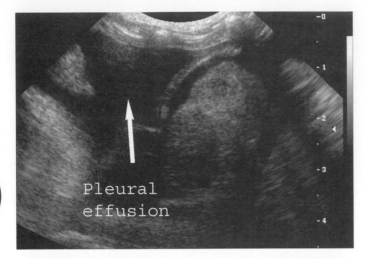

Figure 7-8 Anechoic (black) fluid is seen within the pleural space in a patient with suspected feline infectious peritonitis.

(a)

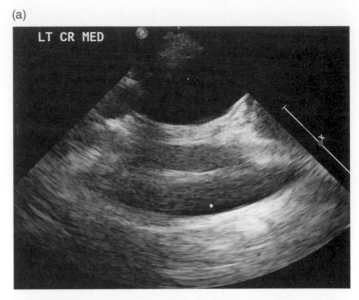

(a)

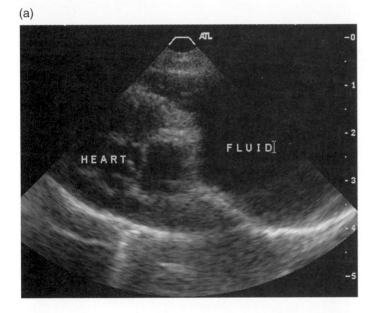

(b)

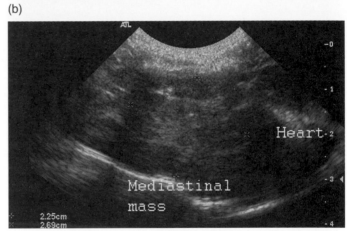

Figure 7-10 (a) Normal cranial mediastinum surrounded by pleural effusion. (b) A mixed echogenic mass is seen cranial to the heart. Lymphosarcoma was the final diagnosis.

(b)

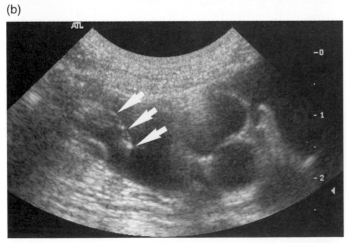

Figure 7-9 (a) A large anechoic fluid pocket adjacent to the heart is consistent with a mediastinal cyst. (b) A mediastinal cyst with a needle (arrows) in place for aspiration.

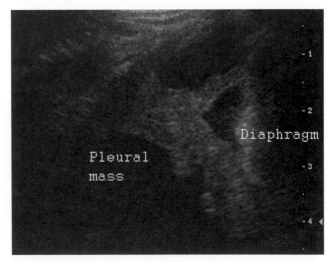

Figure 7-11 An echogenic mass surrounded by fluid is seen extending from the body wall to the diaphragm. The final diagnosis was a neoplastic process.

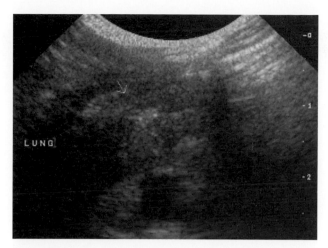

Figure 7-12 A lung mass was identified on thoracic radiographs. Ultrasound can be used to aspirate abnormal lung masses when they are adjacent to the body wall and not surrounded by normal lung. This mixed echogenic mass within the lung was aspirated and the final diagnosis was an adenocarcinoma.

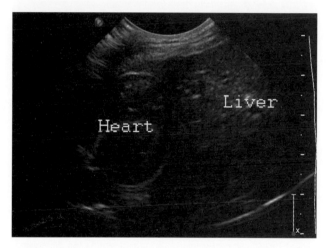

Figure 7-13 A large portion of the liver was found within the pericardial sac adjacent to the heart. A pericardioperitoneal hernia, a congenital malformation, was the final diagnosis.

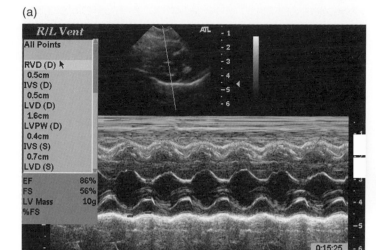

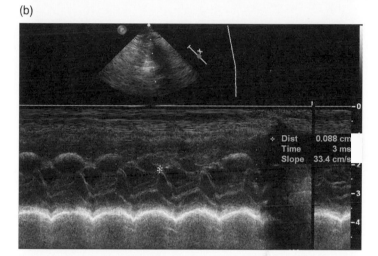

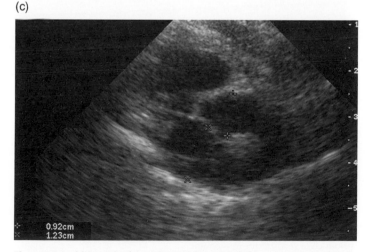

Figure 7-14 (a) M-mode of the right and left ventricle from a right parasternal short-axis view shows normal wall thickness of the interventricular septum and left ventricular free wall. (b) The M-mode of the mitral valve from a right parasternal long-axis view is within normal limits usually less than 2 mm. (c) Measurement of the two-dimensional image of the aorta and left atrium from a right parasternal short-axis view shows the left atrial size less than 1.5 cm.

masses, or lung masses (Fig.7-12). Diaphragmatic or pericardial peritoneal (Fig. 7-13) hernias can be diagnosed by use of ultrasound imaging.

Echocardiograms are more technically difficult to perform in feline patients than in canine patients and are beyond the scope of this text to completely describe. It is best to perform an echocardiogram without sedation and when the patient is not dehydrated or being given intravenous fluids because all of these will alter the cardiac measurements. A normal echocardiogram will typically have the measurements of the interventricular septum and left ventricular free wall less than 6mm in diastole, and the fractional shortening between 45% and 55%. The diameter of a normal left atrium is less than 1.5cm (Fig. 7-14). It is helpful to perform echocardiography in a quiet room with dimmed lighting. Most patients will tolerate these examinations without sedation if the majority of the examination is done while they are in a sternal position. A cardiac table with a cut out will facilitate the probe positioning while the patient is in sternal recumbency. Typically when scanning from sternal, the probe will need to be closer to the sternum to avoid lung interference. Avoid tunnel vision. The structures surrounding the heart are as important to assess as the actual echocardiogram. An abnormal echocardiogram along with fluid accumulation in the pleural space or pericardium can indicate a more advanced stage of heart disease (Fig. 7-15). Increased

(a)

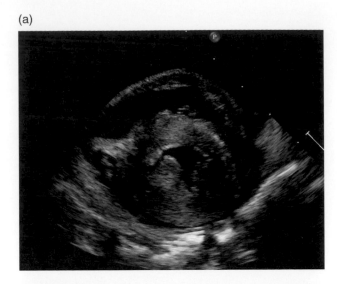

(b)

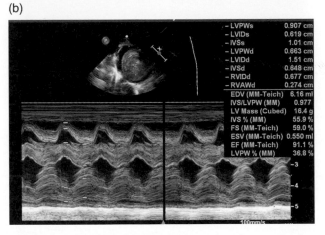

– LVPWs	0.907 cm
– LVIDs	0.619 cm
– IVSs	1.01 cm
– LVPWd	0.663 cm
– LVIDd	1.51 cm
– IVSd	0.648 cm
– RVIDd	0.677 cm
– RVAWd	0.274 cm
EDV (MM-Teich)	6.16 ml
IVS/LVPW (MM)	0.977
LV Mass (Cubed)	16.4 g
IVS % (MM)	55.9 %
FS (MM-Teich)	59.0 %
ESV (MM-Teich)	0.550 ml
EF (MM-Teich)	91.1 %
LVPW % (MM)	36.8 %

100mm/s

Figure 7-15 (a) A two-dimensional image of the heart in a right parasternal short-axis view shows fluid within the pericardial and pleural space. (b) M-mode tracing shows a thickened interventricular septum and left ventricular free wall consistent with cardiomyopathy.

(a)

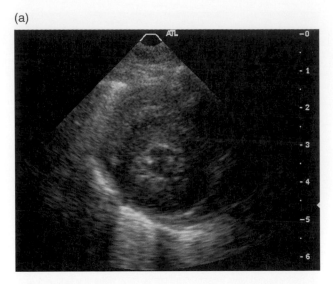

(b)

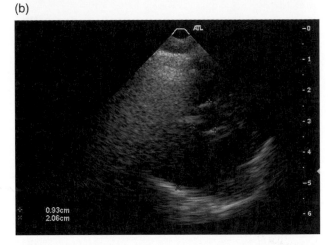

0.93cm
2.06cm

Figure 7-16 (a) A two-dimensional image of the heart in a right parasternal short-axis view shows increased lung interference surrounding the heart. (b) A two-dimensional image of the heart base shows an enlarged left atrium 2.06 cm with increased lung interference.

lung interference during the echocardiogram can be seen with pulmonary edema and is another sign of cardiac failure (Fig. 7-16).

Abdomen

Radiography

Preparation

The abdomen should be properly prepared by having the patient fast and administering an enema to avoid superimposition of fecaloid material over abdominal organs. Adequate chemical or physical restraint should be available to prevent patient movement from causing blurring of the radiographs. A grid should be used if abdominal thickness exceeds 9–11 cm. Although the phase of respiration is less critical than for thoracic radiography, exposure is best made at the expiratory pause to lessen the influence of respiratory movement.

Positioning

At least two projections (VD or DV and lateral) should be obtained. In some instances, additional projections or special projections may be helpful. The diaphragm and pelvic inlet should always be included.

For the VD projection, the cat should be positioned on its back with the hindlegs extended and the front legs held adjacent to the head. The sternum should be superimposed over the spine in the resulting radiograph.

If dorsal recumbency is resisted, the patient can be placed in sternal recumbency (DV view) with the hind limbs in a frog leg position. The forelegs are positioned alongside the head securing both the limbs and the head.

For the lateral view, the cat is rotated slightly so that the ventral midline is at a level even with the spine. The hindlegs are slightly extended to prevent the cat from curling up causing compression of abdominal organs.

Assessment

A well-positioned lateral radiograph (Fig. 7-17a) should show superimposition of the lateral processes of the spine. The abdomen should be straight so that abdominal organs are not compressed.

A well-positioned VD or DV radiograph (Fig. 7-17b) should be symmetrical with the spine being centered in the middle of the radiograph and the spinous processes centered in the vertebrae

Positioning is less critical for the abdomen than for the thorax particularly if the cat is uncooperative and cannot be sedated.

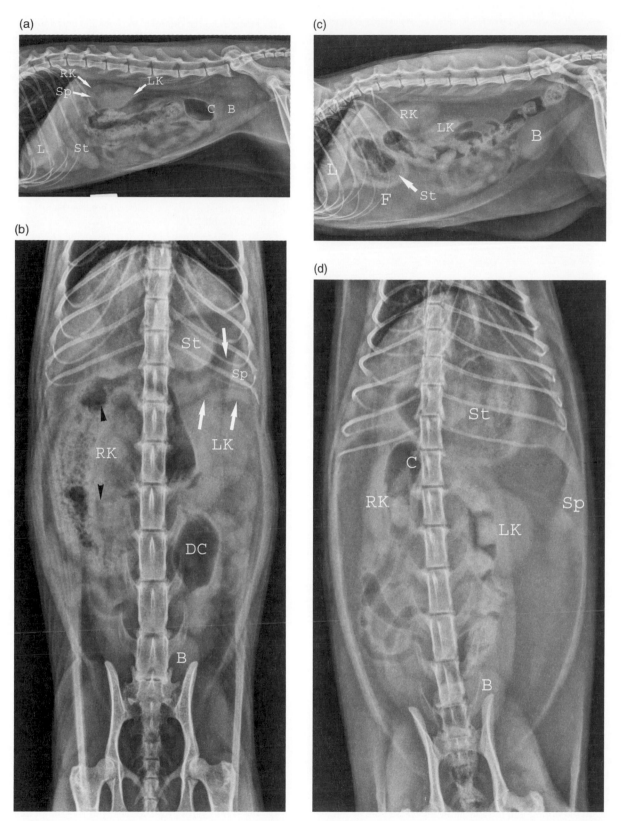

Figure 7-17 (a) Lateral radiograph of the abdomen of a normal thin cat. The small opacity superimposed over the cranial pole of the right kidney is the spleen (Sp). B, urinary bladder; C, colon; L, liver; LK, left kidney; RK, right kidney; St, stomach. (b) Ventrodorsal radiograph. The white arrows indicate the margins of the spleen. The black arrowheads indicate the cranial and caudal margins of the right kidney. DC, descending colon. (c) Lateral radiograph of the abdomen of this less cooperative normal fat cat. The falciform fat (F) separates the liver and stomach from the ventral abdominal wall. The intestines appear "bunched" in the middle of the abdomen in fat cats. Notice the difference between the full stomach in this cat and the cat pictured in Figures 7-17A and 7-17B. (d) Ventrodorsal radiograph.

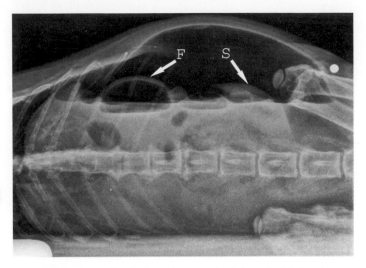

Figure 7-18 A ventrodorsal radiograph was obtained of a cat in right lateral recumbency using a horizontal beam. Air can be seen outside the gastrointestinal track. Left lateral recumbency is preferred to avoid confusing normal gas in the fundus with free gas in the peritoneal cavity. F, gas-filled fundus; S, spleen.

Extra Views

Horizontal beam radiography (Fig. 7-18) can be performed to check for small amounts of extraluminal gas that could indicate perforation of bowel or the presence of gas forming organisms. The patient is placed in left lateral recumbency for 5 to 10 minutes to allow free air to rise to the nondependent side of the body. Left lateral recumbency is preferred so that the gas-filled fundus is dependent. It is important to recognize that gas could also be present for several weeks following abdominal surgery.

Normal

The normal liver (*see* Fig. 7-17) has smooth margins with sharp caudoventral edges. Falciform fat displaces the liver away from the ventral abdominal wall in the lateral projection. The gall bladder is fluid-opaque and cannot be distinguished from the liver.

The spleen is a small opacity cranial to the kidneys in the lateral view. The tail or distal extremity of the spleen is not usually seen ventrally as it is in dogs. In the VD view, the head or proximal extremity appears as a triangular opacity located laterally between the stomach and left kidney. The tail of the spleen may extend caudally along the left body wall.

The kidneys are usually superimposed over each other in the lateral view. The cranial pole of the right kidney is seen separate from the liver unlike in the dog. The kidneys are fluid opaque, smoothly marginated, and surrounded by fat. Each kidney measures about 2.4–3.0 times the length of the second lumbar vertebra except in older cats that may have kidneys that are about two times the length of second lumbar vertebra.

The right lobe and body of the pancreas are found in the mesoduodenum. The left lobe is located in the greater omentum. Lymph nodes are scattered throughout the abdomen associated with abdominal organs and vessels. Each adrenal gland is an oval structure usually located cranial to the kidney on the same side adjacent to the caudal vena cava. Normal pancreas, lymph nodes, and adrenal glands are not radiographically apparent although about 30% of older cats have nonclinical dystrophic mineralization of the adrenals that causes them to be more radiopaque and visible.

The stomach is seen caudal to the liver and may contain fluid or gas. It appears J-shaped in the VD projection with the pylorus being located on or just to the right of the midline. The diameter of the normal small intestine is normally less than 12 mm from serosa to serosa or two times the height of the middle of the body of the fourth lumbar vertebra.

The ovaries and uterus are not seen in the nonpregnant cat. The urinary bladder will be seen in the caudoventral abdomen. Cats have a longer bladder neck than dogs, causing the bladder to be located more cranially.

Contrast Procedures

Contrast Media

Negative contrast media are black (radiolucent) and include air or carbon dioxide (Table 7-2).

Positive contrast media are white (radiopaque) and include barium, ionic organic iodinated contrast, and nonionic organic iodinated contrast. Barium is always administered orally or rectally. There are different organic iodinated contrast media for oral and intravenous use; the label should be checked to determine the correct use. Because nonionic iodinated contrast media are safer and cause fewer side effects than ionic iodinated contrast media, nonionic products should be used in cats. Ionic products are becoming less available (*see* Table 7-2).

Double-contrast procedures can be done, which include both positive and negative contrast procedures. Survey radiographs should always be obtained immediately prior to administration of contrast to obtain a baseline for comparison with contrast radiographs and to check that the technique is correct. In some cases, the diagnosis can be made without the necessity for contrast radiography.

Celiography (Peritoneography)

Celiography can be performed to evaluate for herniation of abdominal contents (Fig. 7-19).

Sterile iodinated contrast medium is injected into the peritoneal cavity at a dosage of 350–400 milligrams of iodine per kilogram. A nonionic iodinated product manufactured for intravenous use can be used.

The injection is made at the level of the umbilicus lateral to the midline with the patient in dorsal recumbency. In a normal celiogram, contrast will be seen smoothly outlining abdominal organs.

Upper Gastrointestinal Series ("Barium Series")

Liquid barium sulfate (30% weight/volume of micropulverized barium suspension) is most commonly used (Fig. 7-20). Nonionic iodinated contrast should be used if gastrointestinal perforation is suspected.

Except in emergency situations, the abdomen should be thoroughly prepared. The patient should be fasted for 12–24 hours and laxatives should be administered. Enemas should be given at least 1–2 hours prior so the colon is as empty as possible. Water should be withheld 1–2 hours before the study so the stomach is not fluid filled.

Barium is administered orally at a dosage of 12–20 mg/kg using a syringe or orogastric tube. The standard abdominal technique should be increased by 6–8 kVp for barium contrast radiography to increase x-ray absorption of the barium and increase contrast between barium and the adjacent soft tissues. Immediately following the administration of contrast, all four views should be obtained (both lateral, VD, and DV).

On the right lateral projection, barium fills the pylorus. Air is usually seen in the pylorus on the left lateral recumbent view. Films should be exposed frequently. Segmental contractions give the duodenum the appearance of a "string of pearls" in approximately 30% of cats. Barium will enter the colon by about 30–60 minutes. By 90 minutes, most of the barium will be in the colon. The cecum is small and has a comma shape.

TABLE 7-2: Examples of Radiopaque Contrast Media. Note that specific manufacturer's instructions and information should be consulted prior to use.

Product Name	Purpose	Contrast Agent	Concentration	Dosage
Isovue-200 (multiple strengths available; number indicates the concentration of iodine)	Angiography, excretory urography, upper GI series, cystography	Iopamidol (nonionic iodide product)	200 mg iodine/ml	For excretory urography: 600–800 mg iodine per kg given intravenously
Omnipaque-180 (multiple strengths available; number indicates the concentration of iodine)	Angiography, excretory urography, upper GI series, cystography	Iohexol (nonionic iodide product)	180 mg iodine/ml	For upper GI series: 600–800 mg iodine per kg diluted to a volume of 10 ml per kilogram Cystography: First infuse 2–3 ml 2% lidocaine to alleviate straining. Place patient in left lateral recumbency when air is infused into the bladder
Hypaque meglumine 30%	Ionic product but can use for cystography	Diatrizoate meglumine (ionic iodide product)	141 mg iodine/ml	Positive contrast cystography: Infuse 2–5 ml/kg iodinated contrast (1 ml/kg or less for fibrotic bladders) Double contrast cystography: Infuse 3 ml iodinated contrast followed by 2–3 ml/kg of iodinated contrast (1 ml/kg or less for fibrotic bladders)
E-Z-Paque	Oral use only	Barium sulfate suspension	96% weight/weight (w/w)	Water is added to bring volume to the 25% w/w fill line (approximately equivalent to 30% weight/volume). Give 12–20 ml/kg orally.
E-Z-Em Barium sulfate	Oral (provided as suspension, paste or tablets) and rectal use (provided as an barium enema kit)	Various formulations of barium sulfate	Variable	Varies with the formulation

GI, gastrointestinal.

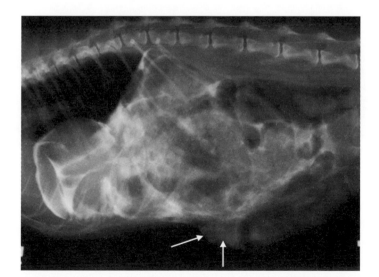

Figure 7-19 Celiography in a cat with multiple ventral hernias. Sterile water soluble nonionic iodinated contrast is injected into the peritoneal space to perform this study. Arrows indicate contrast filling the ventral hernias. Contrast is also seen between the abdominal organs. The diaphragm is bulging cranially into the chest but is not ruptured.

If there is any reason to suspect that there is perforation of the gastrointestinal tract, nonionic iodinated contrast should be given orally instead of barium. The dosage should be calculated to deliver 600–800 milligrams of iodine per kilogram. After the correct amount of iodine is determined, the contrast medium should be diluted to 10 ml/kg. Iodine is not used routinely because it does not coat the intestine as well as barium (*see* Table 7-2).

Pneumogastrography

Air can be instilled into the stomach through an orogastric tube until the stomach is mildly distended so that foreign bodies can be outlined.

Double-Contrast Gastrography

A combination of air and barium can be used to examine the gastric wall for neoplasia or ulcers (double-contrast gastrography). Fasting is necessary prior to this procedure to avoid artifacts. A small amount of barium is administered through an orogastric tube after which air is used to inflate the stomach.

Pneumocolography

Pneumocolography can be performed to check for ileocolic intussusception or cecal inversion or to determine the location of the colon (Fig. 7-21).

A 20- to 30-cc syringe is filled with air and used to infuse air in the colon at a dosage of 5 ml/kg. No preparation is required.

Excretory Urography

Excretory urography is useful for visualizing the kidneys and ureters but can also be used for diseases of the urinary bladder when catheterization

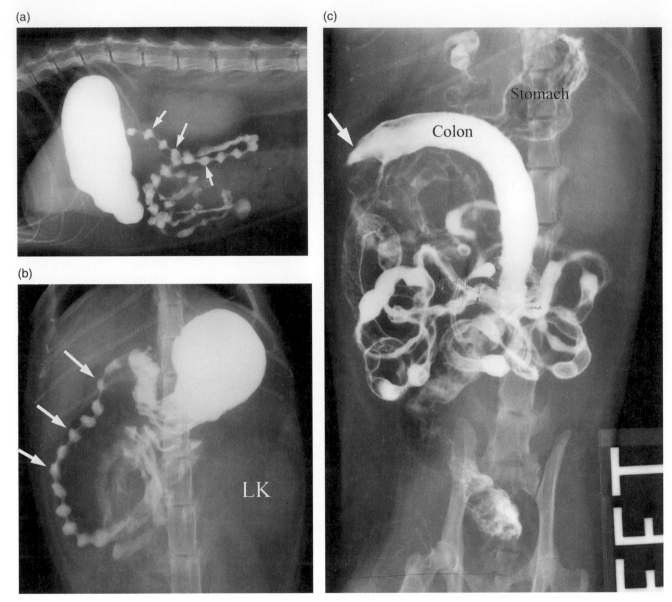

(a)

(b)

(c)

Stomach

Colon

LK

Figure 7-20 Normal upper gastrointestinal series in a cat using liquid barium sulfate. Barium sulfate should only be given orally. (a) Lateral view. (b) Ventrodorsal view. Arrows indicate normal contractions in the duodenum. LK, left kidney. (c) Ventrodorsal view showing that the stomach is now almost empty and most of the barium is in the colon. The white arrow points to the cecum.

is not possible (Fig. 7-22). It is better than ultrasonography for ruptured ureter or bladder or ectopic ureter.

The abdomen should be prepared by having the patient fast and administering cleansing enemas.

Nonionic iodinated contrast is given intravenously at 600–800 milligrams of iodine per kilogram slowly over 1 to 2 minutes.

Vomiting is a common complication, but more serious complications such as pulmonary edema, allergic reactions, and contrast induced renal failure can occur rarely.

In the early part of the study, the kidney becomes radiopaque (nephrogram phase) after which the contrast will be seen in the pelvis and ureter on each side (pyelogram phase), eventually entering the bladder (cystogram phase). Normal ureters are about 1 to 2 mm in diameter, have smooth margins, and appear discontinuous because the contrast moves in waves down the ureter.

Cystography

A catheter is placed into the urethra with the tip positioned in the lumen of the bladder using sterile technique (Fig. 7-23). Injection of 2–3 ml of 2% lidocaine into the bladder can help reduce straining.

Positive- or negative-contrast media or both (double contrast) can be used. Air is most commonly used for negative contrast. Carbon dioxide (CO_2) can be used to avoid air embolism but is rarely used because the incidence of air embolism is rare. Placing the cat in left lateral recumbency with the caudal half of the body elevated may avoid consequences by trapping air in the apex of the right ventricle. Sterile nonionic iodinated contrast should be used to provide positive contrast. A three-way valve is useful to facilitate double-contrast cystography. Possible complications include infection, kinking of the catheter, bladder rupture, trauma to the urethra or bladder, and (rarely) air embolism.

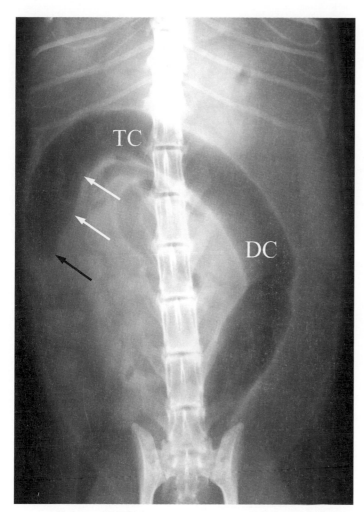

Figure 7-21 Pneumocolography. Air has been placed in the colon to differentiate it from small intestine. white arrows, ascending colon; black arrow, cecum; DC, descending colon; TC, transverse colon.

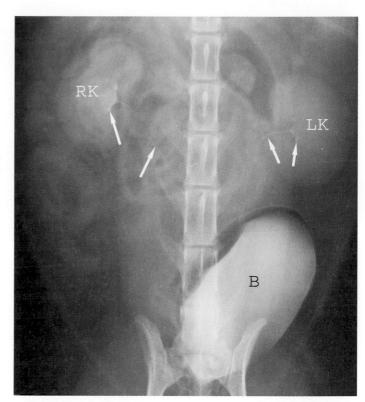

Figure 7-22 Excretory urogram. Nonionic iodinated contrast medium was given intravenously to this cat. Contrast in the right (RK) and left (LK) kidneys is referred to as the nephrogram phase. The arrows indicate the pelvis and ureter of each kidney (pyelogram phase). Contrast in the urinary bladder (B) is referred to as the cystogram phase.

Lateral and oblique views should be obtained to avoid superimposition of the bladder over the spine.

Positive-contrast cystography (Fig. 7-23a) is the procedure of choice for suspected rupture of the bladder because it is easier to visualize radiopaque contrast in the peritoneal cavity than negative contrast. Iodinated contrast medium is diluted 1:1 with sterile water and infused through the catheter at a dosage of about 2–5 ml/kg. Alternatively, iodinated contrast medium can be used that is made specifically for use in the bladder. If resistance is felt, a radiograph should be made to ensure that the bladder is not becoming overly distended. In a normal cystogram, the bladder should appear uniformly radiopaque with no visible radiolucencies.

Double-contrast cystography (Fig. 7-23b) is preferred for evaluation of the bladder mucosa, bladder wall, and mucosal contents because small calculi can be missed when negative or positive contrast is used alone. Infuse 2–3 ml iodinated contrast into the bladder. The patient is gently moved back and forth to coat the bladder wall. Then, 2–3 ml/kg of air are infused into the bladder making sure not to overly distend the bladder. Radiopaque contrast smoothly coats the bladder mucosa and forms a puddle in the dependent side of the bladder. Air surrounds the contrast puddle.

Negative-contrast cystography (pneumocystography) can be effective in localizing the urinary bladder or outlining calculi, but the thickness of the bladder wall can be overestimated and air embolism may be more likely to occur if the bladder wall is ulcerated and nondistensible. Air is

infused into the bladder at a rate of 2–3 ml per kg. A radiograph should be made if resistance is felt to avoid overdistending the bladder.

Urethrography

Urethrography is performed to evaluate urinary tract infection and to check for urethral calculi particularly in males (Fig. 7-24). The catheter is filled with fluid to avoid introduction of air bubbles before catheterizing the cat; 2–3 ml of 2% lidocaine diluted 1:1 with sterile water should be infused into the urethra 1–2 minutes before the infusion of contrast to prevent pain and urethral spasm. A cassette should be placed under the cat and the rotor of the x-ray machine should be started before rapidly infusing 5 ml iodinated organic contrast.

Both lateral and VD projections should be obtained. If catheterization is not possible, the cat can be anesthetized and a voiding urethrogram can be obtained by expressing the urinary bladder following injection of contrast directly into the lumen.

Ultrasonography

Gastrointestinal

Longitudinal and transverse images of the stomach, intestines, and associated lymph nodes should be obtained from both sides of the abdomen. The degree of distension, appearance of the contents, and motility should be evaluated. Decrease depth as much as possible so that bowel loops appear as large as possible on the screen. Applying some pressure can help displace gas in superficial loops allowing visibility of deeper structures. Gastric foreign bodies may be seen more easily if the patient is allowed to stand while the probe is placed on the ventral abdomen. This procedure allows the ultrasound beam to pass through fluid rather than gas.

(a)

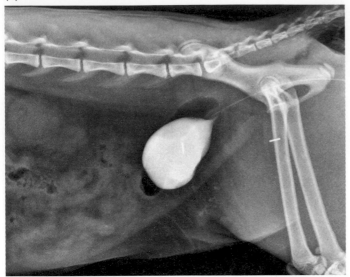

(b)

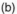

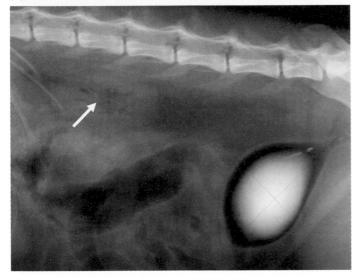

Figure 7-23 Cystography. (a) Positive contrast cystogram performed by infusing iodinated contrast medium into the urinary bladder. (b) Double-contrast cystogram performed by infusing iodinated contrast medium and air into the urinary bladder. Arrow indicates air in the renal pelvis. Reflux from the bladder into the ureter and kidney can occur in normal animals.

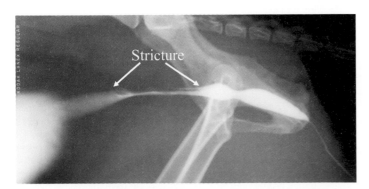

Figure 7-24 Urethrography. A urethrogram was performed by placing a catheter in the urethra and infusing iodinated contrast medium. This cat has a stricture in the urethra.

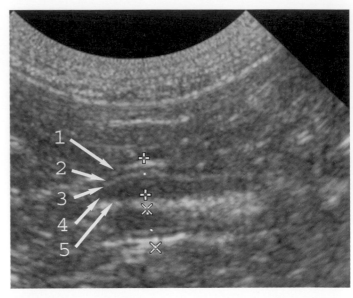

Figure 7-25 Sonogram of small intestine of a normal cat showing normal wall layering. Calipers have been placed to measure the near (+ markers) and far (x markers) walls. 1, subserosa/serosa; 2, muscularis; 3, submucosa; 4, mucosa; 5, mucosal luminal interface.

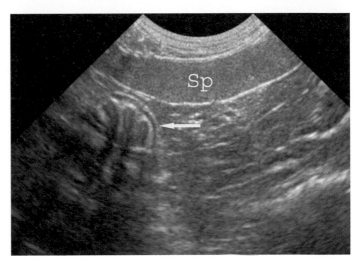

Figure 7-26 Sonogram of an empty stomach of a normal cat (arrow). The cat's head is to the left of the image. The stomach is located at the cranial margin of the spleen (Sp). Compare this to the gas- and fluid-filled stomachs in Figure 7-28.

Normal stomach and intestines have a layered appearance (Fig. 7-25). The outer layer (serosa and subserosa) is hyperechoic. The muscularis is usually hypoechoic but is thicker and almost anechoic in the ileum. The submucosa is a central hyperechoic layer. In the stomach, it is poorly defined and extends into the rugal folds. The mucosa is hypoechoic and is the thickest layer in the duodenum and jejunum. The interface between the wall and lumen (mucosal luminal interface or mucosal surface) is hyperechoic.

An empty stomach has a star-shaped or wagon wheel appearance (Fig. 7-26). These terms have also been used to describe the ileocolic valve imaged in the transverse plane (Fig. 7-27a). The ileum can be distinguished by its thick dark muscularis layer. The colon has a thinner wall than the small intestine due to its thinner mucosa.

(a)

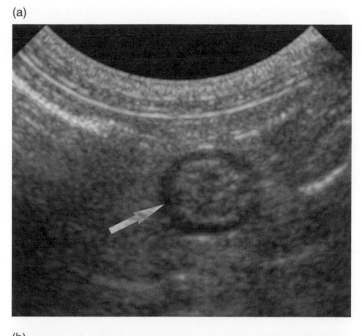

(b)

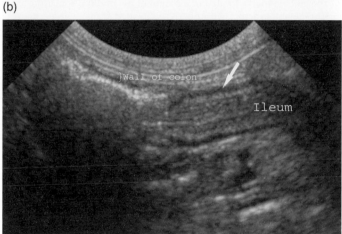

Figure 7-27 (a) Transverse sonogram of the ileocolic valve of a normal cat. The muscularis layer *(arrow)* in the ileum is darker than the muscularis layer of other intestinal loops. (b) Longitudinal sonogram of the ileum of a normal cat. The cat's head is to the left of the image. Gas in the colon causes reverberation artifact that prevents the far wall from being seen. The arrow points to the muscularis layer of the ileum.

(a)

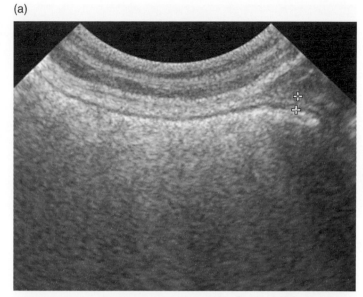

(b)

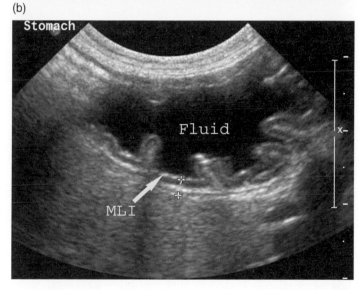

Figure 7-28 (a) Sonogram of the stomach of cat showing reverberation artifact caused by gas in the lumen. Sound passes through the near wall and strikes the gas in the lumen. Echoes reverberate multiple times before returning to the probe to be recorded. The result is that reverberations prevent the far wall (and anything in the lumen) from being seen. Cursors (+ markers) have been placed to measure the wall. (b) Sound readily passes through the fluid in this cat's stomach so that the far wall is clearly visible. Cursors measure the gastric wall from the outside of the serosa to the outside of the mucosal luminal interface (MLI).

The electronic calipers of the ultrasound machine are used to measure gastrointestinal walls from the outside edge of serosa to the outside edge of mucosal luminal interface (see Fig. 7-25).

Gas is hyperechoic and strongly reflective resulting in reverberation artifact, which has been termed a "dirty acoustic shadow" because it prevents visualization of deeper structures (Fig. 7-27). Fluid is anechoic and allows visualization of deeper structures (Fig. 7-28). A large amount of fluid will have fewer interfaces to reflect, absorb, or scatter sound than surrounding tissues. As a result, tissues deep to a fluid-filled stomach or intestinal loop will appear brighter than surrounding structures (acoustic enhancement). A small amount of mucus or ingesta will be hyperechoic but will allow visualization of deeper structures.

Common problems in the gastrointestinal tract include foreign bodies and neoplasia. Foreign bodies vary in appearance. Some are hyperechoic with deep acoustic shadowing whereas the shape of others is visible. If a foreign body causes obstruction, the bowel proximal to the obstruction

will likely be distended. A loss of wall layering or altered wall layering signals infiltrative disease such as neoplasia or severe inflammatory bowel disease (Fig. 7-29).

Kidneys

The most echogenic portions of the kidney are the pelvis, the diverticula, and the capsule. The renal cortex and medulla are hypoechoic but the cortex is more echogenic than the medulla.

The appearance of the kidney varies with plane of the ultrasound beam (Fig. 7-30) as it passes through the kidney. The mid-dorsal plane of the kidney cuts the kidney into two symmetrical halves. The ureter

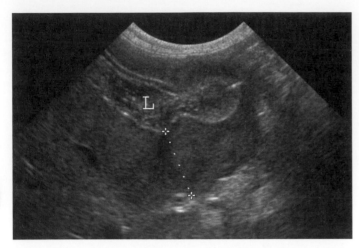

Figure 7-29 The wall of the stomach of this cat is thickened and exhibits a loss of wall layering. This change is usually associated with neoplasia or other infiltrative disease. L, lumen.

enters at the hilus of the kidney; the diverticula can be seen extending from the pelvis toward the cortex. There are three sagittal planes. The medial sagittal plane cuts through the kidney where the ureter enters and expands into the pelvis, giving the kidney a dumb-bell appearance in which the medullary areas appear as two dark circular areas with the hyperechoic pelvis and fat seen centrally. The mid-sagittal plane cuts the kidney centrally through the ventral and dorsal branches of the pelvis, which appear as two hyperechoic bars. The lateral sagittal plane cuts the kidney through the diverticula and medulla causing the kidney to resemble a watermelon with the hypoechoic medulla being divided by the hyperechoic diverticula. In the transverse plane, the kidney is somewhat circular and the branches of the pelvis take the shape of a C.

Urinary Bladder

The urinary bladder has a smooth wall with three or four layers, usually measuring 0.2–0.4 cm (Fig. 7-31a). The lumen is primarily anechoic, although fat, large glucose molecules, or protein can cause the appearance of hypoechoic foci suspended in the lumen even in normal cats.

Tissues deep to the bladder are often more hyperechoic than adjacent tissues because sound is not attenuated as it passes through the fluid in the bladder (deep acoustic enhancement).

If present, urinary cystic calculi are generally hyperechoic and will be found on the dependent side of the urinary bladder (Fig. 7-31b). Larger calculi will often attenuate sound preventing deeper tissues from being seen (deep acoustic shadow). Sound strikes curved surfaces like those of the bladder and kidney at an angle causing sound to be reflected and refracted at the edge of these structures. This can cause the bladder to appear as though there were a hole at the apex. A real hole would not be visible because the bladder would contract as urine flowed from the bladder into the peritoneal cavity. Although ultrasonography would reveal free peritoneal fluid, a ruptured ureter or bladder would be better demonstrated with excretory urography or cystography.

Spleen

The spleen can be found cranial to the left kidney in the craniodorsal abdomen (*see* Fig. 7-26). It is smaller and usually less echogenic than the canine spleen. Compared to the liver, the spleen has a finer, more uniform echotexture. Echogenicity is similar to the liver. The spleen has a well-defined hyperechoic capsule. The splenic vein exits the spleen at several points along the deep surface.

Splenic enlargement or the presence of nodules is more significant in cats than in dogs. Aspiration is recommended for further evaluation (Fig. 7-32).

Liver

The liver is located mostly on the right side. The gastric fundus is at the left caudal border of the liver. A hyperechoic line at the cranial margin of the liver represents the interface between the diaphragm and lung.

Liver may appear to be located on both sides of the diaphragm (mirror image artifact).

Best images are obtained with the probe positioned just caudal to the xiphoid with the beam directed cranially in a sagittal plane (Fig. 7-33a). Sweep the probe from side to side. Then, rotate the probe 90 degrees and image from dorsal to ventral and back to ensure that the entire liver is imaged.

Move the probe to the right of the ventral midline imaging in a sagittal plane medial to the right kidney to visualize the caudal vena cava as it passes through the diaphragm. Hepatic veins may be seen entering the caudal vena cava. The aorta will be located more dorsally and the portal vein will be located more ventrally and to the left.

Intrahepatic branches of the portal vein have hyperechoic walls; the walls of the hepatic veins are poorly seen causing the veins to appear as anechoic tubes.

The gall bladder is located to the right of the midline appearing as an anechoic oval structure with poorly delineated walls. Some echogenic material can be seen in the gall bladder but should swirl around when the cat is repositioned. A bilobed gall bladder is not unusual in cats (Figs. 7-33b and 7-33c). The gall bladder will be larger if the cat is anorexic or has fasted.

Pancreas

The pancreas is found by imaging dorsomedial to the duodenum (right extremity) and between the stomach and transverse colon (left extremity). The pancreatic duct runs centrally through the pancreas as an anechoic tube with thin hyperechoic walls. The pancreatic vein is a larger, more ventral structure that is not seen in all cats (Fig. 7-34). Color Doppler imaging can be useful to distinguish between the two structures.

Adrenal Glands

Feline adrenal glands are small, oval, and almost anechoic. They are usually found by scanning just cranial to the cranial pole of the kidney (Fig. 7-35a), although they are sometimes found more caudally closer to the renal artery.

The left adrenal gland is imaged with the cat in right lateral recumbency with the probe on the left side of the abdomen angled so that the beam passes in a ventrolateral-dorsomedial direction.

The right adrenal gland can be found by placing the cat in left lateral recumbency and scanning in a sagittal plane between the kidney laterally and the caudal vena cava medially. The left adrenal gland may also be visible when scanning in this manner.

Mineralization of the adrenal gland is common in older cats, appearing as a hyperechoic area with deep acoustic shadowing (Fig. 7-35b).

Ovaries

Feline ovaries are usually only visible when the cat is pregnant or in heat. Follicles appear as anechoic structures within the ovary (Fig. 7-36).

Extremities

The radiographic approach to the extremities may require sedation to accurately acquire diagnostic images. Thin rope, tape, or gauze should be used to extend the limbs to avoid exposure of human hands.

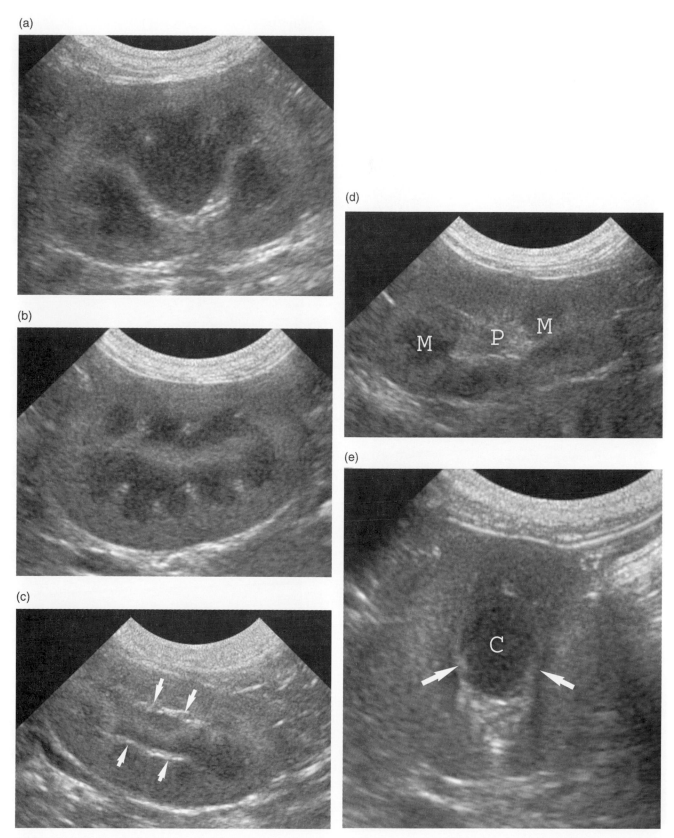

Figure 7-30 The appearance of the kidney varies with the plane of the ultrasound beam. (a) The mid-dorsal plane divides the kidney into two symmetrical halves. (b) In the lateral sagittal plane, the kidney resembles a watermelon. (c) In the midsagittal plane, the two hyperechoic lines (arrows) represent the dorsal and ventral branches of the renal pelvis. (d) In the medial sagittal plane, the pelvis and surrounding fat are seen as a hyperechoic area (P) in the center of the kidney. The medullary areas (M) are hypoechoic. (e) In the mid-transverse plane, the kidney is round. The hyperechoic pelvis (arrows) wraps around the renal crest (C).

(a)

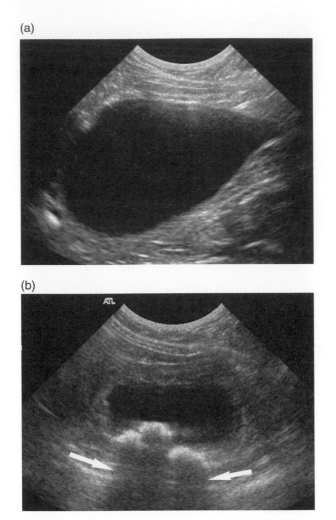

(b)

(a)

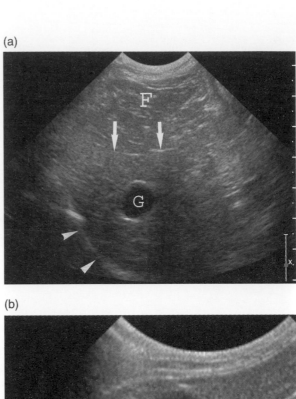

(b)

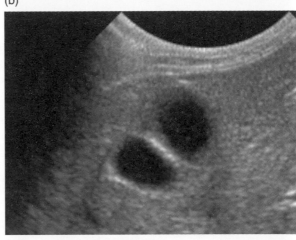

Figure 7-31 (a) The normal urinary bladder of a cat is tear-drop shaped with an anechoic lumen. Some echogenicity at the edge of the walls is a normal artifact caused by imaging of adjacent tissues. (b) Calculi are usually hyperechoic and often exhibit deep acoustic shadowing *(arrows)*.

(c)

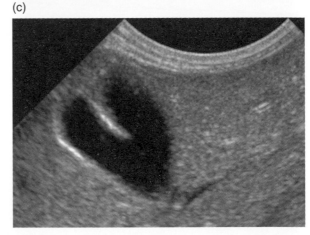

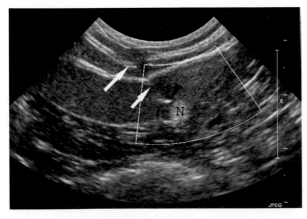

Figure 7-32 Sonographic image showing aspiration of the spleen near the abdominal wall. Nodules in the spleen and enlarged spleens are most often abnormal and should be aspirated. White arrows indicate the path of the needle and the black arrowhead indicates the needle's tip as it approaches a hyperechoic nodule *(N)*.

Figure 7-33 (a) Sonogram of the liver of a normal cat. The probe was placed on the ventral abdomen near the xiphoid with the ultrasound beam directed dorsally and toward the diaphragm. The cat's head is to the viewer's left. Fat *(F)* is seen superficial to the liver. White arrows indicate the ventral margin of the liver. White arrowheads indicate the interface between the diaphragm and lung. G, gall bladder. (b) Transverse image through the liver of a cat revealing two anechoic *(black)* structures that look like cysts. (c) Rotating the probe to obtain a longitudinal image shows that the structures are the two lobes of a bilobed gall bladder. A bilobed gall bladder is not uncommon in cats. Care should be taken to avoid confusing the gall bladder with a true cyst.

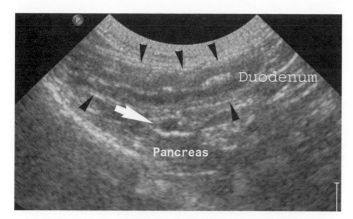

Figure 7-34 The pancreas is difficult to image but can found by imaging deep to the duodenum, outlined by black arrowheads in this sonogram of a normal feline pancreas. The white arrow indicates the pancreaticoduodenal vein, which is a good landmark because it runs through the pancreas ventral to the pancreatic duct *(not shown)*.

(a)

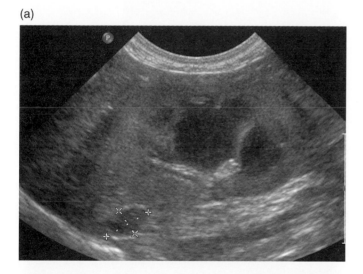

(b)

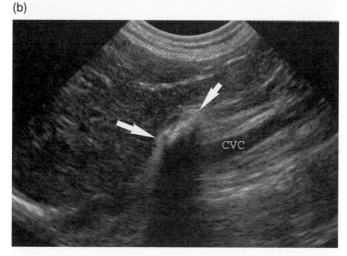

Figure 7-35 (a) Sonogram of a normal cat showing the left adrenal gland cranial to the left kidney. Cursors have been placed to measure the adrenal gland. (b) Arrows indicate mineralization in the adrenal gland of an older cat. The mineralization is hyperechoic with deep acoustic shadowing. CVC, caudal vena cava.

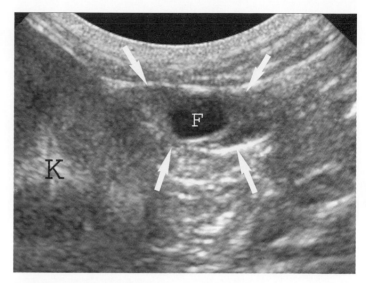

Figure 7-36 Sonogram of an ovary in a normal cat in heat. The ovary is usually found superficially near the caudal pole of the kidney (K). Arrows show the margins of the ovary. F, follicle.

Orthogonal views centered on each joint are important for complete and proper evaluation. A common technical difficulty is achieving proper positioning (not rotated) if the patient is uncooperative or inadequately sedated.

Scapula

See Figure 7-37 for views of the scapula.

Radiographic Views

Lateral and caudocranial are used for imaging the scapula.

Technical Difficulties

Superimposition of the body wall over the scapula can create some imaging problems.

Positioning

Lateral View

The scapula of interest should be closest to the table and pulled back caudally, while the opposite limb is pulled forward. Another method for obtaining a lateral view of the proximal scapula is achieved by pushing the down scapula in a dorsal direction and pulling the opposite limb ventrally.

Caudocranial View

With the patient lying on its back and rotated 15–30 degrees toward the unaffected side, the front limb is pulled forward, and the beam is centrally located over scapula.

Shoulder Joint

See Figure 7-38 for views of the shoulder joint.

Radiographic Views

Mediolateral, caudocranial, or oblique views are used for imaging the shoulder joint.

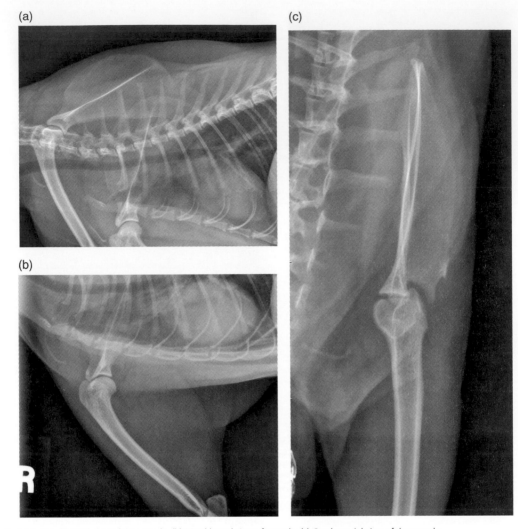

Figure 7-37 Scapula. (a) Proximal lateral view of the scapula. (b) Distal lateral view of scapula. (c) Caudocranial view of the scapula.

Technical Difficulties

Rotation, superimposition of the cervical spine, sternum, or opposite limb on lateral image can cause problems with imaging the shoulder joint.

Positioning

Lateral View

The shoulder of interest should be closest to the table and pulled forward. The beam is centered on the shoulder joint and closely collimated. The opposite limb needs to be pulled in an upward and caudal direction; the head and spine need to be extended to prevent overlap with the shoulder joint.

Caudocranial View

With the patient lying on its back, the front limbs are pulled forward, and the beam is centered on the shoulder joint. If possible keep the front legs at a symmetrical distance from the table so the patient is not rotated.

Humerus

See Figure 7-39 for views of the humerus.

Radiographic Views

Lateral and caudocranial are used for imaging the humerus.

Positioning

Lateral View

The limb of interest should be closest to the table and pulled forward. Proper evaluation includes both the shoulder and elbow joints. The opposite limb is pulled in a caudal and dorsal direction.

Caudocranial View

The patient is lying on its back with the foreleg of interest extended forward. The beam is centered on the mid-humerus and includes the shoulder and elbow joints.

Elbow

See Figure 7-40 for views of the elbow.

Radiographic Views

Lateral, craniocaudal, or oblique views are used for imaging the elbow.

(a)

(b)

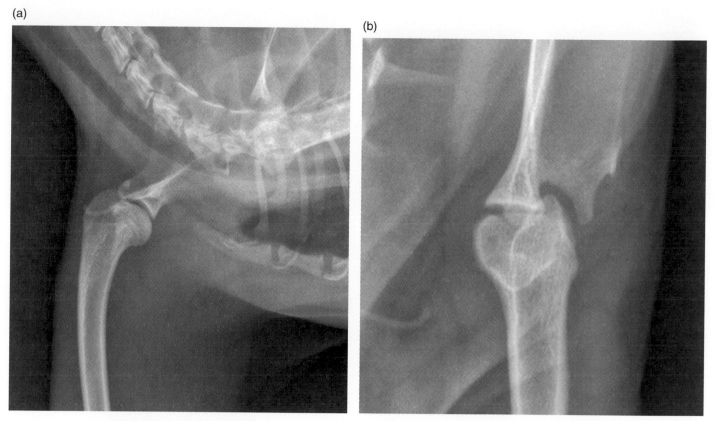

Figure 7-38   Shoulder joint. (a) Lateral view of shoulder joint. (b) Caudocranial view of the shoulder joint.

(a)

(b)

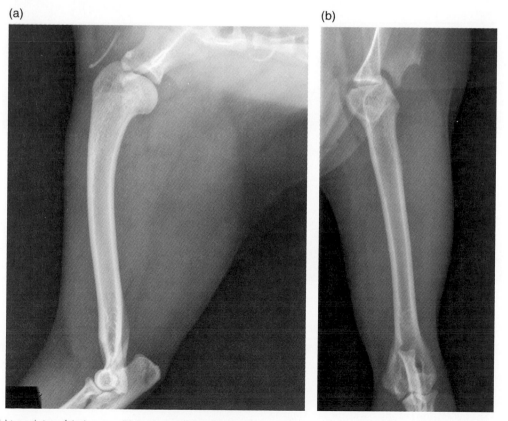

Figure 7-39   Humerus. (a) Lateral view of the humerus. (b) Caudocranial view of humerus.

(a)

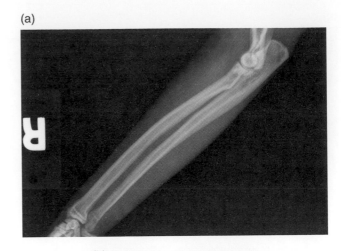

(b)

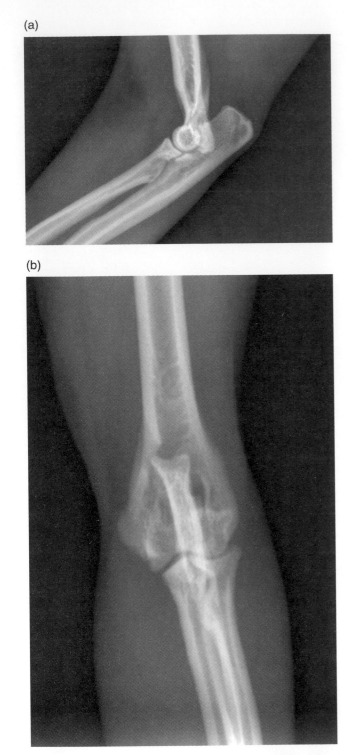

Figure 7-40 Elbow joint. (a) Lateral view of elbow joint. (b) Craniocaudal view of the elbow joint.

(a)

(b)

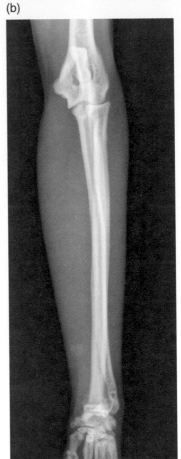

Figure 7-41 Radius/Ulna. (a) Lateral view of radius and ulna. (b) Craniocaudal view of the radius and ulna.

Positioning

Lateral View

The limb of interest should be closest to the table and extended forward; the opposite limb should be pulled upward and back. The head and neck can be a neutral lateral position.

Craniocaudal View

The cat is placed in a sternal position with the limb of interest extended forward. Try to palpate the distal humerus to be sure the limb is not rotated prior to exposing the radiograph.

Radius/Ulna

See Figure 7-41 for views of the radius/ulna.

(a)

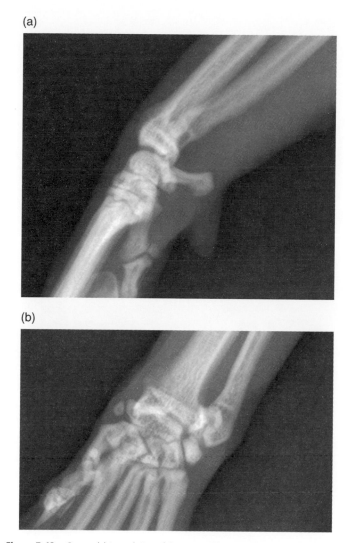

(b)

Figure 7-42 Carpus. (a) Lateral view of the carpus. (b) Dorsopalmar view of the carpus.

Radiographic Views

Lateral and craniocaudal are used for imaging the radius/ulna.

Positioning

For both views, include from the elbow to carpal joints.

Lateral View

The limb of interest should be closest to the table and pulled forward. With the cat's head extended and the nose pointing up, the beam should be centered in the middle of the radius/ulna.

Craniocaudal View

The cat is placed in a sternal position with the limb of interest pulled forward. The head should be directed toward the opposite limb to ensure it is not superimposed of the area of interest.

Carpus/Metacarpus

See Figures 7-42, 7-43, and 7-44 for images of the carpus/metacarpus.

(a)

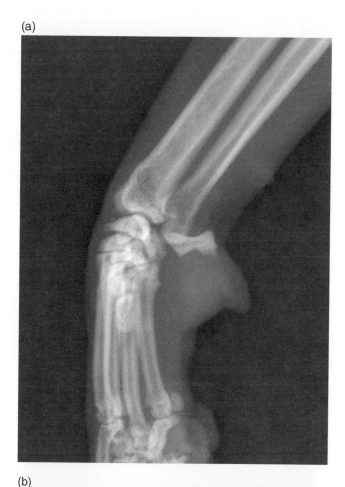

(b)

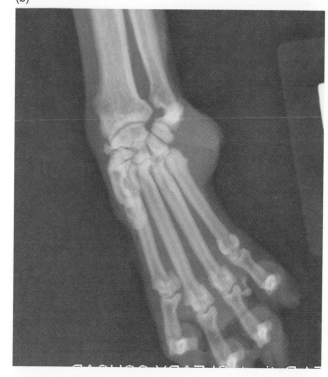

Figure 7-43 (a) Lateral and (b) dorsopalmar views showing soft-tissue swelling is present surrounding the carpus. No bone lysis was evident. A faint periosteal reaction was present along the accessory carpal bone adjacent to the swelling.

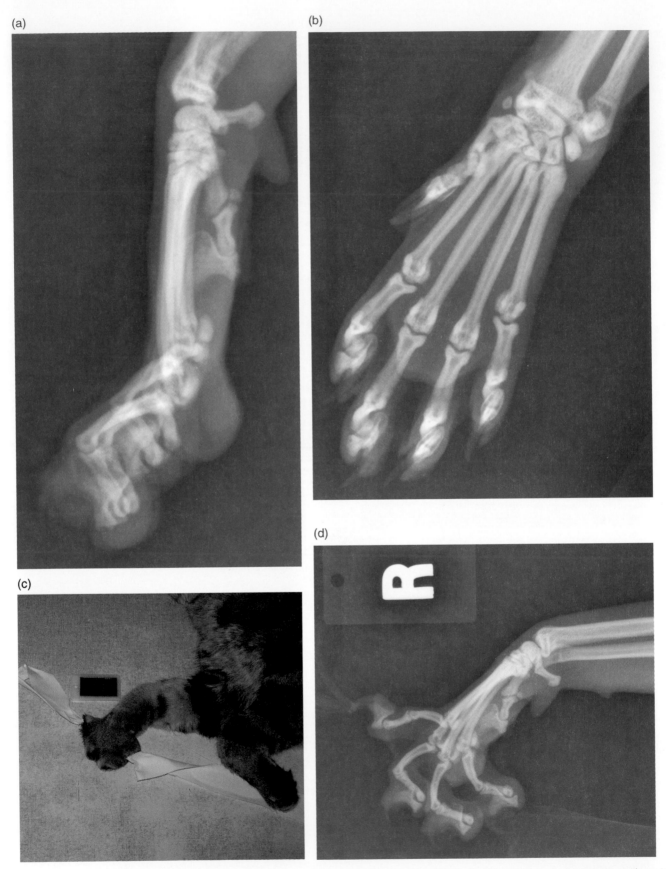

(a)

(b)

(c)

(d)

Figure 7-44 Metacarpus. (a) Lateral view of the metacarpus. (b) Dorsopalmar view of the metacarpus. (c) Cat positioned with digits spread apart using gauze to avoid superimposition of the metacarpal bones and digits. (d) Oblique view of the metacarpus.

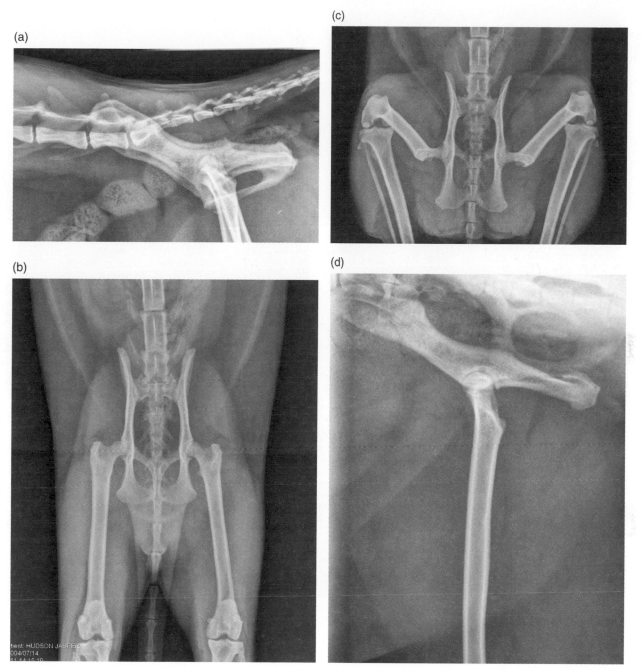

Figure 7-45 Pelvis. (a) Lateral pelvis. (b) Extended ventrodorsal view of the pelvis. (c) Flexed or frog-legged view of the pelvis. (d) Oblique view of the pelvis to visualize the coxofemoral joint.

Radiographic Views

Lateral, dorsopalmar, or oblique views are used for imaging the carpus/metacarpus.

Positioning

Lateral View

The limb of interest should be closest to the table and pulled forward. This can be accomplished by pushing from the elbow joint or by taping the distal limb before pulling it cranially with the tape.

Dorsopalmar View

The cat is placed in a sternal position with the limb either pulled forward after taping the digits or by pushing from the elbow joint. A wooden spoon can be used to fully spread out the digits.

Extra Views

An oblique view may be helpful to isolate a specific digit, typically by applying tape to the first and last digits then pulling them apart. The key is to mark which digit is pulled forward or back to facilitate interpretation.

Pelvis

See Figures 7-45 and 7-46 for images of the pelvis.

(a)

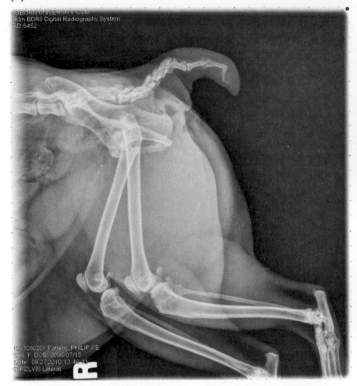

(b)

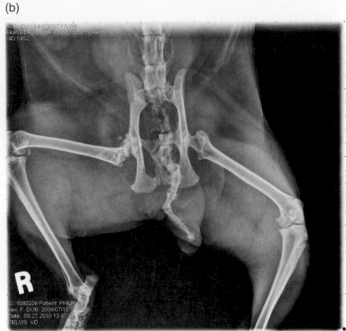

Figure 7-46   Cat with a chronic fracture of the right femoral neck. (a) Lateral view. (b) Ventrodorsal view. A small bone fragment is seen adjacent to the right coxofemoral joint. Congenital malformations of the caudal vertebrae and tail are present.

Radiographic Views

Lateral, VD extended, VD frog legged, or oblique are used for imaging the pelvis.

Positioning

Lateral View

Center the beam over the coxofemoral joints with the limbs in a "scissor-kick" position with the leg closest to the table pulled cranially and other limb caudally. Open collimation to include the caudal lumbar spine and tail.

VD View (Extended)

With the patient lying on its back using a positioning trough, the legs are pulled toward the table with equal force to minimize rotation. Remember to rotate the stifles slightly inward and down toward the table.

VD View (Frog Legged)

With the patient lying on its back in a positioning trough, pressure is equally applied to the feet so the hip joints will now be in a flexed position. This view is essential when a fracture of the femoral head or neck is suspected but is not visualized on the extended view.

Oblique View of the Coxofemoral Joint

The cat is placed in a lateral position with the coxofemoral joint of interest closest to the table. The opposite limb is pulled back

and upward causing the coxofemoral joint of interest to be projected lower (ventral) and preventing superimposition of the two joints. This view is helpful when evaluating for acetabular fractures.

Femur

See Figure 7-47 for images of the femur.

Radiographic Views.

Lateral and craniocaudal are used for imaging the femur.

Lateral View

Positioning is similar to that used for an oblique view of the coxofemoral joint. The limb of interest should be closest to the table with the opposite limb pulled back and upward.

Craniocaudal View

The patient is placed on its back in a positioning trough with the leg pulled toward the table.

Stifle

See Figures 7-48 and 7-49 for images of the stifle.

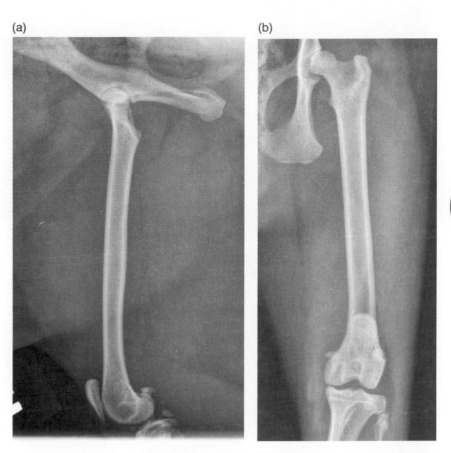

Figure 7-47 Femur. (a) Lateral view of the femur. (b) Craniocaudal view of the femur.

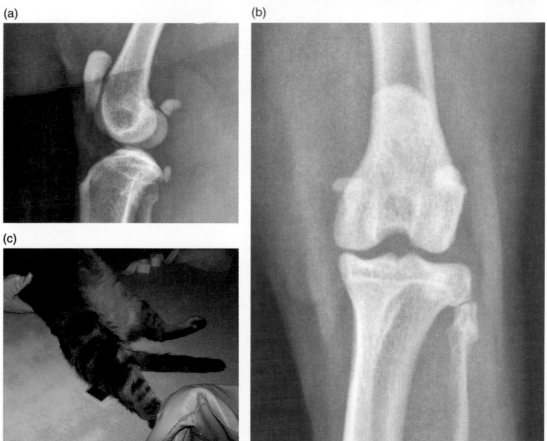

Figure 7-48 Stifle joint. (a) Lateral view of the stifle joint. (b) Craniocaudal view of the stifle joint. (c) The cat can be placed in a "sitting" position for imaging of the stifle and femur.

(a)　　　　　　　　　　　　　　　　　　　　　(b)

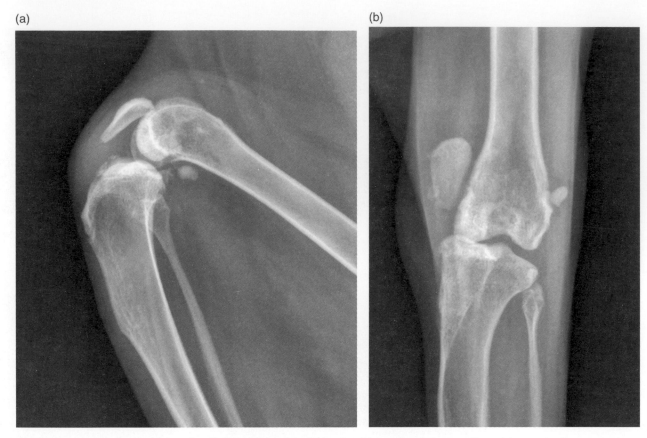

Figure 7-49　　(a) Lateral and (b) craniocaudal views of a stifle joint with chronic medial luxation of the patella. Soft-tissue swelling and degenerative changes are present.

Radiographic Views

Lateral, craniocaudal or oblique views are used for imaging the stifle.

Positioning

Lateral View

The limb of interest should be closest to the table with the opposite limb pulled caudally to prevent superimposition.

Craniocaudal View

Positioning can be done in a V trough with the leg pulled toward the table or while holding the patient in a "sitting" position the limb is pulled toward the table.

Tibia/Fibula

See Figure 7-50 for images of the tibia/fibula.

Radiographic Views

Lateral and craniocaudal views are used for imaging the tibia/fibula.

Positioning

Center the beam on the mid-shaft of the tibia/fibula and include the stifle and tarsal joints.

Lateral View

Positioning of the limb is similar to the stifle.

Craniocaudal View

Positioning is similar to the stifle. While holding the patient in a sitting position, push down on the musculature over the femur to extend the limb.

Tarsus/Metatarsus

See Figures 7-51 to 7-54 for images of the tarsus/metatarsus.

Radiographic Views

Lateral, dorsoplantar, or oblique views are used for imaging the tarsus/metatarsus.

Positioning

Lateral View

Extending the limb from the level of the proximal femur allows your gloved hands to be out of the primary beam. Alternatively tape could be applied around the distal limb to allow extension of the down limb over the table. However, some digital systems may pick up the tape and this may obscure the image. Be sure to leave a tag so the tape can be removed quickly because most awake cats will not appreciate its removal.

(a)   (b)

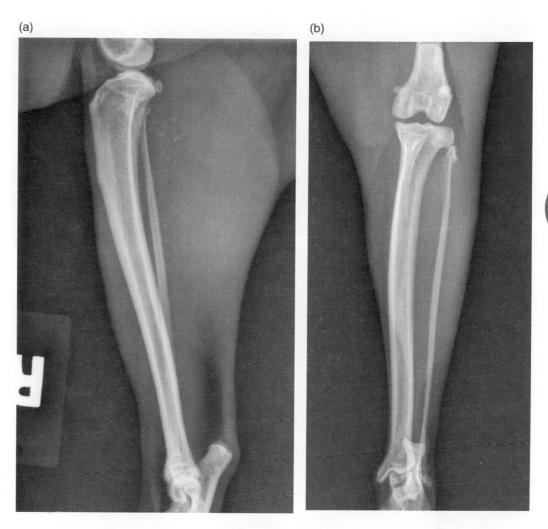

Figure 7-50   Tibia/Fibula. (a) Lateral view of tibia and fibula. (b) Craniocaudal view of the tibia and fibula.

(a)   (b)

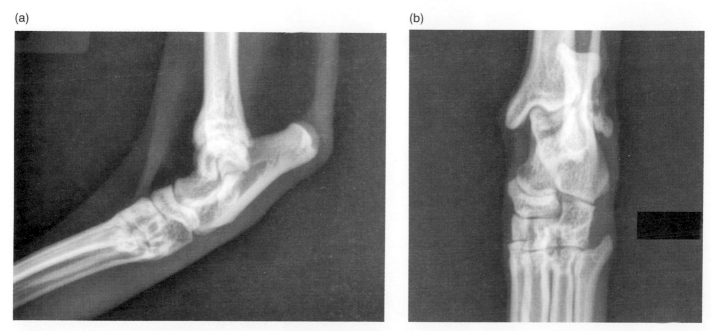

Figure 7-51   Tarsal joint. (a) Lateral view of the tarsus. (b) Dorsoplantar view of the tarsus.

(a)

(b)

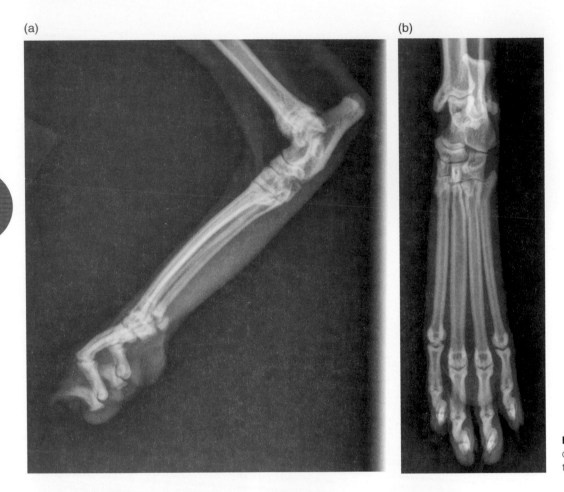

Figure 7-52 Metatarsus. (a) Lateral view of the metatarsus. (b) Dorsoplantar view of the metatarsus.

(a)

(b)

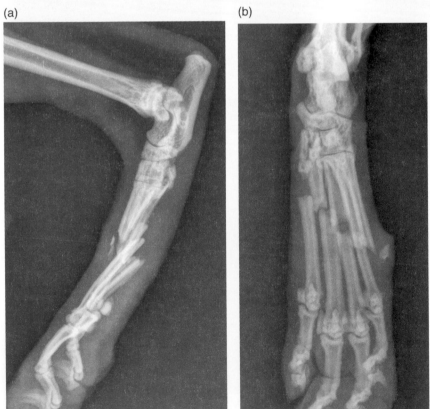

Figure 7-53 (a) Lateral and (b) dorsoplantar views of a patient with multiple fractured metatarsal bones.

(a)

(b)

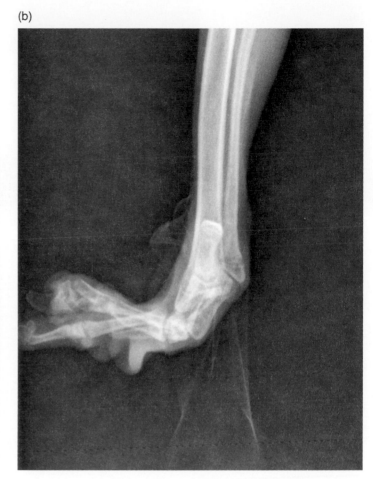

Figure 7-54 (a) Lateral and (b) dorsoplantar views of a kitten with a chronic fracture involving the tarsal and metatarsal bones. Notice the entire foot is displaced almost perpendicular to the proximal limb.

Dorsoplantar View

Place the cat in a sitting position and extend the leg. Alternatively place tape around the distal limb to extend the limb into position.

Extra Views

Use and oblique view similar to front leg for evaluation of the digits.

Skull

Radiographic Views

See Figure 7-55 for images of the skull.

Heavy sedation or general anesthesia is necessary for well-positioned radiographs of the skull, particularly when open mouth and oblique views are included. Lateral and VD or DV views of the skull are standard. Symmetry is important to allow comparison of structures on each side.

The frontal view is useful to evaluate the frontal sinuses. The nasal passages can be seen in the open mouth VD view. Intraoral DV and lateral oblique views are also helpful.

Nasopharyngeal polyps can be visualized most consistently from the lateral projection.

Oblique views are useful for evaluating the upper and lower dental arcade. The mouth is held open using needle caps cut to size while the skull is rotated between 30 and 45 degrees from the lateral position to isolate each arcade of the maxilla and mandible. Intraoral radiographs can also be made with dental plates.

VD and DV views allow evaluation of the temporomandibular joints. Oblique views can be made by positioning the skull for a VD projection and then rotating the skull 20 degrees.

Tympanic bullae can be visualized on open mouth rostrocaudal, left dorsal 20 degrees right ventral oblique, and right dorsal 20 degrees left ventral oblique views.

Spine

A high mAs/low kVp technique should be used to maximize film contrast. Anesthesia should be used to relax the spine and allow correct positioning. If the cat must remain in lateral recumbency because of trauma to the spine, a VD view can be obtained using a horizontal beam.

Sponges should be used to elevate the mid-cervical spine and other areas as necessary so that the spine is parallel to the cassette. For the VD view, sandbags can be used to prevent rotation.

Lateral and VD radiographs (Fig. 7-56) should be made centered over each portion of the spine (cervical, cervicothoracic, thoracic, thoracolumbar, lumbar, and lumbosacral). Additional views can be made centered over the area of interest.

Disease conditions include fracture, disc disease, and neoplasia.

(a)

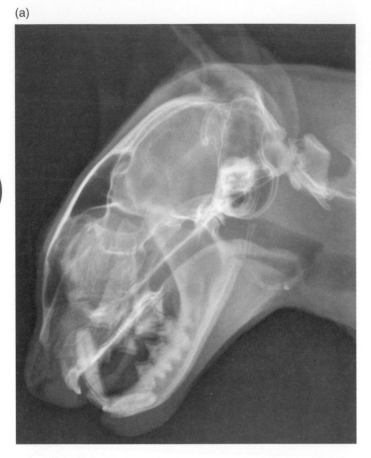

(b)

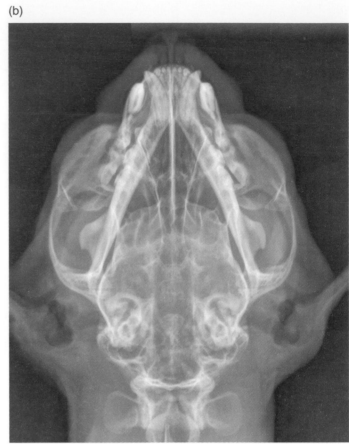

(c)

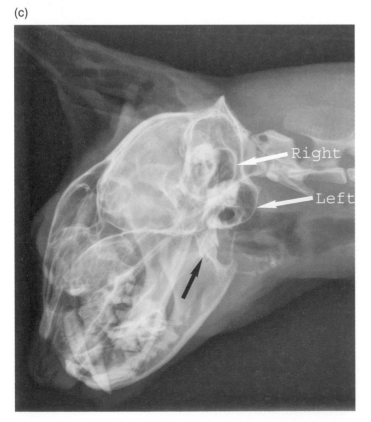

(d)

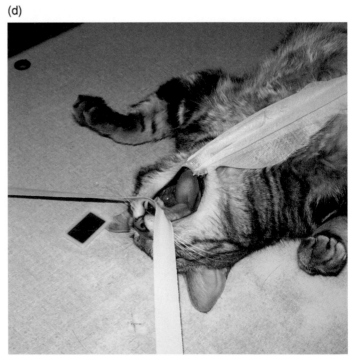

(e)

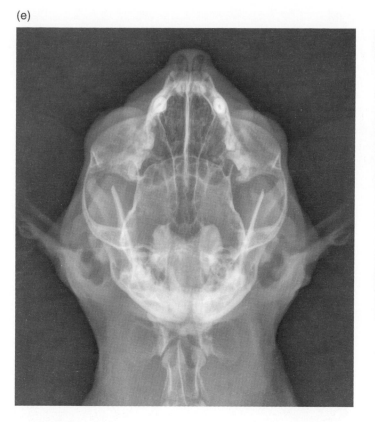

(f)

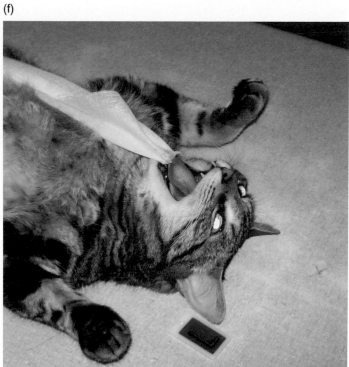

(g)

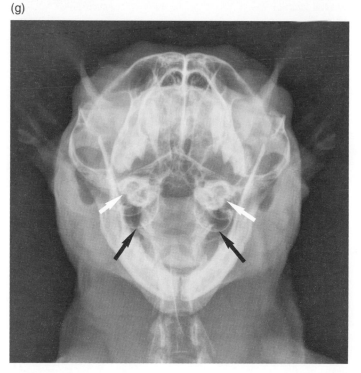

Figure 7-55 Skull radiographs. (a) Lateral view. (b) Ventrodorsal view. (c) Oblique view to demonstrate the left tympanic bulla and temporomandibular joint *(black arrow)*. Although both tympanic bullae *(white arrows)* are seen, the left is more easily visualized. The cat is in left lateral recumbency with the head rotated to the left. (d) Cat positioned to image the nasal passages. Gauze has been used to open the mouth, moving the mandible out of the way. If necessary, tape can be applied to secure the maxilla to the table. (e) Open mouth view showing the nasal passages. (f) Cat positioned to image the tympanic bullae. The mouth is opened with gauze or tape. The x-ray beam is directed vertically so it bisects the angle formed by the jaws. (g) Open mouth view showing the tympanic bullae *(black arrows)* and petrous temporal bones *(white arrows)*.

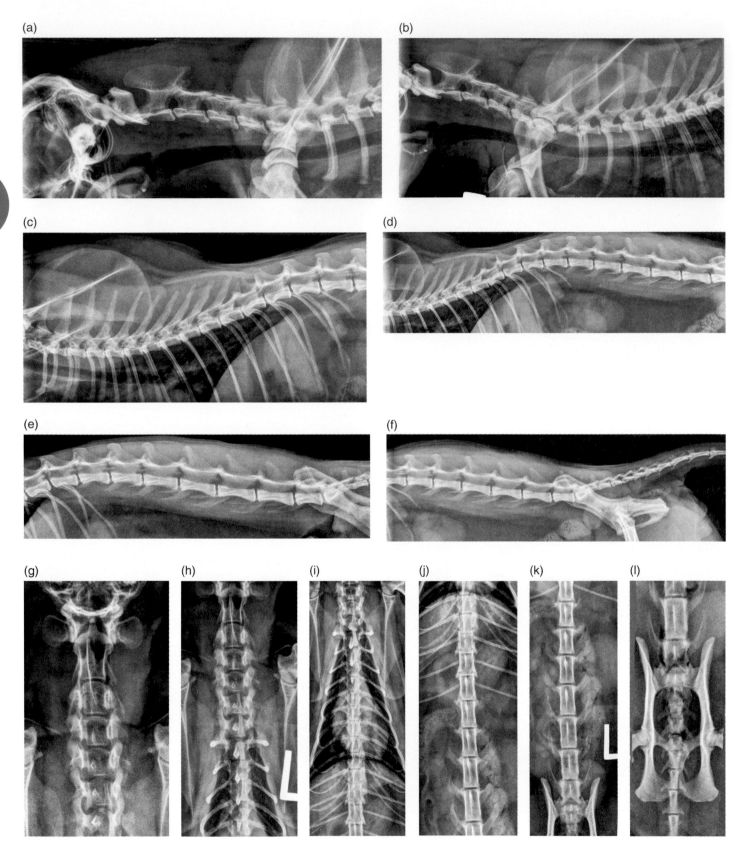

Figure 7-56 Spine radiographs. Radiographs are optimally obtained from the cervical, cervicothoracic, thoracic, thoracolumbar, lumbar, and lumbosacral regions. (a)–(f), Lateral views. (g)–(l), Ventrodorsal views.

Acknowledgment

Special thanks to Leigh Wagner, Catherine Bassett, Kim Bryan, and Betty Files for their assistance in obtaining images and reviewing the text.

Suggested Readings

Bonagura JD. 2000. Feline Echocardiography. *J Fel Med Surg*. 2:147–51.

Feeney D, McClanahan SL, Walter PA. 1999. *Radiography in Veterinary Technology*, 2nd ed. Philadelphia: WB Saunders.

Lavin L. 2006. *Radiography in Veterinary Technology*, 4th ed. Philadelphia: WB Saunders.

Penninck D, d'Anjou M. 2008. *Atlas of Small Animal Ultrasonography.* Ames: Wiley Blackwell.

Morgan JP. 1993. *Techniques of Veterinary Radiography*, 5th ed. Ames: Iowa State University Press.

Slater D. 2002. *Textbook of Small Animal Surgery*, 2nd ed. Vols. 1, 2. Philadelphia: WB Saunders Co.

Thrall DE, ed. 2007. *Textbook of Veterinary Diagnostic Radiology*, 5th ed. Philadelphia: WB Saunders Co.

Wallack ST. 2003. *The Handbook of Veterinary Contrast Radiography.* Solana Beach: San Diego Veterinary Imaging.

Wright M, Spencer D, Stafford C, et al. 2008. Radiation Safety and Non-Manual Patient Restraint in *Veterinary Radiography.* San Diego: Animalinsides.com.

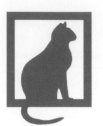

Venipuncture and Cystocentesis

Karen M. Lovelace

Overview

Venipuncture refers to venous (veni-, i.e. vein) puncture using a needle for the drawing of a blood sample. Cystocentesis refers to the puncture of a hollow body cavity such as the urinary bladder (cysto-) for the purpose of drawing out fluid (-centesis), such as urine. There are numerous safe and effective techniques for collecting blood and urine samples from cats using a sterile syringe and needle. Equipment, indications, contraindications, preparation, and procedure will be covered for both in this chapter. Because it is often preferable to collect urine from patients prior to venous sampling in the event that a nervous patient should evacuate his or her bladder, cystocentesis will be covered first.

Cystocentesis

Equipment

A 6- or 12-cc syringe and a 1.0- or 1.5-inch 22- or 25-gauge needle are used. A 1.5-inch needle is preferred for ultrasound assisted cystocentesis. A 25-gauge needle may be preferred for cystocentesis in kittens. Other equipment needed includes isopropyl alcohol and appropriate sterile urine laboratory submission tubes. For learning purposes, it may be easiest to use a 3- or 6-cc syringe.

Indications/Contraindications

Cystocentesis, manual bladder expression, catheterization, or voided "free catch" samples are all means of obtaining urine samples for urinalysis. Diagnostic cystocentesis and sterile catheterization are chosen when a sterile urine sample devoid of contaminants from the lower urinary tract or skin is desired. For example, when a bacterial urinary tract infection is suspected these methods are preferred for obtaining urine for culture. Other than samples naturally voided by the patient, all techniques may result in some degree of physical trauma to the patient. For this reason, cystocentesis is often preferred over catheterization in awake, unobstructed feline patients when an uncontaminated urine sample is desired. Nevertheless, the bladder should always be physically handled in a gentle manner, especially in cases of suspected urethral obstruction in which the bladder may be large, turgid, and painful. Although rare, if the bladder is handled too aggressively, the vagal nerve may be stimulated to elicit a vagal response that may manifest as weakness or collapse. In extreme cases, such as urethral obstruction in which the bladder is very full and very firm, a combination of bladder manipulation and urine leakage into the abdomen from the needle puncture site may result in such pain as to elicit shock, the symptoms of which could include collapse, extreme weakness, vocalizing, pale mucous membrane color, or vomiting. Extreme caution should be used when puncturing a full, turgid bladder and avoided in favor of catheterization whenever possible. Catheterization is chosen in these cases to avoid bladder rupture, tears, or excess pain. Cystocentesis should only be attempted when urinary catheterization is not practical because of high bladder pressures or unsuccessful catheterization and *only* under the supervision of a veterinarian.

Nursing the Feline Patient, First Edition. Edited by Linda E. Schmeltzer and Gary D. Norsworthy.
© 2012 John Wiley & Sons, Inc. Published 2012 by John Wiley & Sons, Inc.

Preparation

Because cats are easily stressed, location is essential. Ideally, urine should be collected in a quiet room away from barking dogs and other loud noises (such as laundry or lobby). Owners, if present, should be encouraged to remain calm. Giving cats a soft, warm, and comfortable area to recline is also helpful. Lowering the lights and whispering may also help to calm a stressed cat. Life stage, body condition, and temperament will help determine patient preparation and technique. For senior or geriatric cats in which arthritis or other painful conditions may be a consideration, pain medication at the veterinarian's discretion should be given ahead of time. For cats that appear apprehensive, feline facial pheromone (Feliway™) or Bachflower Essence (Rescue Remedy™) may be used prior to restraint for their anxiety-relieving effects. Some cats may also be calmed when a muzzle or snap on Elizabethan collar is used to cover or shield their eyes, or the patient may be placed in a "cat bag," although this is generally more likely to be warranted for venipuncture. Finally, a "cat clip," which is a large plastic clip placed at the scruff of the neck, may help to release natural endorphins and relax a cat for minimal restraint.

In the awake, unobstructed feline patient body condition score will affect positioning and needle size. For obese patients in which the bladder is harder to isolate, using a 1.5-inch needle in right lateral recumbency, the two-hand technique (which will be described) can be employed, or the patient can be placed in dorsal recumbency for ultrasound-guided cystocentesis using a 1.5-inch needle. For cats with thin to normal body condition scores, right lateral recumbency is preferred because the bladder can usually be successfully isolated. If the bladder cannot easily be located (for any size cat), it is best to wait several hours for the bladder to fill and become easily identifiable for safety reasons. Isopropyl alcohol can be used to cover the area targeted for cystocentesis regardless of positioning or method.

Right Lateral Recumbency

In this method, the bladder is palpated and isolated dorsally away from other organs, and cystocentesis is performed blind (i.e. without visualization using ultrasound). Some clinicians will advocate visualization of the bladder in all cases, but if the bladder is correctly isolated dorsally against the body wall, the needle will enter only through the body wall and the bladder rather than entering another organ such as the colon, which could result in contamination. An assistant will gently position the cat with its right side down on the table, head facing away. The assistant should gently stretch the cat's hind legs caudal to the abdomen and help keep the cat's spine in a straight alignment by using the forearm to support the cat's back. Supporting the back also aids in calming the cat and reduces struggling (Fig. 8-1). To gently palpate and isolate the urinary bladder in this position using one hand, choose the hand that will not be holding the syringe, which is usually the nondominant hand. Make a C shape with the fingers and thumb of this hand, and starting as caudally as the pelvic inlet, with the thumb positioned dorsally, move the C all the way to the spine until the bottom of the vertebrae is felt. Gently close the fingers and thumb together and move the hand together cranially until light resistance is met and the bladder is felt. If you unsure whether it is the bladder, slightly decrease the distance between them thumb and fingers in the C shape and move the hand both cranially and caudally until the bladder slips swiftly

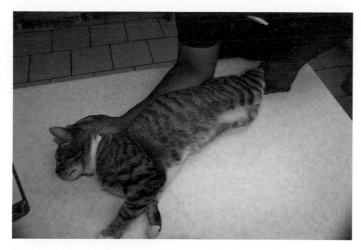

Figure 8-1 Restraint for cystocentesis is accomplished with a technician holding the scruff in one hand with the forearm parallel to the cat's spine. The other hand holds the cat's rear legs.

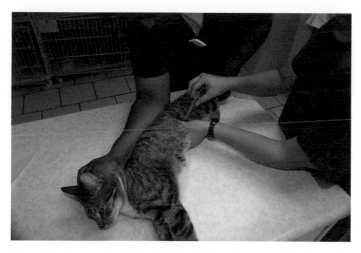

Figure 8-2 The operator stabilizes the cat's bladder with one hand lifting it up to the body wall. The syringe and needle are guided with the other hand until the needle enters the bladder.

through the fingers. Because it is hollow and filled with fluid, the bladder should feel like a water-filled balloon. When the bladder is isolated, keep the thumb and fingers closed and gently position the bladder dorsally (up) and to the spine (away). Gently tap on the bladder with a finger to confirm that it feels bouncy, as if tapping a water balloon. The average-sized bladder will be approximately the size of a large lemon, but it can range from the size of a walnut to grapefruit. Remember that the bladder is most fixed at its base caudally and most mobile cranially. Therefore, isolation will be most successful when starting palpation caudally especially if the bladder is small. Once the bladder is successfully isolated, hold the syringe and needle in the dominant hand and puncture through the skin and directly into the dorsally isolated bladder, ideally at a 45-degree angle (Fig. 8-2). If the bladder is correctly isolated dorsally toward the skin, the needle (especially if using 1.5-inch needle) should not need to be advanced very far. Approximately half an inch should be sufficient. Once the needle has been inserted into the bladder, the syringe should be aspirated to collect urine. Once the syringe is full, *stop* aspiration, *then* withdraw the syringe and needle. Aspirating as the needle is withdrawn can result in urine leakage, hemorrhage, or sample contamination. So when the syringe is full, *stop* aspiration, *then*, after aspiration is stopped, withdraw the syringe and

needle. If the bladder is missed on the first attempt or if blood is noted in the needle hub, *stop* aspiration and withdraw the unit to change needles, but *only* if a second attempt is safely indicated. It is not advisable to continuously redirect the needle blindly. Doing so risks urine leakage, hemorrhage, or sample contamination. A careful new attempt (if safely indicated) using a clean needle will reduce these risks as well as reduce the risk of spreading neoplastic cells in the event that a tumor is discovered in or around the bladder.

For larger or obese cats, a two-hand technique, using a second assistant, may be appropriate. In this method, one assistant gently restrains the cat in right lateral recumbency as previously described. A second assistant uses two hands in a cupped sandwich fashion and starts caudally to try and isolate the bladder. Closing the sandwiched hands at either cranial or caudal ends while attempting to roll over the bladder in a cranial to caudal fashion is used to isolate the bladder. Once isolated, the bladder is again elevated to the skin surface and the person to aspirate taps the bladder prior to puncture and aims the needle through the skin where the bladder is in closest contact with the skin dorsally. This technique will often take more practice because it requires a third person and therefore, better person-to-person communication. Again, if the bladder cannot be easily identified, cystocentesis should be temporarily abandoned.

When palpation is unsuccessful, ultrasound-guided cystocentesis may be preferred. The advantage of ultrasound guidance is that the bladder size, location, and surrounding structures can be visualized, and thus the risk of puncturing unwanted structures is greatly reduced. Bladder identification is generally easier in cats that are thin or have fuller bladders. If the bladder is nearly empty, the needle will "bounce" off of the wall instead of penetrate it; if so, cystocentesis should be abandoned. Position the cat in dorsal recumbency, ideally in a soft trough. Isopropyl alcohol often does not pool caudally over the bladder as it does in some dogs, so visualization is still best for guiding aspiration. However, wetting the skin with alcohol allows good contact with the ultrasound probe and avoids the need for coupling gel. Once the bladder is visualized on ultrasound, the needle should again be introduced in a straight "in and out" fashion, and aspiration employed as described previously. If possible, once visualized the bladder can be gently isolated with a free hand up toward the cat's ventral body wall. If traumatic urinary sampling inadvertently leads to suspected bladder tear, rupture, or abdominal hemorrhage, ultrasound can be used to screen for free fluid in the abdomen.

Once urine is collected, it should be analyzed as soon as possible or refrigerated promptly prior to same day laboratory pick up. Delay of analysis or refrigeration may result in change in some urine parameters (i.e. pH, bacteria, crystal content, turbidity), which can result in the aberration of diagnostic results.

Venipuncture

Equipment

A 6-cc syringe and a ¾-inch 20-gauge needle are used for adult cats. A 1-cc syringe and 25-gauge needle or a tuberculin or insulin swaged 27-gauge needle/syringe is preferred in kittens. Other equipment includes isopropyl alcohol and appropriate sterile laboratory submission tubes. It may be easiest when learning to practice using a 3-cc syringe.

Indications/Contraindications

Venous blood collection is contraindicated when safety to the cat or to veterinary personnel is prohibitive for most feline adults and kittens. If airway or circulation is compromised because of restraint or underlying disease or if the patient would suffer undue pain or stress as determined by the overseeing veterinarian, sedation may be employed or venipuncture abandoned.

Preparation

Preparation can be approached similarly to that of cystocentesis in that any pain, temperament, or life stage related conditions should first be addressed with appropriate analgesic or anxiety relieving treatments as prescribed by a veterinarian. Similar methods of restraint to shield a cat's visual perimeter (i.e. muzzle, snap-on Elizabethan collar), "cat clip," or cat bag, can be used to calm cats and protect veterinary staff. Such restraint devices may be more practically used for venipuncture due to patient positioning. However, for venipuncture, most often a "less-is-more" approach to restraint will be most successful. The environment for feline blood collection is equally (if not more) essential than for urine collection because cats notoriously experience stress-related changes on their leukogram. This can be tempered by collecting blood in a dimly lit, quiet room, away from barking dogs and other loud noises. Owners, if present, should be encouraged to remain a calming influence. Providing cats with a soft, warm, and comfortable towel or pillow to lie on during collection is also helpful, especially if the body condition score is 3/9 or less. Lowering the surrounding room lights and using one directed light source for vein identification may also help to calm a stressed cat.

Blood can be most easily collected from three main sites: the (left) jugular vein, the medial saphenous veins, and the cephalic veins. Ideally, these areas should be sterilely prepared by clipping the hair and applying isopropyl alcohol to cleaned skin. However, preparation will depend on case selection and should be directed by the veterinarian. For example, some cats (and owners) will fare better if hair is not shaved. Regardless of the area chosen, while learning in a teaching setting or if time permits in a clinical more practical setting, local analgesia as when used for intravenous catheterization may be useful. In these instances, after the skin is shaved and cleaned, a topical cream containing 4% or less lidocaine (such as EMLA Cream®) is applied to the skin, covered with a dressing, and venipuncture is delayed for at least 30 minutes. For obvious reasons, in a clinical setting this is not always practical.

For jugular and cephalic blood collection, the cat can be "restrained" in a natural sitting or sternally recumbent "sphinx" position. For medial saphenous collection, lateral recumbency is preferred. For jugular, a technique that places the cat in dorsal recumbency can also be employed. This technique will be described.

Jugular blood collection is often preferred and will be described first. The left jugular vein in most cats is more prominent, so this side is often preferred. To locate the left jugular vein, anatomically draw an imaginary line from the lateral right limbus of the eye (junction of the cornea and sclera) to the thoracic inlet. Place light pressure with the right thumb at the thoracic inlet in this location, and the jugular should appear. Alcohol will help to make the jugular vein more prominent, as will lightly tapping the finger on top of and from right to left over this imaginary line or shaving hair over the area. In addition, having an assistant gently stretch the cat's neck and turn the cat's head to the right approximately 45 degrees may also help make visualization easier. In obese or very dehydrated cats, the jugular may not be seen, and this imaginary line and anatomical landmarks will guide for aspiration. In obese cats, a layer of fat will often surround the jugular vein, and although it may not be seen, the vein is often very flat and superficial. Insert the hub of the needle, bevel *up*, into the jugular vein. Some may find it helpful to first bend the needle at its base at a 30-degree angle. Be deliberate in the needle insertion. While harpooning the vessel is neither necessary nor beneficial, if the needle insertion is too delicate the vein will be pushed away by the needle tip, and the cat will feel the needle tip and be more likely to react with pain. While inserting the needle aspirate the syringe with light but continuous pressure until a flash of blood in the hub is seen. Be careful not to thread the needle to far or deep because penetration through the opposite side of the vein is possible. If you think this has happened, with light negative suction continue to aspirate as you slowly withdraw the needle back into the vein. Once you get a flash of blood, hold the syringe and needle steady and continue to aspirate until the syringe is full. Maintaining anatomical alignment with the needle and syringe to

the vein is helpful. Blood should fill the syringe in approximately 5–6 seconds once you are correctly in the jugular vein. Also remember that veins are low pressure relative to the arterial blood supply, so if you aspirate too forcefully, you may inadvertently collapse the vein. Use light, slow, and steady aspiration. Practice withdrawing the plunger from the needle on room air to become more comfortable holding the needle in one place while drawing back on the syringe. Once blood has been collected, stop aspirating, remove the needle and syringe, and apply pressure to the venipuncture site for 30–60 seconds as sufficient to prevent bruising.

Blood collection from the jugular vein can often be accomplished in cats that are in a seated upright position with no more restraint than lightly directing their jaw dorsally and to the right with little else than a finger. In fact, many cats are more cooperative with minimal restraint and will often allow for one-person venipuncture (with practice). Alternatively, in slightly more nervous cats, situating the cat in dorsal recumbency in a lap over a towel, with the legs bent at a 90-degree angle aids in a calmed patient restraint and good jugular vein visualization. Sit on the floor or in a chair with feet on a step stool, but it is easiest to sit on a countertop (Fig. 8-3). The back of the cat's head rests at the knees, and its rump and feet rest against the abdomen. This technique usually requires two assistants. One assistant extends the neck and directs it in a 45-degree angle to the right as previously described for jugular collection, and the other assistant gently holds the front and back legs together in a cradled position directed caudally.

If only a small amount of blood is indicated or jugular blood collection is prohibitive, the cephalic or medial saphenous veins are frequently used to collect blood in cats. These veins can be prepared as if for placement of an intravenous catheter. For cephalic blood collection using the lightest restraint possible, point the cat's head upward as an easy distraction while keeping the head pointed forward. This relaxes the cat's jaw muscles and can result in calming, as well as keeps the teeth safely away from the phlebotomist. Sometimes the cat will relax more when placed gently in the sternally recumbent Sphinx position. The assistant will use his or her thumb to wrap from medial to lateral across the cephalic vein just distal to the elbow, to occlude the vein. The vein should be apparent centrally and dorsally over the antebrachium. Lightly tapping over the vein and using alcohol will again help the vein to stand up. The needle and syringe are advanced in the same fashion as for the jugular vein,

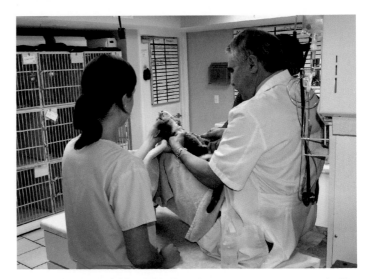

Figure 8-3 An alternative method of jugular blood collection, known as the "lap method," has the operator sitting on a countertop or table and placing the cat in dorsal recumbency on his or her lap with the head near the operator's knees. One assistant holds the cat's head and another holds the cat's feet. After wetting the area with alcohol, the jugular vein stands up more prominently than with other methods.

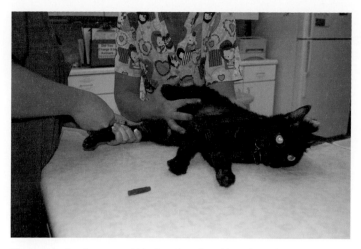

Figure 8-4 Small amounts of blood can be collected from the medial saphenous vein with the assistance of one helper. The helper holds the cat's scruff and supports the cat's spine with one hand and holds the free rear leg and the tail while holding off the vein with the other hand.

except that it may be necessary to use less and slower aspiration because smaller veins tend to collapse more readily. If this is consistently a problem, consider trading to a smaller volume syringe with an extension set or using a 26-gauge butterfly set.

For cats that do not tolerate minimal restraint, seated, or dorsally recumbent positions, the medial saphenous veins may be used. Most often, the patient is positioned in right lateral recumbency as for cystocentesis, except that the assistant uses his or her left hand in a "karate chop" fashion to apply light pressure at the region of the femoral triangle

to occlude the vein (Fig. 8-4). Unlike the jugular or cephalic vein approach, this vein has low pressure and will less often "bounce" or stand up when gently tapped. However, because the skin is very thin in this region, the vein filled with dark blue blood can frequently be seen with ease, especially after alcohol is applied or the hair is shaved. A 25-gauge needle with a 1- or 3-cc volume syringe is recommended.

Conclusion

Careful consideration to the unique needs, history, and temperament of each feline patient, along with patience, loving care, and practice, will result in successful blood and urine collection in feline patients. The skills of venipuncture and cystocentesis will enable the veterinary team to submit the diagnostic tests necessary for the treatment of feline patients. This, in turn, will result in improving the quality of life of our feline patients, and their owners.

Suggested Readings

Buckley GJ, Aktay SA, Rozanski EA. 2009. Massive Transfusion and Surgical Management of Iatrogenic Aortic Laceration Associated with Cystocentesis in a Dog. *J Amer Vet Med Assoc.* 235(3):288–91.

Norsworthy GD. 2011. Jugular Blood Collection. In GD Norsworthy, ed., *The Feline Patient*, 4th ed., pp. 902–903. Ames: Wiley-Blackwell.

Pozza M, Stella J, Wagner S., et al. 2008. Clipnosis Technique. *J Fel Med Surg.* 10(2):82–87. Philadelphia: Elsevier.

Rush JE. 1999. Syncope and Episodic Weakness. In PR Fox, D Sisson, NS Moïse, eds., *Textbook of Canine and Feline Cardiology*, 2nd ed., pp. 446–54. Philadelphia: WB Saunders.

Wagner KA, Gibbon KJ, Strom TL, et al. 2006. Adverse Effects of EMLA (lidocaine/prilocaine) Cream and Efficacy for the Placement of Jugular Catheters in Hospitalized Cats. *J Fel Med Surg.* 8(2):141–44.

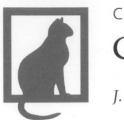

Cytology

J. Scot Estep

Introduction

Cytology is an incomplete art, like looking at a crime scene through a peephole. In the right situation and used in conjunction with clinical information cytology can provide valuable diagnostic data, but in the wrong situation with the wrong technique it can be a waste of time and in some cases misleading as to the actual diagnosis. The goal of this chapter is to empower the technician and clinician with proper cytology collection and slide preparation techniques to get the most out of cytology. Minimal guidance for slide interpretation is offered; Chapter 13 and numerous excellent cytology books are available to guide the systematic evaluation of cytology samples.

Samples can be obtained from almost any tissue and in many different ways: fine-needle biopsy, fine-needle aspiration, impression smear, body cavity fluid, joint fluid, cerebrospinal fluid, transtracheal wash, traumatic urinary catheterization, prostate massage/ejaculation, vaginal swab, eye/ear swab, blood, bone marrow, impressions, and scrapes.

Control Points

Each step of sample collection and slide preparation is critical for the production of diagnostic cytology samples. A photo is only as good as the focus and lighting when the picture is taken; likewise, a cytology sample is only as good as the process that made it. The following are the five fixable pitfalls, which are the critical control points of cytology.

Lack of Identification on the Slides

Failure to identify radiographs or blood samples is considered malpractice, yet most clinicians/technicians do not label cytology slides. Admittedly slides are hard to write on, but without a name and location on the slide, a sample quickly becomes useless. The best way to learn to be a better cytologist is to refer back to the slides once a diagnosis is made; however, without proper identification this is impossible.

Poor Sample Collection

Mastering the right collection technique for the right situation is critical. It takes practice, and in the long run it will improve service to patients.

Poor Slide Prep

Making a good smear, drying and fixing the slides, proper staining, and cover slipping slides are all critical for getting the most out of the sample.

Poor Microscope/Poor Utilization of a Microscope

Microscopes need to be clean and mechanically maintained regularly, and most clinics have a better microscope than they think. Lack of knowledge of how to use the diaphragm and condenser, lack of a coverslip with the high dry (40× or 60×) lens, and contamination of the high dry

lens with oil all contribute to poor image quality and compile the frustration of cytology.

The "Home Run or Nothing" Mentality

On its own, cytology rarely produces a definite diagnosis, but in almost every case it can give some useful clinical information. A monomorphic population of lymphoblasts from a lymph node aspirate is diagnostic, but finding reactive lymphocytes and plasma cells is also clinically useful even if it does not confirm the differential.

Sample Collection

Preparing all the necessary items before beginning sample collection will improve identification and eliminate sample degradation as a result of delays. The supplies that are needed for every sample are (Fig. 9-1):

- Clean dry slides preferably with one frosted end.
- Pencil or slide marker pen. Identify slides before collecting sample.
- Clean fresh cytology stains preferably Diff-Quik® (a modified Romanowsky stain).
- Immersion oil and coverslips.

Fine-Needle Biopsy (FNB)

This technique is gentle on the cells and is ideal for soft masses, lymph nodes, and intra-abdominal organs. It works well for specimens that are fragile and cannot handle the negative pressure of aspiration. Start with this more gentle method and move on to the more aggressive fine-needle aspiration if good cells are not obtained.

Supplies: 18- to 22-gauge needle, 5- or 20-cc syringe, and intravenous extension tube (optional).

- Shave area if necessary for exposure.
- Clean area with alcohol or surgical prep.

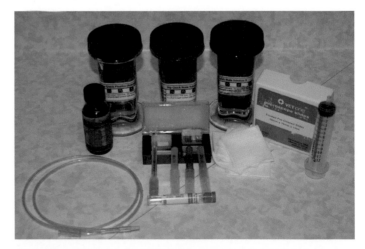

Figure 9-1 Cytology supplies: Frosted slides, 18-gauge 1-inch needle, 12-ml syringe, short intravenous extension set, gauze pads, purple top tube, Diff-Quik® stain set, cover slips, and immersion oil.

Nursing the Feline Patient, First Edition. Edited by Linda E. Schmeltzer and Gary D. Norsworthy.
© 2012 John Wiley & Sons, Inc. Published 2012 by John Wiley & Sons, Inc.

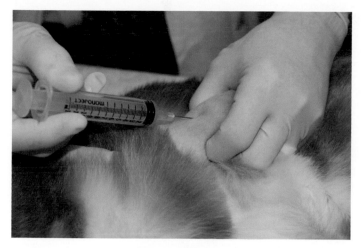

Figure 9-2 A subcutaneous or intra-abdominal mass is immobilized with one hand so a 22-gauge needle can be inserted into the mass with the other hand.

- Stabilize mass or lymph node between fingers.
- Use either a needle only, a needle attached to a plunger-less syringe, or a needle attached to an intravenous extension set that is attached to a syringe (Fig. 9-2).
- Insert the needle into the mass and redirect four to five times with a pecking motion without leaving the capsule of the target tissue.
- Open the syringe plunger and attach to needle and then blow the sample onto a prelabeled slide.
- To prepare a vertical pull-apart smear (drop-spin-pull), place another prelabeled slide upside down and cross ways on top of the sample allowing only the weight of the slide and capillary action to stick the slides together. If they will not stick together a small drop of saline can be added.
- Holding the frosted edges, rotate the slides and pull them vertically apart from each other, producing two good slides (Fig. 9-3).
- Dry the slides. Stain some and leave others unstained.

Fine-Needle Aspiration

This technique is more aggressive and can be used as a follow-up if insufficient cells are retrieved with the FNB. It can be used as a primary technique for fibrous masses. Some choose to start with this technique for intra-abdominal organs.

Supplies: 18- to 22-gauge needle, 5- or 12-cc syringe, and intravenous extension tube (optional).

- Shave area if necessary for exposure.
- Clean area with alcohol or surgical prep.
- Stabilize mass or lymph node between fingers.
- Use either a needle attached to a 5- or 12-cc syringe or an intravenous extension tube that is attached to a syringe.
- Insert the needle into the mass, apply negative pressure with the syringe, and redirect four to five times with a pecking motion without leaving the capsule of the target tissue. Release the negative pressure and withdraw (Fig. 9-4).
- Remove the needle from the syringe, fill the syringe with air, reattach the needle, and blow the sample onto a prelabeled slide.
- Prepare a vertical pull-apart slide (drop-spin-pull) as described previously, producing two good slides.
- Dry the slides, stain some, and leave others unstained.

Impression Smear

This technique is useful for surgical or necropsy samples as well as ulcerated or draining cutaneous lesions. It can be useful to quickly separate

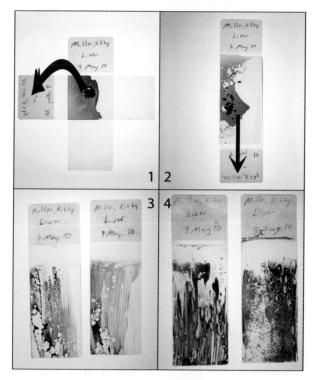

Figure 9-3 (1) A sample is applied to a prelabeled slide and covered with second prelabeled slide placed face down. The top slide is then rotated 90 degrees. (2) The slides are pulled laterally apart. (3) Two stainable smears are produced. (4) Two stained smears containing multiple clumps of cells are seen after staining.

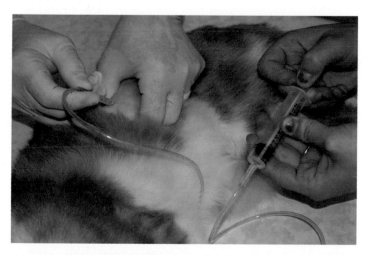

Figure 9-4 A subcutaneous or intra-abdominal mass is stabilized with one hand while the other hand inserts a 20-gauge needle attached to an intravenous extension set and a syringe. An assistant applies negative pressure with a 12-cc syringe.

neoplastic versus inflammatory lesions but can be misleading for any lesion with surface ulceration and secondary infection.

Supplies: Paper towel or gauze pads for blotting and scalpel blade.

- Cut solid samples to get a clean surface or clean the surface of skin lesions.
- Alternate between blotting with a gauze pad and touching the slide (blot, smear, and repeat [Fig. 9-5]).
- Make at least four slides in case special stains are needed.
- Dry the slides, stain some, and leave others unstained.

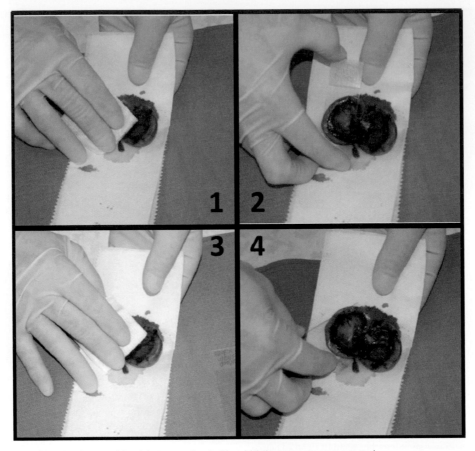

Figure 9-5 (1) A transected mass is blotted with gauze. (2) A slide is pressed on it. (3) and (4) These two steps are repeated.

Swab

This technique is useful for any area with a surface lesion or orifice that cannot be reached for an impression smear. The swab is most frequently used for ear and vaginal samples but is also useful for draining tracts, nasal, eye, anal sacs, and more surfaces or mucocutaneous areas. The biggest downfall of the swab is that the sample is frequently too thick; therefore, be careful to avoid leaving too much material on the slide. If the sample is too thick, another slide can be used with the vertical pull-apart method to produce two smears that are not as thick.

Supplies: Clean, dry swabs and saline.

- Clean and dry the area if possible
- Avoid surface contamination by inserting a dry or saline-moistened swab (do not use lube or ultrasound jelly) into the area of interest and gently spin the cotton tip.
- Remove the swab being careful to avoid contamination.
- Gently roll the swab on the surface of three to four slides, avoiding leaving too much sample on the slide (Fig. 9-6).
- Dry the slides, stain some, and leave others unstained.

Skin Scrape

This technique is useful for superficial cutaneous and follicular lesions that cannot be sampled with an impression smear or fine-needle aspiration. It works for a well with follicular parasites, fungal infections, and flat cutaneous lesions.

Supplies: Scalpel blade and mineral oil or saline.

- Shave the area if necessary.
- Clean the area with alcohol or surgical prep.

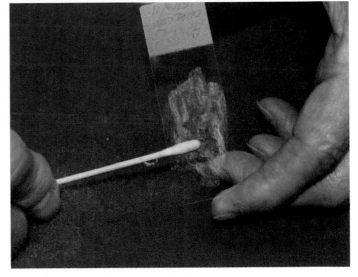

Figure 9-6 A thin layer of material collected from a lesion with a moist cotton-tipped applicator is rolled out on a slide prior to staining.

- Pinch up and elevate skin.
- With fresh prep samples to rule out follicular parasites apply mineral oil to the skin surface; for samples that will be stained before evaluation, use saline.
- Aggressively scrape the skin with the scalpel blade without lacerating the skin.

- Alternate between scraping the skin and squeezing the area until blood and serum exude from the scraped surface (Fig. 9-7).
- Apply the exuded serum and blood to a slide, create a vertical pull-part sample, and either add a coverslip and examine the fresh sample or dry and stain some slides for examination.

Fluid Samples

Fluid samples can be obtained from numerous sources. Subsequent cytologic examination can be useful for determining the origin. Cells within fluids will degrade quickly; therefore, immediately after collection all fluids should be checked with a refractometer for total protein (not specific

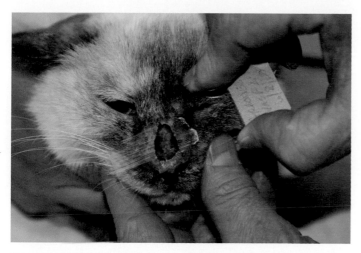

Figure 9-7 After pinching the skin to cause blood or serum to exude, a slide is pressed onto the lesion.

gravity), and three to four smears should be made from the fresh fluid. These two procedures will provide a snapshot of what the cells look like at the time of collection. Fluid samples can be obtained from the thoracic or abdominal cavity, joints, epidural space, cysts, trachea, urinary bladder, and others.

See Table 9-1 for interpretation guidelines.

Supplies: 18- to 22-gauge needle, 12- or 20-cc syringe, purple-topped tube, red-topped tube, refractometer, urine dipstick, intravenous extension set, and stopcock (optional).

- Shave the area if necessary.
- Clean the area with surgical prep. Most fluid samples come from closed compartments, and surgical sterility should be maintained if possible.
- Insert the needle, withdraw fluid, leaving the needle in place, remove the syringe and save some fluid for culture and some in the ethylenediaminetetraacetic acid (EDTA) tube for cytology.
- Immediately invert the EDTA tube several times to mix contents.
- Check and record the total protein level with a refractometer.
- Make three to four blood smear-type slides with the fresh fluid.
- If the sample has low cellularity it can be centrifuged at 1000–1500 rpm for 5 minutes (similar to urine sediment), and slides can be made from this sediment.
- Dry and stain some slides and leave others unstained.

Slide Staining and Preparations

Most clinics use a modified Romanowsky stain kit (Diff-Quik®). This stain will differentiate nuclei from cytoplasm and will stain most bacterial and fungal organisms. Stains used for cytology should be kept clean (not used for fecal or ear stains) and periodically changed out. Many facilities rotate the stains from cytology use for the first 30–45 days then to fecal and ear samples for another 30–45 days. Slides should be stained

TABLE 9-1: Laboratory interpretation of fluid samples

	Chylous Effusion	Transudate	Modified Transudate	Exudate	Fip	Hemorrhage
Refractometer total protein (g/dl)	High lipid content interferes	<2.5 (most below 1.5)	2.5–7.5	>3.0	>4.0	>2.5
Nucleated cell count (cells/μl)	<10,000 sometimes lower	<1500	1000–7000	>10,000	2000–6000	Variable PCV up to 10%
Color	Milky white to pink	Clear	Amber, white, red	White to red, cloudy	Clear, amber to pink	Red
Cells	Lymphocytes, macrophages containing fat droplets	Macrophages, lymphocytes, mesothelial cells, nondegenerate neutrophils	Macrophages, lymphocytes, mesothelial cells, nondegenerate neutrophils, neoplastic cells	Septic: Degenerate neutrophils nonseptic: nondegenerate neutrophils, macrophages, neoplastic cells	Nondegenerate neutrophils, lymphocytes, macrophages	Fresh hemorrhage: RBCs, platelets, peripheral blood >24 hrs post hemorrhage: RBCs, macrophages with erythrophagocytosis and hemosiderin, no platelets
Differential	Idiopathic, cardiomyopathy, neoplasia, mediastinal mass, ruptured thoracic duct	Low oncotic pressure: Hypoalbumin, protein losing diseases	Increased hydrostatic pressure, passive congestion, neoplasia, impaired, lymphatic drainage	Peritonitis, bile peritonitis, ruptured urinary bladder, pancreatitis, bacterial/fungal, abscess, neoplasia	Wet form has a viscous fluid, dry form does not product an effusion	Trauma, neoplasia, coagulation defects, heart disease

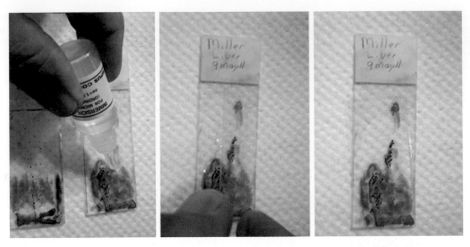

Figure 9-8 *Left to right,* A small drop of oil is applied to a stained slide; a coverslip is placed over slide; and the completed smear is ready for viewing.

by the manufacturer's instructions, but the number of dips or dipping times can be altered based on clinic preference or the age of the stains (I prefer 12 dips in each jar). After staining, slides should be thoroughly dried and covered with a small drop of mineral or immersion oil and a coverslip. The high dry 40× or 60× lens will only work with a coverslip (Fig. 9-8).

Evaluating Slides

Every cytology sample should, at a minimum, be stained and evaluated in house for quality, cellularity, artifacts, and contamination. To improve abilities as cytologist it is also educational to critically evaluate the slide and add a diagnostic impression on the submission form to the pathologist. Most pathologists will consider the differential and will comment on the salient features of the slide in response to comments.

Each step of slide evaluation should be completed systematically; no one feature or cell is enough to support a diagnosis. Follow the "rule of three" to support any diagnosis. Example #1: Bacteria on a slide do not indicate a bacterial infection, but (1) bacteria, (2) inside, and (3) degenerate neutrophils can be diagnosed as a bacterial infection. Example #2: Just the presence of a mitotic figure does not support a diagnosis of neoplasia, but (1) mitotic figures, (2) variation in nuclear size, and (3) nuclear atypia are diagnostic for neoplasia (Figs. 9-9 to 9-15).

The recommended steps are:

- Look at the slide off the stage in the light and get an impression as to cellularity and staining.
- At low power (4×–10×) drive around the slide; find where the best clumps are and evaluate overall cellularity. Do not forget the bottom edge of the slide.
- Evaluate cells at 40× and using the algorithm in Figure 9-16.

Cell Types

The first question of a cytology sample after assessing the quality is "What cell types are present?" The major divisions are between inflammatory cells and tissue cells. The following is a summary of the major cell types (Figs. 9-17 and 9-18).

Neutrophils

Neutrophils are 7–15 μm wide with multilobed nuclei. In the absence of pyogenic bacteria, neutrophil nuclei become hypersegmented and even-

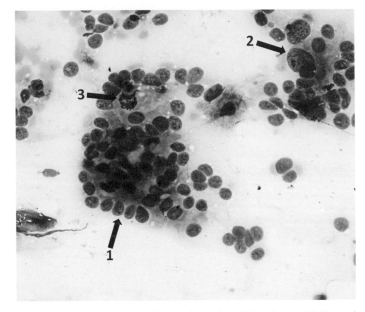

Figure 9-9 Renal cell carcinoma. (1) Normal epithelium. (2) Anisokaryosis. (3) Abnormal mitosis.

tually pyknotic (nondegenerate). *See* Figure 9-16. In infected inflammatory lesions the neutrophils undergo rapid degeneration, vacuolation, and eventual rupture (degenerate). *See* Figure 9-17.

Lymphocytes

Normal lymphocytes are identical to blood smear lymphocytes. They are 7–10 μm wide with a large nuclei and a small amount of blue cytoplasm. Activated lymphocytes have more prominent cytoplasm that often blebs up or extends from the cells like a handle. Immature lymphoid cells (lymphoblasts) are characterized by their large size (10–15 μm) and the presence of a nucleolus.

Plasma Cells

Plasma cells are similar in size to small lymphocytes, but the nuclear chromatin is denser, the cytoplasm is blue and abundant, and a perinuclear clear area (Golgi apparatus) is usually apparent.

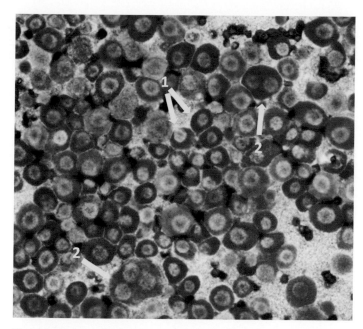

Figure 9-10 Mast cells (round cell tumor). (1) Individual round cells. (2) Multifocal multinucleate cells.

Macrophages

Macrophages range in size from 12–100 μm, have a single or multiple round to oval nucleus that may contain an apparent nucleolus, and have light blue, usually vacuolated cytoplasm. These cells phagocytize cellular debris, foreign material, and bacteria. Neutrophils, cellular debris, erythrocytes, red blood cell pigments, lipids, and phospholipids; however, they are commonly encountered within the cytoplasm of these phagocytic cells.

Eosinophils

Eosinophils appear similar to eosinophils in peripheral blood and are associated with various types of lesions, including allergic inflammation, parasitic inflammation, eosinophilic granulomas, collagen necrosis, and mast cell tumors.

Mast Cells

Mast cells are round cells with a round to oval nucleus and cytoplasm that contains purple granules. The granules occasionally do not stain well with Diff-Quik®. Mast cells may be present in low concentration in many types of inflammatory disorders, but if present in high concentrations, mast cell neoplasia should be suspected (*see* Fig. 9-10).

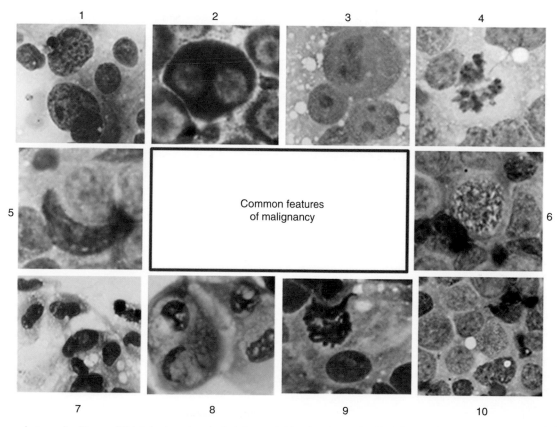

Figure 9-11 Common features of malignancy: (1) Variation in nuclear size (anisokaryosis). (2) Multinucleate cells. (3) Multiple nucleoli and irregular nucleoli. (4) Frequent mitosis. (5) Nuclear molding (hugging). (6) Irregular nuclear chromatin. (7) High yield of spindled cells. (8) Dyskeratosis (keratinizing with intact nucleoli). (9) Abnormal mitosis. (10) Monomorphic cell population.

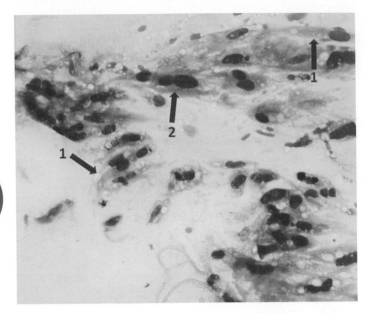

Figure 9-12 Sarcoma. This tumor is characterized by (1) formation of tails by the cytoplasm and (2) anisokaryosis. Note the overall high cell yield typical for a for spindle cell tumor.

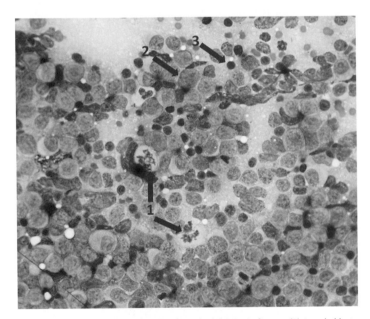

Figure 9-13 Lymphosarcoma in lymph node. (1) Mitotic figures. (2) Lymphoblasts. (3) Normal lymphocytes (size of erythrocytes).

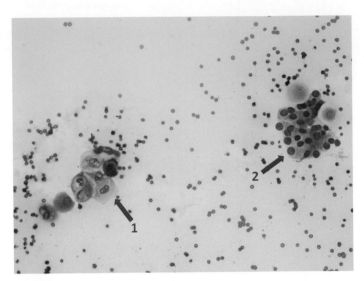

Figure 9-14 Nasal squamous cell carcinoma. (1) Normal nasal epithelium. (2) Atypical squamous cells.

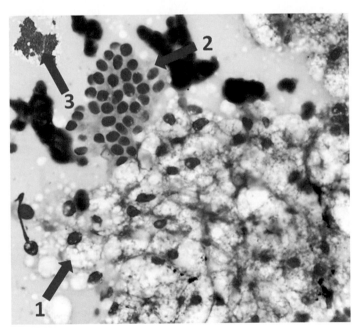

Figure 9-15 Hepatic lipidosis. (1) Large discrete vacuoles that sometimes peripheralize the nuclei. (2) Normal bile duct epithelial cells. (3) If ultrasound gel is used, it will be found in the sample.

Mesothelial Cells

Mesothelial cells tend to proliferate and exfoliate when fluid accumulates in a body cavity. They may appear singly or in clusters and are large (12–30 μm), have light to dark basophilic cytoplasm, and have single or multiple, round to oval nuclei with one or more nucleoli. The cytoplasmic border may appear to have a pink "fringe" around it.

Microorganisms

Bacteria stain blue with Romanowsky stains and must be distinguished from background protein and stain sediment. They are usually somewhat uniform in size, present within the cytoplasm of neutrophils, and if present in large numbers, may be both free and phagocytized. Other types of microorganisms, such as fungal organisms and protozoa, may also be infrequently seen in cytology specimens, including: *Coccidioides*, *Blastomyces*, *Histoplasma*, *Cryptococcus*, and *Toxoplasma gondii*.

Epithelial Cells

Epithelial cells occur in high cell numbers, so they usually exfoliate easily. In addition, they tend to be shed in clusters. Cell shape may reflect that of the specific epithelial type (squamous, cuboidal, or columnar),

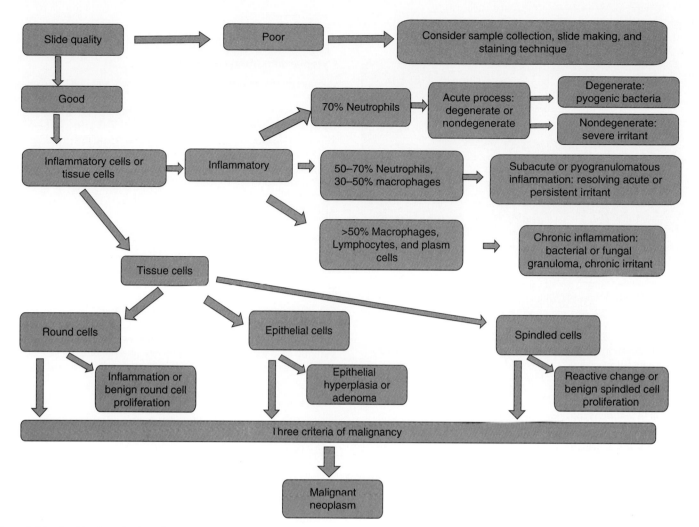

Figure 9-16 Algorithm for evaluating cells.

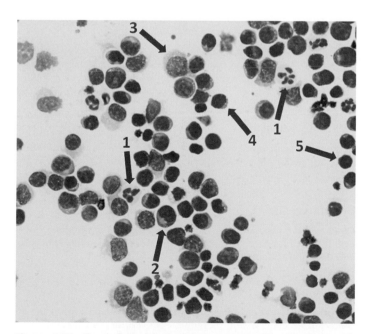

Figure 9-17 Pleural fluid. (1) Nondegenerate neutrophils. (2) Plasma cell. (3) Lymphoblast. (4) Activated lymphocyte. (5) Normal lymphocyte.

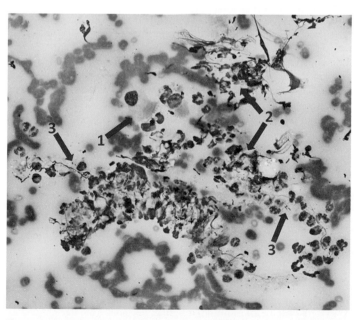

Figure 9-18 Suppurative rhinitis. (1) Respiratory epithelium. (2) Degenerate neutrophils. (3) Bacteria.

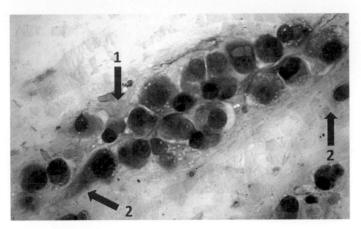

Figure 9-19 Feline osteosarcoma. (1) Clumps of cells are separated by pink "osteoid material." (2) Occasional tails are present.

A single large cytoplasmic vacuole, marked distension of cytoplasm, or acinar-like formations (balls, morulae) indicates glandular epithelial origin. The neoplastic cells tend to be roundish, polyhedral, and large, and their nuclei tend to be round (*see* Figs. 9-9, 9-14, and 9-15).

Spindled (Mesenchymal) Connective Tissue Cells

Spindled connective tissue cells tend to exfoliate poorly (low cell numbers) and are more prone to exfoliate individually, although groups of cells may be closely apposed in highly cellular specimens. Cell shape is elongated (spindle shaped), and nuclei are oval or elongated. Cytoplasm tends to "stream" at the end of the cell making a tail or point. These tails are the best feature to differentiate clumps of spindled cells from epithelial cells and, when in doubt, "tails trump clumps" (Fig. 9-19).

Round Cell Tumors

Round cell tumors exfoliate high numbers of discrete cells. Round cells are previously described with inflammatory cells. The amount of cytoplasm varies with the tumor type. Nuclei are round and often quite uniform. Specimens from these tumors tend to be cellular, and characteristic morphologic features often allow specific cytologic diagnosis (*see* Fig. 9-10).

Criteria of Malignancy

Once a sample is differentiated between inflammatory and tissue cells, the individual cells need to be assessed to determine if there are significant characteristics of malignancy. This requires consideration of the entire clinical picture. Even if the cells are spindled or epithelial, finding multiple characteristics of malignancy can be supportive of surgical excision and further characterization with histology.

General Criteria of Malignancy

The general criteria are uniform population, pleomorphic cells, large cell size, abnormal location, and cell yield.

Nuclear Criteria of Malignancy

Anisokaryosis (most frequent feature of malignancy), variable nuclear to cytoplasmic ratio, multiple/irregular nucleoli, irregular chromatin, irregular nuclear size, frequent mitoses, and abnormal mitoses are the nuclear criteria (*see* Fig. 9-11).

Cytoplasmic Criteria of Malignancy

Cytoplasmic criteria are basophilia, vacuolation, and ill-defined margins.

Clinical Feline Cytology

There are numerous well-written books that will lead the technician/clinician in a systematic evaluation of cytology slides. Several are listed in the suggested readings. The following information is intended as a short list of the major conditions seen in each system, listed in order of frequency.

Skin and Subcutis

Dermatitis

Mixed inflammatory cells are the key to diagnosing dermatitis (*see* Fig. 9-2). Granulomatous aspirates should be stained for fungal of acid fast organisms.

Basal Cell Tumor

These are epithelial tumors, but they often exfoliate as round cells, individually or in groups. They produce one or more bulging skin nodules, often located on the head and neck, and are usually ulcerated.

Mast Cell

This is a common round cell tumor of the skin of cats. Some can be pleomorphic and multinucleate, but despite these malignant features, these masses are almost always benign (*see* Fig. 9-10).

Squamous Cell Carcinoma

This is a common tumor of older cats, especially white cats, and it occurs in various locations including the skin of the ears, nose, and mouth. Touch imprints or fine-needle aspirates contain large cells – greater than 60 μm in diameter – with abundant basophilic to gray cytoplasm, and central to eccentric round nuclei. Usually there are numerous neutrophils present because the tumors have an ulcerated surface (*see* Fig. 9-14).

Sarcoma

There are many categories of sarcomas in the cat, but it is rarely possible to diagnose the cell type with cytology. Most sarcomas have the same poor prognosis so the important feature is being able to diagnose the cytoplasmic tails, elongated nuclei, and multiple malignant features (*see* Fig. 9-12).

Mammary Gland

In the cat, most mammary masses are caused by infection, cysts, diffuse fibroadenomatous hyperplasia, or neoplasia. Mammary neoplasms are usually highly malignant simple adenocarcinomas.

Lymphosarcoma

Cutaneous lymphosarcoma is a difficult diagnosis to make with cytology. It is characterized by a monomorphic population of lymphocytes with multiple malignant features.

Melanoma

Melanoma is found most commonly in the mouth and eyes. It can be characterized cytologically by round, spindled, or epithelial cells that contain brown pigment and have prominent nucleoli and moderate anisokaryosis.

Feline Lymph Node Cytology

Lymphoid Hyperplasia

Normal lymph nodes contain 20% lymphoblasts that are 10–20 μm in diameter and 80% small lymphocytes that 7–10 μm in diameter. Hyperplastic lymph nodes can have up to 45% lymphoblasts but are also accompanied by reactive lymphocytes and significant plasma cells.

Lymphosarcoma

Lymph node aspirates with greater than 50% lymphoblasts are consistent with lymphosarcoma. Many cases of lymphosarcoma have greater than 80% lymphoblasts. Cases with near 50% should either be biopsied and submitted for histology or reaspirated in 4–6 weeks (*see* Fig. 9-13).

Suppurative Lymphadenitis

Lymph nodes near sites of infection will frequently have draining neutrophils, but more than 15% neutrophils are consistent with suppurative lymphadenitis.

Granulomatous Lymphadenitis

High numbers of histiocytes in a cutaneous lymph node is supportive of granulomatous lymphadenitis. If no etiology is seen on the slides, special stains for fungal organisms or acid-fast bacteria should be performed.

Metastatic Neoplasia

Unless there is previous history of carcinoma or melanoma, it is rare to find metastatic neoplasia in lymph node aspirates. But in cases of previous regional malignant tumors, lymph nodes aspirates can be a sensitive test for spread to lymph nodes.

Feline Basal Cytology

The normal cells that you expect to see here are elongated cells of respiratory epithelium, not spindled cells.

Rhinitis, Suppurative

High numbers of neutrophils with or without bacteria (*see* Fig. 9-17).

Rhinitis, Granulomatous

High numbers of macrophages, some multinucleate. Rule out fungal infection with special stains.

Lymphosarcoma

A monomorphic population of lymphoblasts with multiple malignant features.

Carcinoma

Clusters of epithelial cells with multiple features of malignancy (*see* Fig. 9-14).

Feline Liver Cytology

Hepatic Lipidosis (Fatty Liver)

This is by far the most common finding in feline liver biopsies. It is characterized by large discrete vacuoles that expand the cytoplasm of over half of the hepatocytes. Some fat is seen in almost every liver aspirate, so

it is important not to overinterpret the sample just because there is some intercellular lipid.

Bile Stasis

This is also common in sick cats. It is characterized by green-black pigment that is within the cytoplasm and occasionally filling the bile canaliculi, causing bile plugs to form between some hepatocytes (*see* Fig. 9-15).

Lymphosarcoma

This neoplasm is often associated with anorexia and is therefore accompanied by hepatic lipidosis and bile stasis in many cases. It features moderate numbers of large lymphocytes, particularly lymphoblasts with multiple malignant features (*see* Fig. 9-15).

Hepatitis, Acute or Suppurative

Suppurative hepatitis can be challenging cytologically. It is characterized by degenerate hepatocytes with neutrophils associated directly with the hepatocytes. Cytologic signs of hepatocyte degeneration include cell swelling, disruption of the cell membranes, and fragmenting of the nuclei.

Hepatitis, Lymphoplasmacytic

Peripheral blood is expected with liver aspirates, but reactive lymphocytes, and especially plasma cells that are associate with the hepatocytes clumps, are supportive of chronic hepatitis.

Hepatitis, Granulomatous

As with skin and lymph nodes, granulomatous inflammation is generally secondary to fungal or bacterial and special stains should be performed to rule out organisms.

Carcinoma

Clusters of epithelial cells with multiple features of malignancy.

Suggested Readings

Cowell RL. 2008. *Diagnostic Cytology and Hematology of the Dog and Cat.* Philadelphia: Mosby.

Cullen JM. 2009. Summary of the World Small Animal Veterinary Association Standardization Committee Guide to Classification of Liver Disease in Dogs and Cats. In JM Cullen, ed. *Vet Clin North Am Small Anim Pract.* 39(3):395–418.

Dean R, Adams V, Whitbread T, et al. 2006. Study of Feline Injection Site Sarcomas. *Vet Rec.* 159(19):641–42.

Dempsey SM, Ewing PJ. 2011. A Review of the Pathophysiology, Classification, and Analysis of Canine and Feline Cavitary effusions. *J Am Anim Hosp Assoc.* 47(1):1–11.

Latimer SK, Mahaffey EA, Prasse KW, et al. 2003. Cytology. In JR Duncan, KW Prasse, eds., *Duncan & Prasse's Veterinary Laboratory Medicine: Clinical Pathology*, pp. 304–30. Ames: Iowa State Press.

Rothuizen J. 2006. *WSAVA Standards for Clinical and Histological Diagnosis of Canine and Feline Liver Disease.* World Small Animal Veterinary Association. Liver Standardization Group. Philadelphia: WB Saunders.

Tyler RD, Cowell RL. 1989. Evaluation of Pleural and Peritoneal Effusions. *Vet Clin North Am Small Anim Pract.* 19(4):743–68.

Withrow SJ, Vail DM. 2007. *Withrow and MacEwen's Small Animal Clinical Oncology.* Philadelphia: Saunders Elsevier.

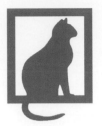

In-Office Methodology and Quality Assurance Assessment

Craig M. Tockman

Introduction

As a veterinary technician or veterinary nurse you will likely use in-house or point-of-care laboratory equipment designed to measure blood chemistry, hematology, blood gases, and some combination of these tests and others. Laboratory evaluation of the patient is a critical component of not only diagnosing illness but also assessing patient health at the routine visit.

Benefits of In-House Testing

Technology now provides the ability to perform a large percentage of tests in the veterinary hospital. Today's analyzers are accurate, precise, and extremely competitive in cost to run and maintain. There are many advantages to performing these tests in the veterinary office. This is known as point-of-care testing, and the immediate results provide information that allows the doctor to rapidly determine the health status of the patient. The doctor can discuss the results with the pet owner during the visit, allowing for a better understanding of the results, as well as creating time savings for both the doctor and the pet owner. If additional tests are indicated from the results those tests can be performed immediately, again providing better medical care for the patient and cost and time savings for both the practice and the owner. Monitoring of the patient is improved, especially when hospitalized. Critical care patients benefit greatly from immediate results. Preanesthetic tests can be performed the same day providing real-time information that is far more valuable than older information. This is only a partial list of the benefits of in-house testing.

Need for Quality Control

Part of operating these analyzers, however, requires that they be maintained properly and that their accuracy and precision be checked or verified on a regular basis, if not on every patient. This is true for all analyzers including those far more expensive ones used in veterinary university reference laboratories and commercial labs. In addition, it is best when running blood analyzers that knowledge of the operating principles of the equipment be understood. In that way, problems that occur are understood, and quality of patient care is maintained.

This chapter will not attempt to provide details on any particular product or equipment. The goal is to understand the important concepts required to obtain the optimal, accurate, and precise laboratory results for patients.

Quality Control versus Quality Assurance

On a Monday morning, a technician runs a quality control panel on the chemistry analyzer. All the results are within the appropriate ranges. As per the manufacturer's instructions, the quality control analysis is performed 30 days later and the results for three of the analytes are not within range. These tests have been performed on 90 patients between these quality control analyses. What do you know about the results from

those 90 patients? When did the analyzer start producing inaccurate results, or is it really even producing inaccurate results now? What should you tell the owners of those cats?

The same scenario can occur with a hematology analyzer or any other analyzer. In addition to performing quality control as recommended by the manufacturer, it is important to have a true quality assessment program in the practice to ensure accurate and precise results. This does not have to be difficult or extensive, and it should not make one fearful of using in-office point-of-care analyzers. For optimum use, understand how analyzers work, what they can and cannot do to ensure quality results, and what to look for in results. Therefore, some definitions important to the process need to be understood.

Analyte

Analyte is the chemical being evaluated. Examples are blood urea nitrogen (BUN), creatinine, and glucose.

Quality Control

This term usually refers to the use of solutions with a known value to be used in the analyzer. The analyzer should produce a result within a certain range provided with the solution. Two examples are the BUN on the chemistry analyzer should fall between 10 and 15 mg/dl, and a white blood cell (WBC) count on the hematology analyzer should be between 6,000 and 6,500 $10^3/mm^3$.

Quality Assurance

This term usually refers to the entire process of monitoring the accuracy and precision of results.

Accuracy

This term refers to how close the value is to the true value. Graphically, if shooting arrows at a target, you will hit the bull's eye every time. This is an accurate shot (Fig. 10-1a).

Precision

This is the repeatability of the test. If the test is repeated, the same (or similar result) will occur every time (Fig. 10-1b).

Clearly, for a truly accurate result, both good precision and good accuracy are needed so that a clinician is confident that the results are correct and repeatable.

Calibration

This provides the proper mathematical formulas to the analyzer to calculate the result from the data provided. This is usually provided in software from the manufacturer and is specific to each lot of reagents, and in the best analyzers, specific to each species. When an instrument is calibrated, it has the mathematical computations to meet the standard for which the analyzer was designed.

Nursing the Feline Patient, First Edition. Edited by Linda E. Schmeltzer and Gary D. Norsworthy.
© 2012 John Wiley & Sons, Inc. Published 2012 by John Wiley & Sons, Inc.

(a)

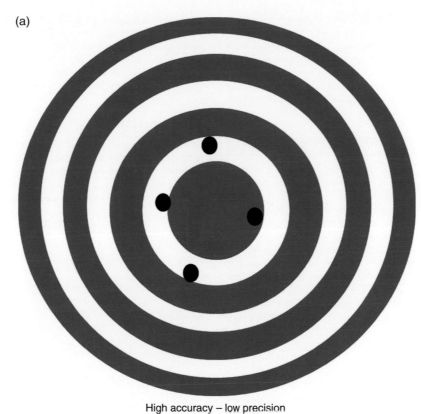

High accuracy – low precision

(b)

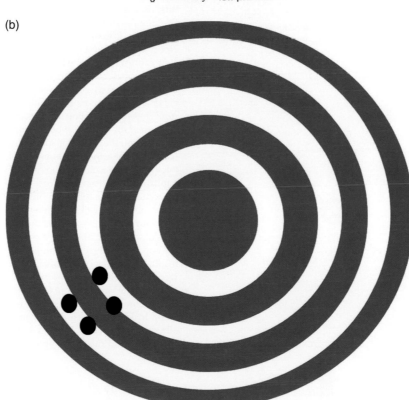

Low accuracy – high precision

Figure 10-1   (a) Accuracy refers to how close the value is to the true value. The four shots are close to the bull's eye. (b) Precision is the repeatability of the test. The four shots are clustered close to one another.

The goal in performing a quality control and a quality assurance program is to ensure that results from the analyzer are as accurate as possible for best patient evaluation. Because quality control with external materials cannot be performed prior to every analysis there must be a way to evaluate every result. This means we need to understand how the analyzer works, what information it provides on every analysis to evaluate its accuracy, what its limitations are, and how it is calibrated.

Quality Assessment with a Chemistry Analyzer

Chemistry analysis performed in private veterinary practice is most commonly performed using a spectrophotometer, an instrument that reads changes in color. Most of these analyzers use either liquid reagents or dry slides. In either case, the analyte in question is part of a chemical reaction that causes a color change to occur in the solution or on the slide. The instrument then measures either the change in the intensity of the color at a certain time point (called end point reaction) or the rate of change of the color (called rate reaction).

Color change is used to obtain a result using Beer's Law. In the simplest terms it means that the change in color of the reaction is proportional to the concentration of the analyte in questions (Fig. 10-2).

Many things can affect the results of a chemistry reaction. The major ones will be addressed.

Environment

Chemistry reactions should take place at an appropriate temperature. For most tests, the temperature should be close to the body temperature of the patient. Therefore, it is most desirable if the analyzer has a controlled temperature that allows the reactions to occur near body temperature. If not it should at least be placed where the ambient temperature is fairly consistent and close to body temperature. Keep analyzers away from vents and windows.

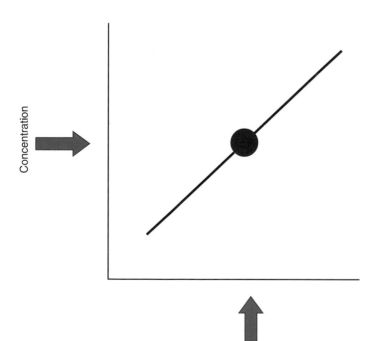

Figure 10-2 Color change is used to obtain a result using Beer's Law. In the simplest terms it means that the change in color of the reaction is proportional to the concentration of the analyte in questions.

In addition, the air in veterinary practices usually contains hair and other debris. However, hair and dust can get into instruments or contaminate samples and affect the reaction or the absorbance. Instruments that run in a closed environment will minimize this effect. This is even a bigger problem for hematology instruments because they count particles. It is critical that hematology instruments be kept clean.

Poor Sample Handling

Sample handling should be one of the most important areas of concern, whether performing the testing in the office or sending it to a reference or commercial lab. It is also a factor that can be directly controlled. How the sample is drawn, how it is placed in the tubes, and how it is handled after it is placed in the tubes can all affect the results.

Important Tips

Some important tips regarding sample handling and the effects include:

- Difficult blood draws with a struggling patient can cause hemolysis or rupture of the red blood cells (RBCs). This will be discussed in detail later in the chapter.
- Blood transfer: Transferring blood into the tubes can be a source of sample damage. Blood is a tissue or organ system and must be handled accordingly. If you are not using a one-way vacuum system (Vacutainer®) it is imperative to remove both the needle and the cap of the blood tube prior to dispensing the blood. The vacuum inside vacuum tubes is determined so it will not harm the blood; however, pushing blood back through the needle can easily cause cells to rupture. Blood contains a great deal of protein and is quite sticky. Pushing blood back through a needle is like running it over sandpaper. It is important that you prepare your tubes prior to the blood draw by removing the caps to insure good sample quality.
- Tube filling order: Some blood tubes, such as green and purple (lavender) top tubes, contain an anticoagulant to keep blood from clotting. Purple top tubes contain ethylenediaminetetraacetic acid (EDTA) either as a sodium or potassium salt. EDTA essentially prevents blood from clotting by binding all the calcium in the sample because calcium is required for clotting. If blood from this tube is used in the chemistry analysis or if the syringe is contaminated with EDTA because that tube was filled first, the results of the blood chemistries will likely have fallaciously low calcium and high potassium values. This could cause a misdiagnosis or lack of trust in the analyzer. Therefore, always fill blood tubes in the following order: red (or tiger), green, and purple.
- There are many available references to remind you of these important procedural concepts, such as the one shown in Figure 10-3.
- Fill volume: If the blood tube containing anticoagulant is not filled to the appropriate level the sample may be diluted. This will cause the results to be inaccurate because the concentration of the analytes would be affected.
- Mixing of the blood: Except for purple top tubes to be used for complete blood counts (CBC) tubes should not be placed on a rocker or shaken. Blood rockers are designed only for the CBC; hemolysis occurs when other tubes are placed on them. If whole blood is the desired sample, it should be hand-mixed by gentle inversion ten times prior to use.

Sample Integrity

Sample integrity evaluates three common interferents that cause poor results: hemolysis, lipemia, and icterus. These affect results on *all* analyzers regardless of what any manufacturer or literature states. These can cause either an increase or decrease from the real result, depending on the analyte and the interferent. Sample integrity is vitally important to obtain accurate results. Reports from laboratory instruments costing more than $100,000

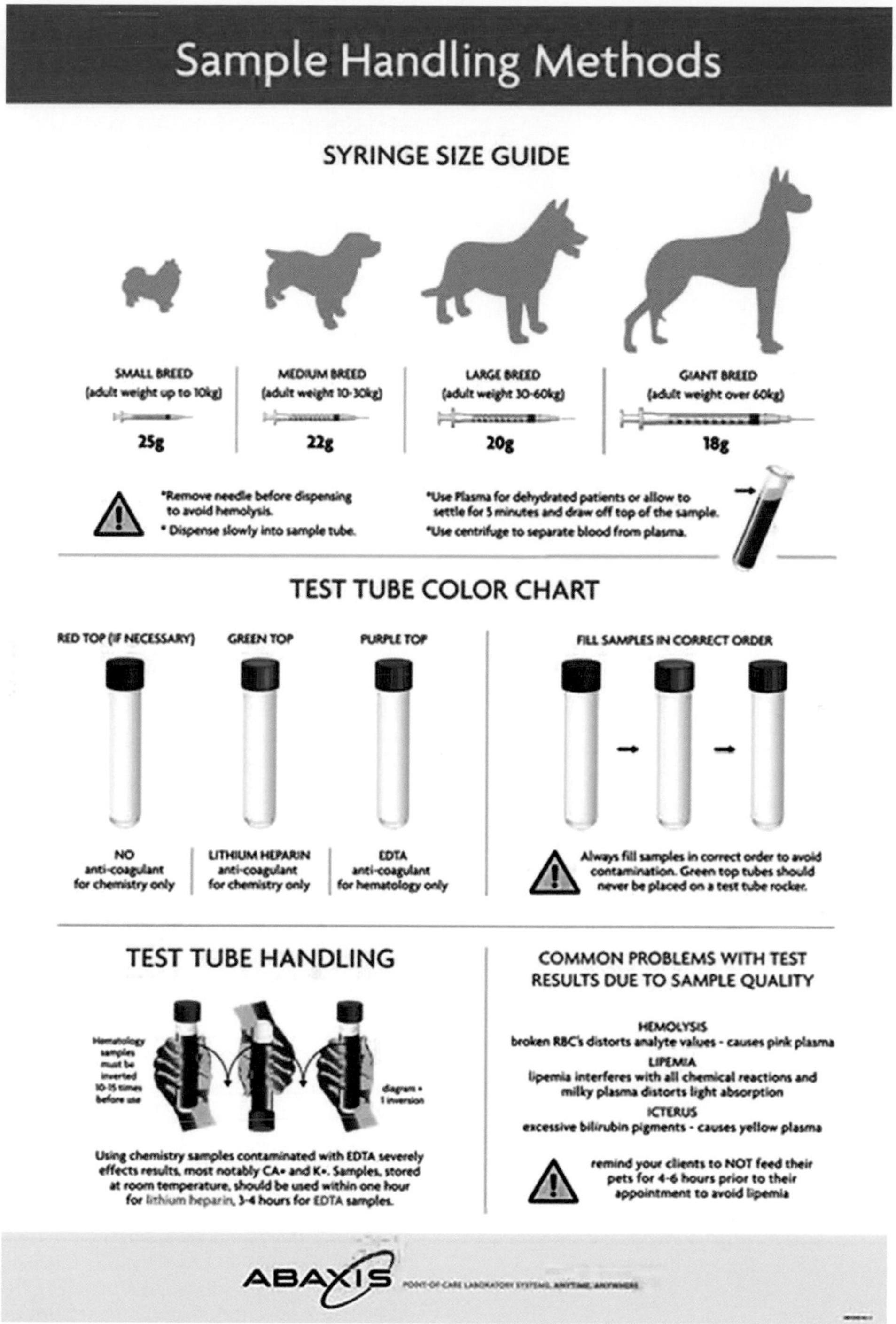

Sample Handling Methods

SYRINGE SIZE GUIDE

SMALL BREED	MEDIUM BREED	LARGE BREED	GIANT BREED
(adult weight up to 10kg)	(adult weight 10-30kg)	(adult weight 30-60kg)	(adult weight over 60kg)
25g	22g	20g	18g

⚠ *Remove needle before dispensing to avoid hemolysis.
* Dispense slowly into sample tube.

*Use Plasma for dehydrated patients or allow to settle for 5 minutes and draw off top of the sample.
*Use centrifuge to separate blood from plasma.

TEST TUBE COLOR CHART

RED TOP (IF NECESSARY)	GREEN TOP	PURPLE TOP	FILL SAMPLES IN CORRECT ORDER
NO anti-coagulant for chemistry only	LITHIUM HEPARIN anti-coagulant for chemistry only	EDTA anti-coagulant for hematology only	⚠ Always fill samples in correct order to avoid contamination. Green top tubes should never be placed on a test tube rocker.

TEST TUBE HANDLING

Hematology samples must be inverted 10-15 times before use

diagram = 1 inversion

Using chemistry samples contaminated with EDTA severely effects results, most notably CA+ and K+. Samples, stored at room temperature, should be used within one hour for lithium heparin, 3-4 hours for EDTA samples.

COMMON PROBLEMS WITH TEST RESULTS DUE TO SAMPLE QUALITY

HEMOLYSIS
broken RBC's distorts analyte values - causes pink plasma
LIPEMIA
lipemia interferes with all chemical reactions and milky plasma distorts light absorption
ICTERUS
excessive bilirubin pigments - causes yellow plasma

⚠ remind your clients to NOT feed their pets for 4-6 hours prior to their appointment to avoid lipemia

ABAXIS POINT-OF-CARE LABORATORY SYSTEMS, ANYTIME, ANYWHERE

Figure 10-3 This chart shows proper tube selection and the order in which blood is to be split between different tube types.

will clearly state the likelihood of interferents. The level of hemolysis, lipemia, and icterus is measured, and the potential effect on each analyte is reported. In some cases the results can change by 50% or more (Fig. 10-4).

Hemolysis

When a sample is hemolyzed, the RBCs have broken apart or lysed, and the hemoglobin that carries oxygen has been released from the cell. This creates a red color to the serum or plasma. Because almost all the measurements are based on a color change read by the instrument, the red color can cause significant problems. In addition, hemoglobin can interfere with the reactions themselves with high amounts.

Common effects of excessive hemolysis are:

- Addition of constituents to the sample: aspartate aminotransferase (AST), potassium (minor), and adenylate kinase (can affect creatine kinase [CK] results).
- Alteration of the following (not a complete list):
- Mild changes: alkaline phosphatase (ALP), total protein, calcium, albumin, and bilirubin.

Examples of the effects of lipemia and
hemolysis on sample integrity.

Lipemia, 1+

Lipase increased by 10–20%.

Hemolysis, +2

ALT increased up to 45%

AST increased upto 20%

LDH increased up to 50%

Total bilirubin increased up to 30%

Potassium increased by 20–25%

Direct bilirubin decreased up to 90%

Triglyceride decreased up to 10%

Figure 10-4 Mild lipemia and hemolysis can have significant effects on several values in the chemistry profile.

- Moderate changes: alanine aminotransferase (ALT) and CK.
- Marked changes: potassium and AST.

Hemolysis can occur naturally with some disease states that cause the RBCs to break apart. However, it is usually caused by poor sample handling, either because of a difficult blood draw or because the needle and cap were not removed prior to transferring blood into the tube.

Lipemia

Lipemia is caused by excessive fat in the blood, usually in the form of triglycerides (not cholesterol). When blood is centrifuged the liquid part looks like a milkshake. Pancreatitis and a few other diseases may cause lipemia; however, the most common cause of lipemia is a recent meal. This is why fasting is recommended prior to blood collection. Fortunately, this is not as common a problem with cats as with dogs. Lipemia affects all chemistry instruments and every effort should be made to reduce its level. Because lipemia is essentially fat in the blood it causes light to scatter or can completely block light from passing through the sample. It also can affect the actual chemical reaction. In addition it takes up physical volume, so for analytes such as electrolytes, it can cause a major problem. It also causes hemolysis thus complicating the integrity of the sample even further.

Commonly affected analytes (not a complete list) include:

- Bilirubin, glucose, and creatinine.
- Electrolytes measured with an isoelectric method: Dilutional >> Nondilutional.

Icterus

Icterus is caused by a yellow pigment in the blood. When it stains the tissues it is called jaundice. There are many potential causes of icterus, but the most common causes are liver disease and disease that affects bile flow in the liver or through the bile duct. It can also be caused by prolonged fasting and by disorders that cause red cells to rupture.

Because icterus changes the color of the plasma or serum it interferes in a manner similar to hemolysis, but the color is different. The most affected analytes are bilirubin and creatinine.

Application

It is important to know if these interferents are present in the sample. One chemistry analyzer (Abaxis Vetscan® and Vetscan VS2®, Abaxis Inc, Union City, CA) used for point-of-care testing measures sample integrity and reports the levels to the user. This provides either a correction of the value based on the level of the interferents or the instrument alerts the user that the result was affected. As of this writing, no other point-of-care analyzer displays this information. If the analyzer used does not measure these interferents, it is important at least to visually inspect the sample prior to the analysis. Although this cannot provide quantitative or numerical information, it can be determined that the sample may be affected and result in spurious data. If the sample appears compromised, it is best to either redraw the sample (hemolysis) or fast the patient (lipemia). A compromised sample can not be uncompromised.

The Chemistry Reaction

Sometimes chemistry reactions simply do not run correctly. There are many factors that can cause this. A quality assurance program should identify when this occurs.

First, always remember that patients are being treated, not values or chemistry results. If a value does not match the clinical picture question the validity of the results. More expensive instruments, such as those at reference or commercial laboratories, can identify when these reactions do not run properly. The laboratory automatically repeats the analysis without even indicating this was performed. Some in-house point-of-care analyzers also are capable of monitoring each chemistry reaction. It is vitally important that as part of the quality assurance program you understand if your analyzer is capable of this and to what extent.

There are two basic types of chemistry reactions: rate reactions and end-point (often involving dye binding) reactions (Figs. 10-5 and 10-6).

Some analyzers can accurately monitor these reactions and others cannot at least not to any appreciable degree. It is important to understand the capabilities of the analyzer used so the frequency and the need for quality control analysis can be determined. In 1988, a congressional law was passed to regulate and standardize protocols in human laboratories. This law – the Clinical Laboratory Improvement Act of 1988 (CLIA 88) – set standards for quality control and quality assurance in human laboratories. It requires that analyzers be evaluated for their ability to perform advanced quality assurance. If the analyzer or test is deemed to have significant internal quality control checks the frequency of performing actual quality control is either greatly reduced or in some cases eliminated. For example, a human pregnancy test has waived status, meaning anyone can run it without specialized training. There are many levels of waived status, but some chemistry analyzers have been assigned this level. This means the frequency of quality control runs are required at a far less level than other analyzers because of the redundant internal quality control systems they contain.

Although this law does not apply to veterinary laboratories, equipment suppliers should do everything possible to meet those standards. It is important to ask sales representatives or technical service representatives about how the analyzer used performs these internal control checks. It is important to obtain this information prior to analyzer purchase. Some veterinary systems are used in human medicine and therefore, have this type of status; others do not. This should be a major determinant in the level of comfort with results.

Quality controls should be performed at a minimum based on the manufacturer's recommendations. Some hospitals prefer to run them more frequently, and some hospitals do not need to run them at all because of the internal quality control systems on their analyzers. The frequency depends on the clinician, but some guidelines to consider:

- Follow manufacturer's recommendations.
- Perform controls if questionable results are occurring.
- Perform controls to individual comfort level.

(a)

L-Alanine + α-Ketoglutarate ⟶ L-Glutamate + Pyruvate

LDH

Pyruvate + NADH + H⁺ ⟶ Lactate + NAD⁺

The rate of change of the absorbance at 340 nm relative to the change at 405 nm is due to the conversion of NADH to NAD⁺ and is directly proportional to the amount of ALT present in the sample.

(b)

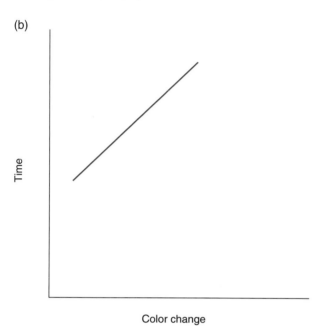

Color change

Figure 10-5 Example of a rate reaction. (a) The analyte in question catalyzes a reaction that converts NADH to NAD+. (b) This is measured over time at two different wavelengths to determine the rate of color change. The difference between the two wavelengths is converted to a value for the analyte.

Sometimes everything appears to run correctly, but a value is reported that does not correlate with the clinical picture. This is called a flier, and it can occur on any analyzer. Remember that chemistry is a science, and sometimes chemistry reactions do not work correctly. Always look at the patient, and be sure the results make sense. Fliers do not mean the instrument is bad, they simply occur once in a while and they need to be understood.

Calibration of Chemistry Analyzer

For blood chemistry testing, calibration is the process of setting the instrument to provide results based on factory-derived testing for each analyte. Analytes with a known value based on a gold standard used by the company are tested against the analyzer, and the appropriate mathematical models are loaded into the software. In addition, some chemistry tests are different for different species, especially those dye-binding tests discussed previously.

Some companies provide software updates on a regular schedule that includes calibration information for a defined set of upcoming lots of reagents. If the software update is not loaded, calibration data and results will be inaccurate. The instrument may not even run the analysis if the lot on site does not match the software. For companies using this model, ask if the calibration data also includes species variability and how far in advance the lots of reagents will be valid.

(a)

$$\text{BCG + Albumin} \xrightarrow[\text{Acid pH}]{\text{Surfactants}} \text{BCG-Albumin complex}$$

Bound albumin is proportional to the concentration of albumin in the sample. This is an endpoint reaction that is measured as the difference in absorbance between 630 nm and 500 nm.

(b)

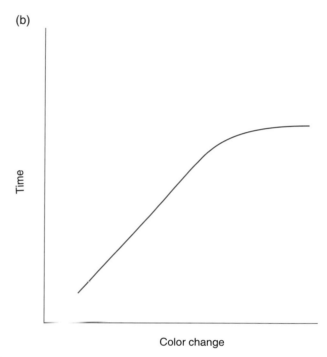

Color change

Figure 10-6 Example of an end-point reaction. (a) The analyte in question binds to a dye to form a complex, which creates a color change. (b) This is measured at the end of the reaction, when no more color change occurs.

Although most systems have barcodes on the tests to identify what they are to the analyzer, one company (Abaxis) includes calibration data for the specific lot and species differences on the barcode to remove variability in different lots as well as to provide specific calibration data for species. This is part of the CLIA 88 standards discussed previously. Many people feel this provides a higher level of quality assurance over other systems.

Sample Dilutions

Sometimes an analyzer will report a value greater than the linear range of the analyzer (i.e. BUN >130), so the actual value is not known. Some practices will dilute the sample with saline and repeat the test to get a value and then multiply the value by the dilution factor to get a result. If this is done in your practice it is important to realize that you are not receiving a completely accurate result, only a possible estimate of the value. There are two reasons for this:

1. Few practices have the precision pipetting instrumentation to do this accurately.
2. The diluent used may have an affect on the chemistry reaction causing a result change.

Using analyzers with as wide a linear range as possible can minimize the number of dilutions needed.

Quality Assessment with a Hematology Analyzer

Quality assessment with a hematology analyzer follows many of the same rules as with a chemistry analyzer. Quality controls should be run at a minimum based on the manufacturer's recommendations or to individual comfort level. There are things to consider when planning and implementing a quality assessment and assurance program in a hematology analyzer that differ from a chemistry analyzer:

1. Calibration can often be performed in the office if needed.
2. Understand methodology and limitations.
3. Identify issues through histograms or dot plots.
4. Hematology instruments run whole blood through the analyzer, so they must be able to be cleaned.

5. Live cells sometimes need human evaluation with a microscope; this can be part of the quality assessment program.

Quality Control and Calibration

Figure 10-7 is an example of a package insert from a quality control material for a hematology analyzer. Notice that there are two tables. The lower table is what should be used to run a quality control. It provides ranges that the analyzer should produce when running this sample. If the quality control run has values falling outside these ranges follow the manufacturer's instruction or contact the technical service department for the company. In most cases, either clean the analyzer (which is not difficult but also not an option on many analyzers) or perform a calibration on the instrument.

VetScan® **HM5 Control Package Insert**

3240 Whipple Road, Union City, CA 94587

FOR CALIBRATION
Normal Level Control LOT # 91042

Please use the assay table below for instrument calibration (when the default choice MCV & MPV calibration is selected).

Control Parameter	Assay	Units
RBC	4.34	M/µl
MCV	85	fl
RDWc	15.6	%
PLT	235	K/µl
MPV	11.9	fl
HGB	12.1	g/dl
WBC	8.0	K/µl
EOS	4.4	K/µl

HM5 Control Values for Quality Control

If you use these controls to perform quality control, please refer to the assay and gap values in the table below.

Parameter	Low: Lot # 91041 Assay	Gap	Normal: Lot # 91042 Assay	Gap	High: Lot # 91043 Assay	Gap	Units
Expires:	05/02/2011		05/02/2011		05/02/2011		
WBC	3.8	± 0.4	8.0	± 0.8	19.2	± 2.0	K/µl
RBC	2.39	± 0.15	4.34	± 0.2	5.03	± 0.25	M/µl
HGB	5.0	± 0.4	12.1	± 0.5	16.0	± 0.6	g/dl
HCT	15.1	± 2.0	36.9	± 2.5	48.3	± 3.0	%
MCV	63	± 4	85	± 4	96	± 4	fl
MCH	20.9	± 2.4	27.9	± 2.8	31.8	± 2.8	pg
MCHC	33.1	± 3.0	32.8	± 3.0	33.1	± 3.0	g/dl
PLT	82	± 15	235	± 30	528	± 55	K/µl
PCT	0.09	± 0.04	0.28	± 0.06	0.64	± 0.10	%
MPV	11.4	± 2.0	11.9	± 1.5	12.2	± 1.5	fl
PDW-CV	35.5	± 12.0	36.7	± 6.0	36.8	± 4.0	%
RDW-CV	18.0	± 3.0	15.6	± 3.0	14.8	± 3.0	%
LYM	1.4	± 0.5	3.2	± 0.6	10.6	± 1.5	K/µl
MON	0.2	± 0.2	0.6	± 0.6	1.4	± 1.4	K/µl
NEU	2.2	± 0.8	4.2	± 1.0	7.2	± 2.5	K/µl
EOS	2.3	± 0.3	4.4	± 0.6	6.8	± 1.2	K/µl

Figure 10-7 This is an example of a package insert from a quality control material for a hematology analyzer. The upper table is the calibration table. In this case, there are no ranges, but rather, exact values for the analyzer to measure. The lower table is what should be used to run a quality control. It provides ranges that the analyzer should produce when running this sample.

The upper table is the calibration table. In this case, there are no ranges, but rather, exact values for the analyzer to measure. These values are placed into the analyzer before the calibration is run, and the instrument is recalibrated to meet these known values.

Calibration should not need to be performed often, but if the analyzer can be calibrated in house it provides a distinct advantage for the quality assessment program.

Understanding Methodology and Limitations

Although quality controls and calibration are important to keep an analyzer functioning properly, there are several other important things that can and should be done to ensure that the quality and accuracy of every individual patient is understood. An important first step is to understand the methodology of the hematology analyzer and to remember that no hematology instrument can do everything. If an instrument requires no maintenance or that it gives all the values needed every time, you are probably being misled.

There are two main methodologies used in the veterinary point-of-care instruments.

Impedance Technology

This is sometimes known as the Coulter method and was developed many years ago for the Coulter Counter®. Current analyzers have taken this reliable technology and improved it to be accurate and precise. The cells pass through an electronic current. The size of the deflection of the current determines the size of the cell. There are two separate counts that occur with an impedance analyzer; these are shown in Figure 10-8.

There are some important points about the analysis in Figure 10-8.

1. Hemoglobin (HgB) is actually measured, whereas hematocrit (HCT) is calculated. HCT is an estimate of the packed red cell volume. This makes the HgB a more reliable indicator of anemia as well as monitoring its progression. HgB is the molecule that carries oxygen in the RBCs and is what should be truly monitored. Veterinarians have typically used the HCT value, but with the accurate hemoglobin measured by these instruments, the latter is a more reliable value. In general, three times the HgB value will equal the HCT or packed cell volume (PCV). HCT and PCV will rarely match on any analyzer because HCT is a calculation, whereas PCV is a manual measurement. However, the PCV can be inaccurate because of human error, plasma viscosity, inconsistent spin times and speeds, or other causes. It is desirable for these two values to be nearly identical (within 4%–5%), but to expect better correlation is

not realistic. Consider HgB as the primary value for evaluation of the RBC mass.

2. Mean cell hemoglobin concentration (MCHC) is determined from both the HgB and the HCT. Therefore, this is an important part of a quality assessment because it requires that both sides of the analysis have proceeded normally.
3. The mean cell volume (MCV) or mean red cell volume is measured. This is important especially in the anemic patient in determining the cause of the anemia.

Laser Flow Technology

This has also been used for many years. This technology uses a light beam to read the reflectance of each cell. In this methodology there is no lysis of cells to separate the cell types. In most cases with in-house systems a chemical is mixed with the cells to make the RBCs round instead of concave. This allows the cells to be more uniform and able to be evaluated. A stain is often used, usually one similar to new methylene blue, to help identify components within the cell and help differentiate them. Some differences in laser flow technology from impedance include:

1. Laser flow technology calculates MCV in many cases.
2. HgB is calculated as well because there is no cell lysis.
3. HCT is a calculation, as for impedance analyzers.
4. Some companies do not offer external controls for these analyzers.

Both of these technologies have positives and negatives because no system is perfect. Impedance instruments tend to be more efficient and effective in counting cells while providing good differentials. Laser flow instruments do not seem to count as well, but the differential WBC analysis seems to work better. The bottom line is that neither type of system can provide everything necessary for a complete blood analysis. Reference lab instruments often incorporate both technologies, but this is not economically feasible for most veterinary practices. Therefore, understanding the limitations and taking the next step when an analysis shows abnormalities is important to patient care.

Utilizing Histograms or Dot Plots

A complete description of how to read histograms or dot plots is beyond the scope of this chapter. However, examples of each will be presented so an understanding of their use in a quality assessment program can be developed. These graphs are pictorial representations of what the analyzer is seeing. They give the operator a patient-by-patient analysis of the accuracy of the run.

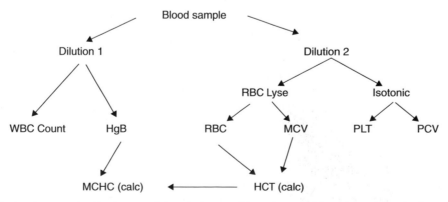

Figure 10-8 Typical procedure for impedance complete blood count analysis. In the first part of the analysis, a sample is taken and diluted and mixed with a lyse solution to remove all the red blood cells. This allows the white blood cells count to occur and the hemoglobin to be measured. Another aliquot of the sample is then diluted with a different solution to count the red blood cells and platelets as well as to determine their size. A calculation then is made to determine the mean cell hemoglobin concentration as well as the hematocrit. HCT, hematocrit; HgB, hemoglobin; MCHC, mean corpuscular hemoglobin concentration; MCV, mean corpuscular volume; PLT, platelet; PCV, packed cell volume; RBC, red blood cell; WBC, white blood cell.

The histogram, provided with impedance analyzers, is divided into an RBC/platelet, WBC, and eosinophil (if the instrument is capable of a five-part differential) graph (Figs. 10-9a,b). The WBC histogram shows how the WBCs were separated by size into lymphocytes, monocytes, and granulocytes. If it is a five-part analyzer, the eosinophil graph is also shown. The RBC/PLT graph shows where the

analyzer stops counting platelets and starts counting RBCs. Studying several of these graphs will equip you to recognize normals and abnormals.

In a similar manner, dot plots evaluate the cell populations, but this is based on reflectance rather than physical size. A typical dot plot is shown in Figure 10-10.

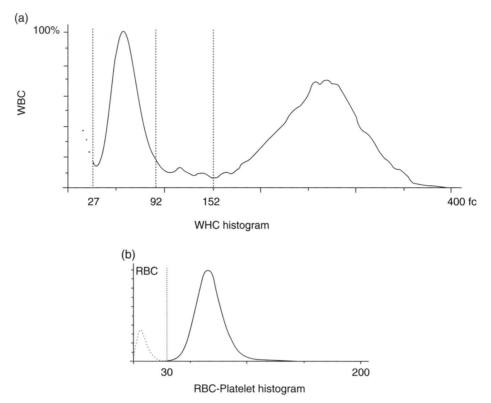

Figure 10-9 The histogram, provided with impedance analyzers, is divided into a RBC/platelet, WBC, and eosinophil (if the instrument is capable of a 5 part differential) graph. (a) The WBC histogram shows how the WBCs were separated by size into lymphocytes, monocytes, and granulocytes. If it is a five-part analyzer, the eosinophil graph is also shown. (b) The RBC/PLT graph shows where the analyzer stops counting platelets and starts counting RBCs. RBC, red blood cell; PLT, platelet; WBC, white blood cell.

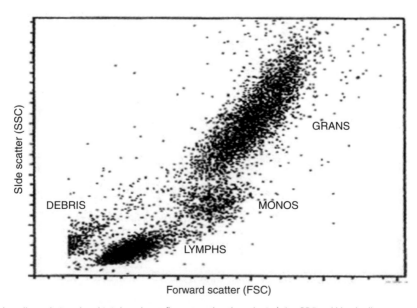

Figure 10-10 Dot plots evaluate the cell populations, but this is based on reflectance rather than physical size. RBC, red blood cell.

A company representative should provide information regarding the use of these important graphs to best assure quality in results.

Maintaining a Clean Analyzer

Blood is a living tissue. It contains live cells, proteins, electrolytes, and wastes. Cells and proteins, when placed directly into a mechanism such as a hematology analyzer, will leave residue and particles that can interfere with accurate counting. It is therefore important that the analyzer remain clean.

The analyzer should be a closed system. This means nothing internally in the analyzer is exposed to the clinic environment. This is helpful in keeping an analyzer clean, but it also means far more. Analyzers have different ways of staying clean, some better than others. Most have a detergent cycle after and analysis to remove debris. Automatic back flushing and electronic cleaning of the cell aperture also occurs on some analyzers.

No matter what an analyzer does after each run, it needs to be cleaned as per the manufacturer's instructions. If the analyzer can be cleaned on a regular basis, this will provide the best possible situation. This cleaning should only take a few minutes and will provide the best results possible. If an analyzer cannot be cleaned manually, then it should be sent into the factory on a regular basis to ensure it is clean and providing good results.

Manual Blood Smears

Performing manual blood smears in the veterinary practice intimidates many technicians and veterinarians. However, there are many benefits to performing these smears in house. Better information about a patient is obtained, and smears can be an important part of a good quality assurance program.

The process begins by preparing a good blood smear. It takes a drop of blood, two slides, and a good technique (*see* Fig. 12-1).

As part of a quality assessment protocol manual smears are important in several areas. See Chapter 12.

Evaluation of Anemia

If a CBC analysis shows the patient to be anemic, examination of the blood smear will help confirm this. RBCs are numerous and in contact with each other until the outer feathered edge is reached; this is the area of the slide to be evaluated. If the patient is anemic, a decrease in the concentration of the red cells will be noted.

Evaluation of WBC Count

Evaluation of a low or high white count is done in the same manner. Patients with elevated WBCs will have more WBCs per field than those with normal or low counts. This is another means for confirming the WBC count.

Evaluation of WBC Differential

The CBC analyzer counts thousands of cells, but confirmation of this is always prudent, especially if the WBC count is elevated or if the histogram or dot plot seems illogical. Either visually scan the slide to estimate the cell differential or count 100 cells and differentiate them. Alternatively, the slide can be sent to a clinical pathologist for confirmation.

Evaluation of Platelet Count

Platelets stick together to form a plug and stop bleeding. Platelets are activated the moment a needle is placed in the vein of a patient. Because of this, accurate platelet counts are difficult to obtain. Even analyzers in reference labs report that platelets are clumped and cannot be accurately counted. Therefore, platelet counts should be regarded as the *minimum* count, not the absolute count. The platelets are then reported as "Adequate," "Increased," or "Decreased" on these reports. This can only be determined by evaluation of the blood smear. If an analyzer reports a count that is below normal, a quick scan of the blood smear is the best method to determine if the platelet count is adequate. Adequate is defined as 6–10 platelets per high-power field.

Visual Inspection of Cell Morphology

No instrument can evaluate cell morphology. There are many morphological changes that are important in determining disease process, cause, and prognosis. See Chapter 12. There are many excellent texts and online classes as well as classes at veterinary conferences to help in this area. In addition, the use of a clinical pathologist may be needed, even when running a sample in-house.

Identification of Cellular Parasites

Many cases of anemia are caused by blood-born parasites; no analyzer can identify them.

Conclusion

Quality assessment for the point-of-care laboratory is an important part of ensuring accurate and precise values for patient care evaluation. This goes well beyond running occasional quality controls. Implementing a true quality assessment protocol, based on the strengths and weaknesses of an analyzer, is an important part of a quality practice. Quality assessment need not be difficult or time consuming and should be evaluated even if all or a majority of the blood tests are sent to a commercial lab because many of the same issues causing problems for the in-house lab cause problems at the commercial lab as well.

Suggested Readings

Latimer SK, Mahaffey EA, Prasse KW, et al. 2003. Quality Control, Test Validity, and Reference Values. In JR Duncan, KW Prasse, eds., *Duncan & Prasse's Veterinary Laboratory Medicine: Clinical Pathology*, pp. 331–42. Ames: Iowa State Press.

Schembri CT, Burd TL, Kopf-Sill AR, et al. 1995. Centrifugation and Capillarity Integrated into a Multiple Analyte Whole Blood Analyzer. *J Automat Chem.* 17(3):99–104.

Stockham SL, Scott MA. 2002. *Fundamentals of Clinical Pathology.* Ames: Blackwell Publishing.

Thrall MA, Baker DC, Campbell TW, et al. 2006. *Veterinary Hematology and Clinical Chemistry.* Ames: Blackwell Publishing.

U.S. Food and Drug Administration. 2009. *Clinical Laboratory Improvement Amendments.* http://www.fda.gov/MedicalDevices/DeviceRegulationandGuidance/IVDRegulatoryAssistance/ucm124105.htm.

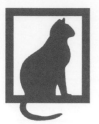

Interpretation of Common Feline Laboratory Values

Keith DeJong

Introduction

The availability of diagnostic tests for feline diseases has soared in the past two decades. Tests for diseases not discovered two decades ago are now often part of routine blood or urine panels. The purpose of this chapter is to give a brief description of how to interpret the commonly used laboratory tests.

This chapter will be organized by the test group then the individual analytes within that group. The common reasons for an increase and a decrease of each analyte will be listed.

Complete Blood Count

The complete blood count (CBC) is the cornerstone of hematologic evaluation and provides information about the presence and cause of disease, monitoring disease progression and severity, and evaluating response to treatment. The CBC can be broken down into three main parts: leukogram, erythrogram, and thrombogram.

Leukogram

Evaluation of leukocytes consists of total white blood cell (WBC) count and differentiation and enumeration of the five types of leukocytes. Leukogram analysis often does not provide a specific diagnosis but does give information about the pathologic processes that may be occurring.

Neutrophils

Neutrophils are the most common circulating leukocytes observed in health (*see* Fig. 12-12). Their primary responsibility is to migrate into tissues to sites of inflammation and participate in phagocytosis of infectious organisms and other material.

Increased neutrophil numbers, termed neutrophilia, are commonly observed and can occur due to physiologic and glucocorticoid stress and acute or chronic inflammation. Differentiating between these conditions is important because they are associated with different etiologies, severities, and prognoses and can lead veterinarians to formulate different medical and treatment decisions. Physiologic stress caused by epinephrine is often seen in young, frightened, or excited cats and can also cause lymphocytosis. Glucocorticoid stress is caused by an increase in endogenous or exogenous corticosteroids and can also cause lymphopenia, monocytosis, and eosinopenia. Acute inflammation is caused by infections and other sources of tissue inflammation and is characterized by a left shift. A left shift is the presence of immature neutrophils: bands (*see* Fig. 12-19e), metamyelocytes (*see* Fig. 12-19d), or myelocytes (*see* Fig. 12-19c). A left shift indicates that tissue demand for neutrophils currently exceeds the current productive ability of the bone marrow. Chronic inflammation, also caused by infections and tissue inflammation, is observed when bone marrow productive ability is increased and meets the body's demand for neutrophils. It takes about a week for the bone marrow to up-regulate its productive ability. Generally, chronic inflammation is not associated with the presence of a left shift, but

Lymphocytosis, monocytosis, eosinophilia, or basophilia may be observed. Stress-related and inflammatory conditions can occur simultaneously, sometimes making differentiation difficult, but the presence of a left shift always indicates acute inflammation.

Decreased neutrophil numbers, termed neutropenia, are observed with overwhelming, rapidly developing tissue inflammation, or decreased, ineffectual bone marrow production and generally carry a poorer prognosis than neutrophilia. Inflammatory neutropenia in which immature neutrophils outnumber mature neutrophils is termed a degenerative left shift and carries a poor prognosis. Neutropenia due to decreased bone marrow production can be caused by chemotherapeutic agents, chloramphenicol toxicity, other medications, or from infectious diseases such as panleukopenia, feline leukemia virus (FeLV) diseases, and toxoplasmosis.

Lymphocytes

Lymphocytes are often the second most common circulating leukocyte in cats (*see* Fig. 12-14). Their primary responsibilities are to act in adaptive immune response through the production of immunoglobulins and cytokines.

Increased lymphocyte numbers, termed lymphocytosis, are commonly observed with physiologic stress, chronic inflammation, and the leukemic phase of lymphoma, which can be associated with FeLV.

Decreased lymphocyte numbers, termed lymphopenia, are most commonly observed with glucocorticoid stress and acute inflammation, especially as a result of bacterial or viral infections. Lymphopenia is also seen with repeated drainage of chylous effusions and lymphoma.

Monocytes

Monocytes are immature cells in peripheral blood circulation that differentiate into macrophages or dendritic cells after migrating into tissues (*see* Fig. 12-15).

Increased monocyte numbers, termed monocytosis, are commonly observed with acute and chronic inflammation, tissue necrosis, and glucocorticoid stress.

Decreased monocytes numbers, termed monocytopenia, are not recognized as a clinical entity in cats.

Eosinophils

Eosinophils are leukocytes that are responsible for combating multicellular parasites and certain bacterial and fungal infections (*see* Fig. 12-13a).

Increased eosinophil numbers, termed eosinophilia, are commonly observed with allergic disorders (flea-bite dermatitis), parasitism (especially lungworms and lung flukes), and the idiopathic conditions of hypereosinophilic syndrome, eosinophilic granuloma complex, and eosinophilic enteritis.

Decreased eosinophil numbers, termed eosinopenia, can be difficult to recognize because the low end of many reference intervals are zero or close to zero. Acute inflammation and glucocorticoid stress can cause eosinopenia.

Nursing the Feline Patient, First Edition. Edited by Linda E. Schmeltzer and Gary D. Norsworthy.
© 2012 John Wiley & Sons, Inc. Published 2012 by John Wiley & Sons, Inc.

Basophils

Basophils are the least common circulating leukocytes and are thought to participate in specific kinds of inflammatory and allergic reactions (*see* Fig. 12-13b).

Increased basophil numbers, termed basophilia, are not commonly observed in cats but have been associated with parasitic disease, allergic disease, and mast cell neoplasia.

Decreased basophil numbers, termed basopenia, are not recognized as a clinical entity in cats.

The Hemogram

Hemoglobin/Red Blood Cell Count/Hematocrit (HgB/RBC/HCT)

These three analytes are often evaluated together because they essentially measure the same attribute.

An increase is termed polycythemia and is most commonly observed secondary to dehydration and can also be seen with splenic contraction as a result of physiologic stress.

A decrease is termed anemia and can be observed as the result of many etiologies. One of the most important determinations regarding anemia is characterizing it as being regenerative or nonregenerative. This differentiation leads down two different diagnostic paths.

Nonregenerative anemia is observed more frequently than regenerative anemia, and specifically, anemia of inflammatory disease (AID) is the most common cause of anemia in feline patients. Sometimes also called anemia of chronic disease (ACD), AID/ACD causes decreased RBC survival, iron sequestration, decreased erythropoietin production, and decreased bone marrow response. Other common causes of nonregenerative anemia are renal and liver disease and FeLV infection.

Regenerative anemia is characterized by the presence of increased numbers of aggregate reticulocytes and is often observed secondary to external or internal blood loss and hemolysis.

Occasionally an anemia can be termed "pre-regenerative" because it takes time for the bone marrow to respond and increase RBC production. This often occurs 3 to 4 days after the onset of blood loss or hemolysis.

Reticulocytes

Reticulocytes are immature RBCs that have been released from the bone marrow and contain small amounts of ribonucleic acid (RNA). This RNA can be identified by special staining, usually new methylene blue (NMB) stain, and is lost as the cells mature over the next 7–10 days. Aggregate reticulocytes (*see* Fig. 12-5c) have large aggregates of reticulum on NMB staining and mature into punctate reticulocytes in less than 24 hours. Punctate reticulocytes (*see* Fig. 12-5d) have few small scattered punctate specks of reticulum and become mature RBCs within several days. Aggregate reticulocytes correspond to the polychromatophils observed in peripheral blood (*see* Fig. 12-7c) and are the only cells counted for enumeration of reticulocytes.

Mean Cell Volume

Mean cell volume (MCV) is the average size of RBCs. Increases, termed macrocytosis, are most often observed secondary to moderately to markedly regenerative anemia. Decreases, termed microcytosis, can be observed with iron deficiency and portosystemic shunts.

Mean Cell Hemoglobin Concentration/Mean Cell Hemoglobin

Mean cell hemoglobin concentration (MCHC) and mean cell hemoglobin (MCH) are measurements of the concentration of hemoglobin or quantity of hemoglobin per average RBC. Increases, termed hyperchromasia or hyperchromic, are artifactual changes and occur due to lipemia,

hemolysis, or oxidative damage to RBCs (Heinz bodies, *see* Figs. 12-5b, 12-9d). Decreases, termed hypochromasia or hypochromic, are seen in iron deficiency or regenerative anemias.

Red-cell Distribution Width

Red-cell distribution width (RDW) is a calculation of the variation in RBC volumes, a mathematical measurement of anisocytosis (*see* Fig. 12-7b). Increases are most commonly observed with moderate to marked regenerative anemias as the result of the presence of increased numbers of reticulocytes. Decreases are not often observed but indicate a lack of variation in RBC volume.

Nucleated Red Blood Cell

Nucleated red blood cells (nRBC; *see* Fig. 12-7d) are immature nucleated RBC precursors. They can be observed with marked regenerative anemia, bone marrow injury or neoplasia, extramedullary hematopoiesis, or disrupted splenic function. nRBCs are counted as WBCs by all automated hematology analyzers, and corrected WBC counts derived from manual blood smear review are required for accurate WBC enumeration.

Platelet

Platelets (PLTs; *see* Figs. 12-17a,b) are small anucleate cells formed from bone marrow megakaryocytes. These cells often contain small fine pink granules and are integral participants in hemostasis.

High numbers of platelets, termed thrombocytosis, can be seen with inflammatory conditions or the result of splenic contraction secondary to physiologic epinephrine stress.

Low numbers of platelets, termed thrombocytopenia, can be observed with decreased production resulting from chemotherapy or infection, increased consumption as a result of disseminated intravascular coagulopathy (DIC), or from a variety of infections.

Mean Platelet Volume

Mean platelet volume (MPV) is the average volume of platelets; this measurement is provided by most hematology analyzers. Increases in MPV can be seen in platelet regenerative responses and platelet clumping and can also be seen in clinically normal cats.

Platelet-Crit

Platelet-crit (PCT) is analogous to hematocrit and is a measurement of the percentage of the plasma volume that is comprised of platelets. This is a relatively new value that is reported by some hematology analyzers, and its utility is still under investigation.

Platelet Distribution Width

Platelet distribution width (PDW) is a measurement of the anisocytosis of platelets. Its increase could signal the presence of a population of large or small platelets.

Clinical Chemistry

Clinical chemistries are biochemical tests that measure the concentrations or activities of various components of bodily fluids, usually blood, serum, or plasma. These tests can provide information concerning organ function, tissue damage, and acid-base, endocrine, electrolyte, and mineral status.

Total Protein

Total protein is the total combined concentration of albumin and globulins in the plasma or serum.

Increases in total protein, termed hyperproteinemia, are caused by dehydration or inflammation. Decreases in total protein, termed hypoproteinemia, are most often observed as a result of blood loss, exudation, renal disease, or secondary to liver disease.

Albumin

Albumin is a protein that is made by the liver. It is a major contributor to plasma oncotic pressure and the primary plasma carrier protein.

Increases in albumin, termed hyperalbuminemia, are only caused by dehydration because overproduction of albumin by the liver has not been documented. Decreases in albumin, termed hypoalbuminemia, are seen with decreased production as a result of liver disease, starvation, or inflammation or from an increased loss from bleeding, exudation, or renal disease.

Globulin

Globulins are a diverse group of proteins produced by the liver and B-lymphocytes. Globulins are most commonly measured as the difference of total protein minus albumin but can also be measured and quantified more specifically by plasma or serum protein electrophoresis.

Increases in globulin, termed hyperglobulinemia, are caused by dehydration and inflammation.

Decreases in globulin, termed hypoglobulinemia, are caused by loss from bleeding or decreased production from acquired immunodeficiencies secondary to FeLV or feline immunodeficiency virus (FIV) infection.

Blood Urea Nitrogen

Blood urea nitrogen (BUN), sometimes called urea, is a molecule synthesized by the liver from the ammonia produced during the metabolism of amino acids. It is one of the analytes used to measure glomerular filtration rate (GFR) of the kidneys because urea is mainly excreted by the kidneys into the urine.

Increases in BUN, termed azotemia, are caused by decreased GFR as a result of dehydration, kidney insufficiency or failure, postrenal obstruction, high protein diets, and gastrointestinal bleeding.

Decreases in BUN are not commonly observed but can be caused by liver failure or insufficiency. Low normal BUN concentrations are commonly observed in young growing animals.

Creatinine

Creatinine is a muscle breakdown product that is produced at a constant rate in the body. It is predominately filtered into the urine and excreted by the kidney. It is the arguably the best commonly used analyte to measure GFR because it is not actively secreted or resorbed by the kidney.

Increases in creatinine, also termed azotemia, are caused by decreased GFR resulting from dehydration, kidney insufficiency or failure, or postrenal obstruction.

Decreases in creatinine are not commonly observed but can be the result of decreased muscle mass secondary to starvation or cachexia. Low normal creatinine concentrations can be observed in young growing animals.

Sodium

Sodium (Na) is the major extracellular cation (positively charged electrolyte) and is the major contributor to extracellular fluid concentration and osmolality. Therefore, knowledge of patient hydration status is necessary for proper interpretation of sodium values.

Increased sodium, termed hypernatremia, is fairly uncommon in cats but can be seen with dehydration, water loss as a result of hyperventilation or fever, and administration of hypertonic saline or sodium bicarbonate.

Normal sodium, termed normonatremia, occurs in normally hydrated cats. In dehydrated cats, normonatremia occurs as a loss of free water in excess of sodium due to vomiting, diarrhea, renal disease, or osmotic diuresis (diabetes mellitus). In cats with edema, normonatremia occurs secondary to heart, liver, or kidney disease.

Decreased sodium, termed hyponatremia, can be observed as a loss of sodium from vomiting, diarrhea, or renal disease. Hyponatremia can also be seen with heart disease, hyperglycemia, and from repeated drainage of chylous effusion.

Potassium

Potassium (K) is the major intracellular cation and is the major contributor in maintaining the resting membrane potential of body cells. Only approximately 5% of the body's potassium concentration is in the blood.

Increased potassium, termed hyperkalemia, is commonly observed with urinary tract obstructions and acute renal failure. Hyperkalemia is also observed with some acid-base disturbances, repeated drainage of chylous effusions, and can be falsely increased with potassium ethylenediaminetetraacetic acid (EDTA) contamination.

Decreased potassium, termed hypokalemia, is commonly observed with anorexia, vomiting, diarrhea, chronic renal failure, and aggressive administration of intravenous fluids.

Chloride

Chloride (Cl) is the major extracellular anion (negatively charged electrolyte) and is important in acid-base maintenance. Chloride, along with sodium, is also important for osmolality, and, given this relationship, changes in chloride should always be interpreted with knowledge of sodium and patient hydration status.

Increased chloride, termed hyperchloridemia, is fairly uncommon in cats but can be seen with dehydration, water loss as a result of hyperventilation or fever, and administration of hypertonic saline. Hyperchloridemia can also be observed with metabolic acidosis resulting from loss of bicarbonate secondary to diarrhea.

Decreased chloride, termed hypochloridemia, can be observed as a result of a concurrent loss of sodium or loss of chloride from vomiting. Hypochloridemia can also be seen with ketoacidosis and lactic acidosis.

Total Carbon Dioxide

Total carbon dioxide (TCO_2), sometimes called bicarbonate or represented as HCO_3^-, is the major extracellular buffer base of body acids and, although it does not replace direct pH and blood gas measurement, it can be used as an indicator of acid-base status.

Increases in TCO_2, often termed metabolic alkalosis, occurs as a result of loss of acid from the body from vomiting or renal loss or from a gain in base from treatment with sodium bicarbonate.

Decreases in TCO_2, often termed metabolic acidosis, occur as a result of increased acid from lactic acidosis, ketoacidosis, and decreased acid secretion resulting from kidney disease, urinary tract obstruction, or increased loss of base due to diarrhea.

Calcium

Calcium (Ca) is essential for cells primarily as a signal for intracellular processes. Calcium in the plasma is present in three forms: ionized, protein bound to albumin, and complexed. The majority of body calcium is stored in the bone, absorbed from the gastrointestinal tract, and excreted by the kidneys. Calcium and phosphorus are controlled through many of the same metabolic processes, and assessment of calcium and phosphorus values should be performed concurrently. Most chemistry analyzers measure total calcium, but ionized calcium determination is also available and can be useful to further describe and diagnose calcium abnormalities.

Increased calcium, termed hypercalcemia, is caused by neoplasia, hyperparathyroidism, and rarely, from renal disease. Idiopathic hypercalcemia, hypercalcemia resulting from an unknown cause, has been reported commonly in cats and is the most common form of hypercalcemia seen clinically.

Decreased calcium, termed hypocalcemia, can be caused by low albumin, hypoparathyroidism, and chronic renal failure. Hypocalcemia has also been reported with acute pancreatitis.

Phosphorus

Phosphorus (P) is the major intracellular anion and is a component of deoxyribonucleic acid (DNA), RNA, adenosine triphosphate (ATP), and cell membranes. It is stored in the bone, absorbed from the gastrointestinal tract, and excreted by the kidneys.

Increased phosphorus, termed hyperphosphatemia, can be caused by decreased GFR resulting from dehydration, kidney insufficiency or failure, or urinary obstruction. Hyperphosphatemia also occurs secondary to hyperthyroidism and from treatment with phosphate-containing enemas.

Decreased phosphorus, termed hypophosphatemia, is most commonly observed as a result of anorexia or phosphorus-deficient diets. Hypophosphatemia has also been observed secondary to diabetes mellitus and hepatic lipidosis.

Magnesium

Magnesium (Mg) is the second most abundant intracellular cation and an important intracellular enzymatic catalyst. It is stored primarily in the bone, and only relatively small amounts are found in the blood.

Increased magnesium, termed hypermagnesemia, can be observed with decreased GFR from acute or chronic renal failure and urinary obstruction.

Decreased magnesium, termed hypomagnesemia, can be observed with hypoproteinemia, hyperthyroidism, diabetes mellitus, and diabetic ketoacidosis.

Serum Enzymes

Serum enzymes are proteins that catalyze intracellular chemical reactions. Leakage enzymes are enzymes that "leak" from cells during states of cellular stress or damage, and induced enzymes are those that have increased production during cholestasis. Knowledge of tissue specificity and plasma half-lives of these enzymes gives information of the location, extent, and time course of disease, especially with serial testing. The magnitude of serum enzyme increases can give some indication of the severity of the disease processes but cannot differentiate mild diffuse disease from marked focal disease or reversible and irreversible cellular damage. Decreases in enzyme activities are not clinically relevant, and enzymes have no physiologic purpose in the blood.

Alanine Transaminase or Alanine Aminotransferase

Alanine transaminase or alanine aminotransferase (ALT) is a cytoplasmic enzyme that is found in high concentrations within hepatocytes, lower concentrations within skeletal muscle, and has a half-life of less than 24 hours. ALT is considered a liver leakage enzyme and increases in ALT are associated with liver damage. Liver damage could be the result of hypoxia, hepatic lipidosis, diabetes mellitus, hyperthyroidism, neoplasia, infectious causes (including feline infectious peritonitis [FIP]), steroid hepatopathy, and trauma. Although ALT is also found within skeletal muscle, only mild increases in ALT are observed with marked skeletal muscle damage.

Aspartate Transaminase or Aspartate Aminotransferase

Aspartate transaminase or aspartate aminotransferase (AST) is a cytoplasmic and mitochondrial enzyme that is found in high concentrations within hepatocytes, skeletal muscle cells, and RBCs and has a half-life of less than 2 hours. AST is considered a liver leakage enzyme and increases in AST are associated with the same processes as observed with ALT. Additionally, skeletal muscle damage, and in vivo and in vitro hemolysis will also cause increases in AST.

Sorbitol Dehydrogenase and Glutamate Dehydrogenase

Sorbitol dehydrogenase (SDH) and glutamate dehydrogenase (GLDH) are cytoplasmic (both) and mitochondrial (GLDH) enzymes that are found in high concentrations primarily within hepatocytes. These enzymes have not been widely available in the United States, but their use is increasing. They are considered liver leakage enzymes, and increases are associated with liver damage. Liver damage could be the result of hypoxia, hepatic lipidosis, diabetes mellitus, hyperthyroidism, neoplasia, infectious causes (including FIP), steroid hepatopathy, and trauma.

Creatine Kinase

Creatine kinase (CK) is a cytoplasmic enzyme that is found in high concentrations within skeletal and cardiac muscle. CK is considered a muscle leakage enzyme, and increases in CK are associated with muscle damage. Muscle damage could be due to hypoxia, saddle thrombus, and trauma.

Alkaline Phosphatase

Alkaline phosphatase (ALP) is an inducible membrane-bound enzyme that is found within many tissues, but the highest concentrations are found within hepatocytes, biliary epithelial cells, and osteoblasts. Intestinal, placental, and mammary gland epithelium also contain ALP but generally do not contribute to measured plasma concentrations. Increases in ALP are specific for liver disease in cats because the half-life of ALP is less than 8 hours. Therefore, any and all increases in ALP are clinically relevant. Increases in ALP commonly occur as a result of cholestasis, hepatic lipidosis, induction by certain drugs, steroid hepatopathy, and hyperthyroidism.

γ-glutamyltransferase or γ-glutamyltranspeptidase

γ-glutamyltransferase or γ-glutamyltranspeptidase (GGT) is an inducible membrane-bound enzyme that is found in highest concentrations within biliary epithelial, renal tubular cells, and exocrine pancreatic acinar cells. Increases in GGT are caused by cholestasis, biliary hyperplasia, and induction by certain drugs. GGT generally increases before ALP in many instances of liver disease, with the exception of hepatic lipidosis.

Bile Acids

Bile acids are produced by the liver from cholesterol, stored in the gall bladder, and released into the small intestine to aid in fat digestion. The vast majority of bile acids are then absorbed into the portal circulation and recycled by the liver. Bile acid are often considered to be the most sensitive indicator of hepatic dysfunction but do not have good specificity for the determining the cause of dysfunction. Paired pre- and postprandial samples are often performed to aid in the diagnosis of portosystemic shunts. Increases in bile acids are observed with portosystemic shunts, diffuse hepatocellular disease, hepatic cholestasis as a result of hepatic lipidosis, diabetes mellitus, infectious diseases, and posthepatic cholestasis.

Bilirubin

Bilirubin is the yellow pigmented breakdown product of heme catabolism from hemoglobin. Increases in bilirubin, termed hyperbilirubinemia, are observed with hemolytic disease, hepatic and posthepatic cholestasis, fasting, and anorexia. Increased bilirubin can cause jaundice, a yellow discoloration of the skin, conjunctiva, and mucous membranes. Cats can become jaundiced before increases in ALP and GGT are observed, especially with obstructive cholestasis.

Cholesterol

Cholesterol is a steroid metabolite that is an important constituent of cell membranes and a precursor for steroid hormones and bile acids. The liver is responsible for the synthesis of the majority of circulating cholesterol, but other tissues also contribute.

Increases in cholesterol, termed hypercholesterolemia, are observed as a result of obstructive cholestasis, diabetes mellitus, nephrotic syndrome, and protein-losing enteropathy. Hypercholesterolemia commonly occurs after eating (postprandial), with a peak a few hours after eating and a return to a basal cholesterol concentration in 8–16 hours. Decreases in cholesterol, termed hypocholesterolemia, are observed with portosystemic shunting and protein-losing enteropathy.

Triglycerides

Triglycerides are lipids that are the major constituent of fat and are made by the liver, small intestine, adipose tissue, and mammary glands. Triglyceride concentration is representative of the balance of absorption by the small intestine, synthesis and export by the liver, and uptake into fat tissue. Increases in triglycerides, termed hypertriglyceridemia, are commonly observed postprandially and with acute pancreatitis and diabetes mellitus. Decreases in triglycerides, termed hypotriglyceridemia, are not a clinical entity in cats.

Amylase and Lipase

Amylase and lipase are cytoplasmic enzymes found in high concentrations within pancreatic acinar cells. Increases in amylase or lipase are often associated with pancreatitis or decreased GFR. However, because it is relatively rare to see an increase in amylase or lipase with pancreatitis, amylase and lipase evaluation is of little to no clinical utility.

Feline-Specific Pancreatic Lipase Immunoreactivity

Feline-specific pancreatic lipase immunoreactivity (fPLI) is an enzyme that is specific to feline pancreatic acinar cells. Increased concentrations are associated with leakage from the pancreas, typically from inflammation, and are associated with pancreatitis. This test has a greater sensitivity and specificity for the diagnosis of pancreatitis than any other single blood test; however, it is recommended that this test be used only as one of several criteria for diagnosing pancreatitis.

Total Thyroxine

Thyroxine is a hormone synthesized by the thyroid gland that is released into circulation and regulates basal metabolism. Total thyroxine (TT_4) is the total thyroxine concentration of the blood, composed principally of protein-bound thyroxine plus a small amount of free, unbound, biologically active thyroxine (fT_4). Increased TT_4, termed hyperthyroxemia, is produced by thyroid neoplasia and is the cause of the most common endocrine disease of cats, hyperthyroidism. Decreased TT_4, termed hypothyroxemia, is a rare clinical disease in

feline medicine and is most often observed secondary to treatment for hyperthyroidism, namely surgical removal of the thyroid gland or radioactive iodine therapy.

Urinalysis

Urinalysis, the so-called "liquid biopsy of the kidney," is a component of the minimum database and is essential for proper interpretation of CBC and blood chemistry results. The majority of in-house urinalysis is performed using commercially available urine reagent strips, refractometry, and microscopy.

Color/clarity

Evaluation of the color and clarity of the urine is the first step in urinalysis. The color (clear, yellow, straw, orange, red, brown, other) and clarity (clear, cloudy, flocculent, opaque) of urine can provide essential initial information into the clinical state of the patient.

Urine Specific Gravity

Urine specific gravity (USG) is a measure of the concentrating ability of the kidneys. It is the ratio comparing the density of urine to water and is measured by refractometry. "Normal" USG values can be highly variable, even in healthy cats, and are often dependent on the hydration status of the cat. However, the normal USG range for normally hydrated cats is generally accepted as being 1.035 or greater. Evaluation of USG values in combination with hydration status and BUN/creatinine values is vital in the proper assessment of prerenal, renal, or postrenal disorders. The inability to concentrate urine, a USG of ~1.007–1.013, is often the first sign of renal insufficiency and occurs before azotemia or other clinical signs.

pH

pH is the hydrogen ion concentration of the urine and is not an indicator of body pH. Urine pH in health is most affected by the diet, and cats, being obligate carnivores, normally produce acidic urine. Knowledge of urine pH can aid in urine crystal identification, can give insight into whether the patient can correct an acid-base abnormality, and can indicate the presence of bacteria.

Glucose

Normal urine does not contain glucose. The renal threshold for glucose in cats is around 280–300 mg/dL, and when plasma glucose concentrations exceed that level, glucose will enter the urine. Increased urine glucose, termed glycosuria, can occur due to physiologic stress, intravenous glucose therapy, and diabetes mellitus.

Protein

Normal urine has undetectable protein concentrations, although trace amounts can occasionally be observed in very concentrated urine. Increases in urine protein, termed proteinuria, can occur as a result of preglomerular, glomerular, or postglomerular causes. Preglomerular proteinuria occurs when small proteins, mainly hemoglobin and myoglobin, pass through the glomerulus during intravascular hemolysis and muscle damage, respectively. Glomerular proteinuria occurs when the glomerulus is damaged and plasma proteins (albumin and globulins) leak into the urine. Postglomerular proteinuria, the most common cause of proteinuria, occurs when inflammation of the urinary tract allows exudation of plasma proteins into the urine.

Heme

Normal urine does not contain heme proteins. Increases in heme can be the result of RBCs, hemoglobin, or myoglobin in the urine. RBCs in the urine, termed hematuria, occurs as a result of hemorrhage into the urinary tract from trauma, inflammation, or neoplasia and can also occur because of a traumatic urine collection. Hemoglobin in the urine, termed hemoglobinuria, occurs during intravascular hemolysis. Myoglobin in the urine, termed myoglobinuria, occurs as a result of muscle damage or necrosis. Differentiating the cause of a positive heme reaction often requires urine sediment and plasma evaluation because hematuria has RBCs in the sediment and hemoglobinuria is associated with hemoglobinemia. Marked amounts of heme in the urine generally yield trace to 1+ proteinuria on urine reagent strips.

Bilirubin

Normal urine does not contain bilirubin. Increase in bilirubin, termed bilirubinuria, is evidence of cholestasis.

Other Urine Reagent Test Strip Analytes

Urobilinogen, nitrite, leukocytes, and USG on urine reagent test strips are not clinically useful in veterinary medicine.

Sediment Evaluation

A properly performed sediment examination can lead to the identification and enumeration of RBCs, WBCs, epithelial cells, casts, crystals, spermatozoa, lipid droplets, infectious organisms, and neoplastic cells. Normal urine should have no to rare RBCs, WBCs, epithelial cells, and no to moderate numbers of crystals. Lipid droplets are common in feline urine. The presence of infectious organisms, increased numbers of RBCs, WBCs, epithelial cells, crystals, casts, or abnormal cells can lead to further evaluation of the urine through culture and sensitivity, imaging studies, further urine biochemical testing, or pathologist review.

Feline Leukemia Virus

Feline leukemia virus (FeLV) is a retrovirus and one of the most common feline infectious diseases. Common in-house FeLV screening tests rely on detection of the p27 viral core antigen. Negative test results in asymptomatic cats are highly accurate, but positive test results in all cats should be confirmed given the serious consequences of positive results and the possibility of false-positives. Common confirmatory testing modalities include a second p27 antigen test, ideally one that was produced by a different manufacturer than the initial test, laboratory-performed immunofluorescent antibody (IFA), or a polymerase chain reaction (PCR) test.

Feline Immunodeficiency Virus

Feline immunodeficiency virus (FIV) is also a retrovirus and is also one of the most common feline infectious diseases. Common in-house FIV screening tests rely on detection of antibodies directed against several different viral antigens. Negative test results in asymptomatic cats are highly accurate, but positive results in all cats should be confirmed given the serious consequences of positive results and the possibility of false-positives. Common confirmatory testing modalities include a second antibody test, ideally one that was produced by a different manufacturer than the initial test or send-out PCR testing. Western blotting, IFA, and virus isolation testing are also available but are not performed as frequently. FIV vaccination or circulating maternal antibodies will produce positive FIV antibody screening test results, and although there is currently no gold standard method of differentiating natural versus vaccination exposure, IDEXX now offers a PCR test with about 80% sensitivity and 100% specificity for FIV. It is accepted as a reasonably good (80% sensitivity) test for differentiating between infection and vaccine or maternal antibodies. Therefore, all kittens with positive FIV antibody screening test results should tested by PCR or retested after 6 months of age.

Heartworm Antibody and Antigen

Heartworm disease is caused by the parasite *Dirofilaria immitis*. Tests for heartworm antigen (HWAg) detect the presence of sexually mature female heartworm antigen. Tests for heartworm antibody (HWAb) detect the presence of antibodies produced against either male or female heartworms. Positive antigen tests are compatible with a diagnosis of active heartworm infection; however, given the possibility of male-only infections, immature worm-only infections, and infections with only one or two female worms, false-negatives can commonly occur. Positive antibody tests indicate that an infection has occurred, but by itself, cannot confirm the presence of active disease because antibody presence may persist about 4 months following resolution of an infection. False-negatives can occur because some larval stages may not produce a detectable antibody response. Therefore, these tests are often performed concurrently, and clinical signs and thoracic imaging analysis may also be necessary for definitive diagnosis of heartworm disease. These tests should be considered "rule in" tests but not "rule out" tests.

Feline Coronavirus

Feline infectious peritonitis (FIP) is caused by a virulent biotype of feline coronavirus (FCoV). There are currently no testing modalities that can differentiate the virulent biotype that causes FIP, the highly infectious and common enteric coronavirus (ECV), and relatively avirulent biotypes. A positive FCoV antibody test occurs as a result of infection by the ECV or as a result of infection by the FIP virus. Therefore, clinical signs and other testing are needed for further characterization. A negative FCoV antibody test suggests that it is highly unlikely to be clinical disease resulting from ECV or FIP infection; however, cats in the terminal stage of FIP will often have a negative FCoV titer.

Toxoplasmosis

Toxoplasmosis is caused by the protozoal parasite *Toxoplasma gondii*. Felids are the only known definitive host for this zoonotic parasite and can shed infectious oocysts in their feces.

A positive immunoglobulin G (IgG) or immunoglobulin M (IgM) test in any cat is an indication that the cat has been, or is currently, infected. A positive IgG test generally indicates prior infection, that oocyst shedding is unlikely, and that the cat is likely immune to reinfection, especially in healthy cats. However, a positive IgM test is more supportive of a recent or active infection as IgM antibodies are only present for about 12 weeks postinfection. Most cats with positive IgM tests are also not currently shedding oocysts. Negative IgG and IgM tests suggest that the cat is susceptible to becoming infected and shedding oocysts if infected.

Suggested Readings

Giori L, Giordano A, Giudice C, et al. 2011. Performances of Different Diagnostic Tests for Feline Infectious Peritonitis in Challenging Clinical Cases. *J Sm Anim Pract*. 52:152–57.

Levy J. 2008. 2008 American Association of Feline Practitioners' Feline Retroviral Management Guidelines. *J Fel Med Surg.* 10:300–316.

Osbourne CA, Stevens JB. 1999. *Urinalysis: A Clinical Guide to Compassionate Patient Care.* Pittsburgh: Bayer Corporation.

Paul A, ed. 2010. 2010 Feline Guidelines. American Heartworm Society. http://www.heartwormsociety.org/veterinary-resources/feline-guidelines.html.

Stockham SL, Scott MA, eds. 2010. *Fundamentals of Veterinary Clinical Pathology*, 2nd ed. Ames: Wiley-Blackwell.

Thrall MA, ed. 2004. *Veterinary Hematology and Clinical Chemistry.* Baltimore: Lippincott Williams & Wilkins.

Vollaire MR, Radecki SV, Lappin MR. 2005. Seroprevalence of *Toxoplasma gondii* Antibodies in Clinically Ill Cats in the United States. *Amer J Veter Res.* 66(5):874–77.

CHAPTER 12

Hematology

Laura V. Lane and Rick L. Cowell

Introduction

A complete blood count (CBC) and microscopic blood film review are excellent diagnostic tools for evaluation of the feline patient's erythrocytes (red blood cells [RBCs]), leukocytes (white blood cells [WBCs]), and platelets (thrombocytes). The CBC is generated either in the clinic or at an outside reference laboratory by automated hematology analyzers. Blood film review on every CBC is mandatory because it provides quality control on the hematology analyzer (to verify the values on the CBC) and provides additional information that is not detected by analyzers (immature leukocytes, toxic change, cell morphology, and parasites). This chapter will cover basic hematology techniques and provide a brief description of normal morphology of RBCs, WBCs, platelets, and their bone marrow precursor cells as well as common abnormal findings.

Hematology Techniques

Sample Collection

The CBC may be artifactually affected by lipemia (excess fat in the blood), hemolysis (ruptured RBCs), traumatic collection (platelet clumps), and stress (alterations in RBC and WBC numbers). Therefore, fasting the patient (~12 hours), minimizing stress, and proper collection technique are important. Use of the appropriately sized syringe and needle (range 20- to 25-gauge) for the vein and patient will help reduce hemolysis.

Blood from the syringe is transferred to a labeled lavender top ethylenediaminetetraacetic acid (EDTA) anticoagulant blood tube that contains a preset vacuum. The preset vacuum will allow the tube to be properly filled (two-thirds to three-quarters full); select the size of the tube to fit the sample. If multiple types of blood tubes are filled from the same syringe, the EDTA tube should be filled last to avoid the chance of accidentally transferring a small amount of EDTA to the other tubes resulting in artifactual changes to other test results. A blood film should be made soon after collection and can be made from the syringe or EDTA tube. In-clinic CBCs should be performed within 2 hours or stored in the refrigerator until analyzed. Send-out CBCs need to be stored in the refrigerator and shipped with an ice pack. Be sure to send a premade blood film along with the EDTA tube; the blood film does not need to be stained and should not be stored in the refrigerator.

Blood Film Preparation

A blood film is made soon after collection to prevent cell deterioration. The materials needed include EDTA anticoagulated blood, frosted edge glass slides, and a microhematocrit tube, wooden applicator stick, or pipette. The following steps are recommended:

- Label the frosted end of the glass slide with patient identification. Pencil is preferred for labeling because it will not fade or wash off during staining.

- Using a microhematocrit tube, wooden applicator stick, or pipette, place a drop of blood on the glass slide just in front of the frosted edge.
- Place the bottom edge of a second slide (pusher slide) in front of the drop of blood (Fig. 12-1a).
- Back the pusher slide into the drop of blood. Allow the blood to wick across the bottom edge of the pusher slide (Fig. 12-1b).
- In one smooth, quick motion move the pusher slide forward at a 45-degree angle along the length of the bottom slide without applying downward pressure (Fig. 12-1c). Increase the angle of the pusher slide to avoid running off the end of the slide with anemic (thin) samples. Decrease the angle of the pusher slide to spread out the cells for thick samples.
- Allow the slide to air dry completely for about 10 minutes (Fig. 12-1d); a hairdryer may be used to shorten the time.

Bone Marrow Aspirate Preparation

Slides from bone marrow aspirates must be made at the time of collection to avoid deterioration of the cells. Frosted edged glass slides are required; if available, a Petri dish or watch glass and pipette for picking out bone marrow particles can be used. The following steps are recommended:

- Label the frosted end of several glass slides with patient identification. Pencil is preferred for labeling because it will not fade or wash off during staining.
- Dispense one to two drops of aspirated material from the syringe in the middle of a slide. Alternatively, dispense the aspirated material into a Petri dish and use a pipette to remove a bone marrow particle (dull white spec; glistening specs are fat) from the blood and place it in the middle of a slide (Figs. 12-2a,b).
- Place a spreader slide perpendicularly on top of the slide with the aspirated material to spread the bone marrow particles without applying downward pressure (Fig. 12-2c).
- Without applying downward pressure, gently pull the slides apart (Fig. 12-2d).
- Stand slides on end to drain excess blood and allow to completely air dry.

Stains

Quick Romanowsky Type Stains

For routine staining of blood film/bone marrow aspirate slides before microscopic evaluation quick Romanowsky type stains (e.g., Diff-Quik®) are commonly used because they are fast, easy to use, and require minimal equipment (glass or plastic containers). The following steps are recommended:

- Prepare a blood film/bone marrow aspirate slide, and allow it to completely air dry.
- Dip the blood film in the fixative (usually methanol) 10–15 times (according to the manufacturer's instructions), remove the slide, and blot the end on a paper towel (Fig. 12-3a).
- Repeat step 2 with the eosinophilic (orange) stain.

Nursing the Feline Patient, First Edition. Edited by Linda E. Schmeltzer and Gary D. Norsworthy.
© 2012 John Wiley & Sons, Inc. Published 2012 by John Wiley & Sons, Inc.

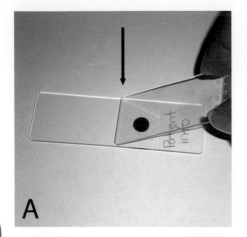
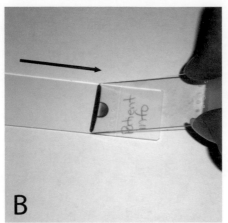
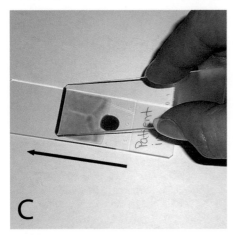
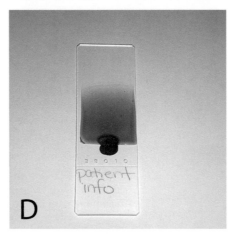

Figure 12-1 Blood film preparation. (a) After a drop of EDTA anticoagulated blood is placed on a labeled glass slide a second pusher slide is placed in front of the drop of blood. (b) The pusher slide is backed into the drop of blood and the blood is allowed to wick across the bottom edge of the pusher slide. (c) In one smooth, quick motion the pusher slide is moved forward at a 45-degree angle along the length of the bottom slide without applying downward pressure. (d) Allow the slide to air dry completely before staining. EDTA, ethylenediaminetetraacetic acid.

Courtesy of Dr. L. V. Lane.

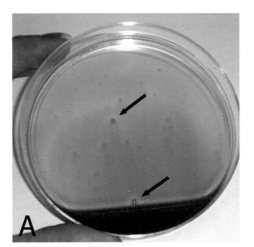
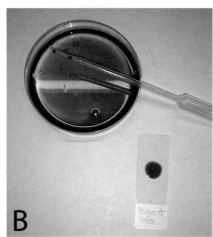
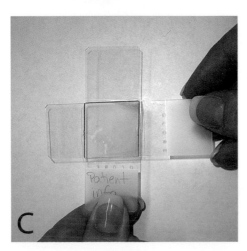
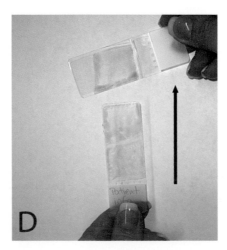

Figure 12-2 Bone marrow aspirate preparation. (a) Aspirated bone marrow material is dispensed into a Petri dish. Bone marrow particles (spicules) are seen as dull white specs *(arrows)*. (b) Using a pipette the spicules are harvested and placed in the middle of a labeled glass slide. (c) A spreader slide is placed perpendicularly on top of the slide with the aspirated material to spread the bone marrow particles. Avoid applying downward pressure. (d) Slides are gently pulled apart without applying downward pressure.

Courtesy of Dr. L. V. Lane.

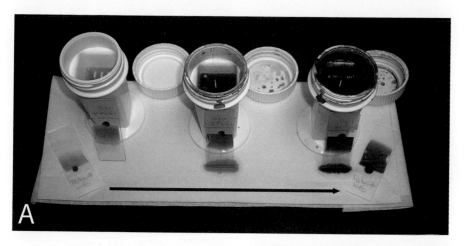

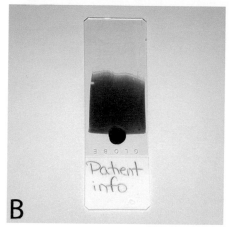 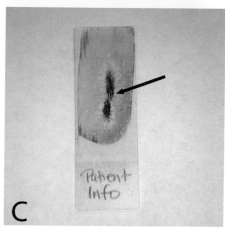

Figure 12-3 Quick Romanowsky type stains. (a) Moving from left to right a prepared blood film is dipped sequentially in the fixative, eosinophilic stain, and basophilic stain. Slides are blotted between stains and rinsed after the last stain. (b) A stained blood film. (c) A stained bone marrow aspirate preparation. The bone marrow particles are seen as the blue material in the center of the slide *(arrow)*.

Courtesy of Dr. L. V. Lane.

- Repeat step 2 with the basophilic (blue) stain, then gently rinse the slide with tap water.
- Place the slide upright to drain the water, and allow it to air dry (Figs. 12-3b,c).

Artifacts

Several common artifacts of improper staining should be recognized and remedied before interpretation is made on the blood film.

- Note that basophil and mast cell granules may not stain well and polychromasia may not be distinctive.
- Pale and unstained nuclei indicate inadequate staining time or aged stain (Fig. 12-4a). To correct, increase the number of dips in each solution or replace the stains.
- Uneven staining is often the result of water pooling on the surface of the slide after staining and rinsing. Always place the slide upright to dry.
- Excessive pink staining is a result of too many dips in the eosinophilic stain or not enough dips in the basophilic stain. Adjust the number of dips.
- Excessive blue staining results from prolonged time in the basophilic stain or a thick blood film. Adjust the number of dips or make a thinner blood film.
- Stain precipitate (not to be confused with infectious organisms) is an indication to change aged stains.
- Water artifact is a result of incomplete drying of blood films or moisture in the fixative (Fig. 12-4b). To avoid, completely dry blood films, change stains as recommended by the manufacturer, and recap stain containers when not in use.

- Staining may reveal WBC aging artifacts that are most often noted as distinct holes in the cytoplasm and nucleus of neutrophils (Fig. 12-4c).
- In addition, rare ruptured, unidentifiable cells are seen on most blood films (Fig. 12-4d).

New Methylene Blue Stain (NMBS)

Required material consists of a small glass or plastic test/culture tube, a pipette, and frosted edge glass slides (Fig. 12-5a). This stain is used to identify Heinz bodies (RBC inclusions; Fig. 12-5b) and reticulocytes (immature RBCs; Figs. 12-5c,d). The following steps are recommended:

- Label a test/culture tube with patient identification. Mix one to two drops of EDTA anticoagulated blood with equal parts of NMBS.
- Allow the mixture to sit for a minimum of 15 minutes.
- Remix the blood/stain mixture, make a blood film, allow it to air dry, and examine it microscopically. No additional staining is needed. If reticulocytes or Heinz bodies are pale and difficult to distinguish allow the blood/stain mixture to sit for additional time.

Two types of reticulocytes are reported in cats. Aggregate reticulocytes have clumps of blue/black dots (Fig. 12-5c). Punctate reticulocytes contain a few separate small blue/black dots (Fig. 12-5d). One thousand RBCs are counted and the number of punctate and aggregate reticulocytes are recorded; alternatively, a Miller square placed in the microscope eyepiece can be used to facilitate reticulocyte counting per manufacturer's instructions. Punctate and aggregate numbers are reported as a percentage by dividing the number of each type by 10. Some hematology analyzers will provide an automated reticulocyte count.

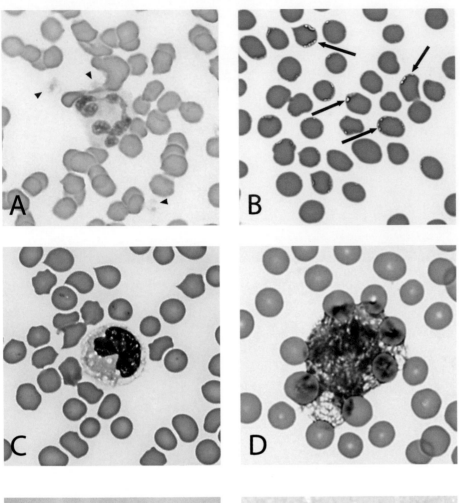

Figure 12-4 Common blood film artifacts. (a) Poorly stained blood cells. Note that all cells are pale and platelets lack visible granulation *(arrowheads)*. (b) Water artifact is seen as refractile dots on the edge of the RBCs *(arrows)*. Incompletely dried blood films or water in the stain are common causes. (c) WBC aging artifacts are noted as distinct holes in the cytoplasm and nucleus of this neutrophil. (d) Ruptured, unidentifiable cell. Aqueous Romanowsky stain (a–d) original magnification 1000x. RBCs, red blood cells; WBC, white blood cell.

Courtesy of Dr. L. V. Lane.

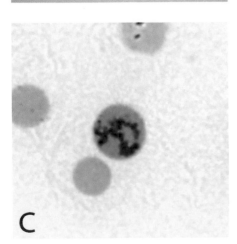

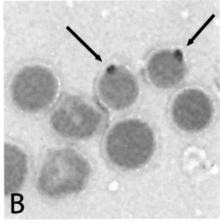

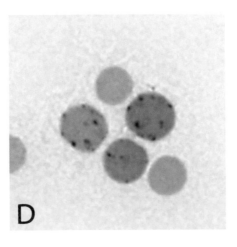

Figure 12-5 New methylene blue stain. (a) Equal parts of EDTA anticoagulated blood and NMBS are allowed to sit for a minimum of 15 minutes in a labeled test/culture tube. A blood film is made from the blood/stain mixture. (b) Heinz bodies (RBC inclusions) stain dark blue *(arrows)*. (c) Aggregate reticulocytes (immature RBCs) have clumps of blue/black dots (center cell). (d) Three punctate reticulocytes contain a few separate small blue/black dots. NMBS (b-d) original magnification 1000x. EDTA, ethylenediaminetetraacetic acid; NMBS, new methylene blue stain; RBCs, red blood cells.

Courtesy of Dr. L. V. Lane.

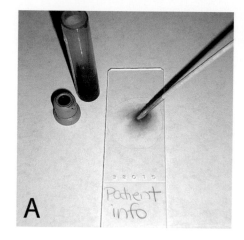

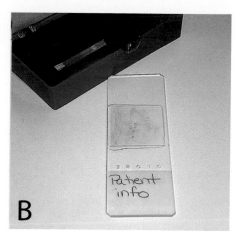

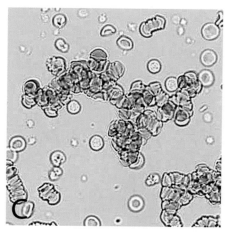

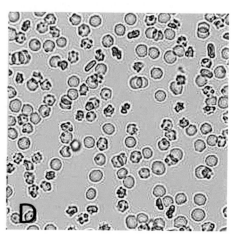

Figure 12-6 Saline dilution/dispersion test. (a) Two to three drops of saline (0.9% NaCl) are placed in the middle of a labeled glass slide. A wooden applicator stick is dipped into the EDTA anticoagulated blood tube and swirled around in the saline. (b) A coverslip is placed over the saline/blood mixture. (c) Under microscopic examination agglutination is seen as clumping of RBCs in the saline/blood mixture. (d) If RBCs disperse and no clumping is seen in the saline/blood mixture rouleaux is confirmed. Unstained (c and d) original magnification 200x. EDTA, ethylenediaminetetraacetic acid; RBCs, red blood cells.

a and b courtesy of Dr. L. V. Lane. c and d courtesy of Dr. T.E. Rizzi, Oklahoma State University.

Saline Dilution/Dispersion Test

This test is used to differentiate agglutination (antibody interaction) of RBCs from rouleaux (charge interaction). The equipment needed includes EDTA anticoagulated blood, frosted edge glass slides, coverslips, saline (0.9% NaCl), a pipette, and a wooden applicator stick. The following steps are recommended:

- Label the frosted end of two glass slides with patient identification. On one slide place a single drop of EDTA anticoagulated blood in the middle (control). On the second slide place two to three drops of saline in the middle.
- Dip the wooden applicator stick into the EDTA anticoagulated blood tube and then swirl it around in the saline on the second slide (Fig. 12-6a).
- Place a coverslip over the single drop of blood and another over the saline/blood mixture (Fig. 12-6b).
- Examine both slides microscopically with the substage condenser of the microscope lowered. If clumping of RBCs is seen in both the drop of blood and the saline/blood mixture agglutination is confirmed (Fig. 12-6c). If the RBCs disperse and no clumping is seen in the saline/blood mixture rouleaux is confirmed (Fig. 12-6d).

Blood Film Evaluation

A well-made blood film is made up of a feathered edge, monolayer, and body. The feathered edge is the end of the blood film furthest from the blood drop. In the monolayer, the RBCs are shoulder to shoulder but not overlapping. The monolayer is the best place to perform a differential cell count and evaluate cell morphology. The body of the blood film is the back portion of the blood film closest to the blood drop where cells are thick and piled on top of each other. Every blood film should be approached in the same manner to avoid missing important changes. The following steps are recommended:

- Scan the entire feathered edge using the 10× or 20× objective to identify platelet clumps, large parasites, or large atypical cells.
- Find the monolayer in relation to the feathered edge using the 10× objective. If RBC density is normal, the monolayer (cells are shoulder to shoulder) begins one to two microscope fields behind the feathered edge and extends to the body of the film. If it takes more fields to reach the monolayer a decreased density is suggested supporting the presence of an anemia. Anemia is an indication to perform a NMBS to evaluate reticulocyte numbers.
- Using the 40× objective evaluate the WBC number by taking the average number of WBCs in ten fields and multiplying by 2,000 to give a "rough" estimate of WBCs/microliter. Placing a drop of oil on the slide with a coverslip over the oil may sharpen the image when using this objective.
- On the 100× oil objective estimate the platelet number by taking the average number of platelets counted in ten fields and multiplying by 20,000 to give a "rough" estimate of platelets/microliter. This equates to a minimum of ten platelets per 100× field to indicate adequate numbers (typically the low end of the reference interval).
- On the 100× oil objective perform a 100 leukocyte differential count by counting 100 consecutive WBCs and categorize them according to type (neutrophil, lymphocyte, monocyte, eosinophil, and basophil).

Start near one edge of the monolayer and move through it in a pattern to avoid counting the same cells twice. Finally evaluate the morphology of all three cells lines (RBC, WBC, and platelets).

- Report the absolute numbers/microliter of each type of WBC by multiplying the percentage of each leukocyte type by the total WBC. For example, for a patient with a WBC count of 12,500/µL and 55% neutrophils the absolute number of neutrophils is: 12,500 x 0.55 = 6,875/µL.

Review of Blood Cells

Erythrocytes

Review Figures 12-7 to 12-10. Normal feline RBCs are round biconcave discs that stain orange-red with quick stains and often do not contain a pale center (Fig. 12-7a). Although RBCs with pale centers may be found as an artifact on blood films made from stored EDTA anticoagulated blood, they may be significant when present in numbers high enough to be readily recognized in most fields of freshly made blood smears. Common changes that should be recognized and reported include:

- Anisocytosis: Variation in size between cells (Fig. 12-7b).
- Poikilocytes: Abnormally shaped cells (Fig. 12-8a); when possible, these should be further classified:

- Acanthocytes: RBCs with multiple, irregular, unevenly spaced blunt spicules; in contrast to echinocytes (Fig. 12-8b).
- Codocytes (target cell): RBCs with a central area of hemoglobin surrounded by a clear ring separating it from the hemoglobin around the edge of the cell.
- Eccentrocytes: RBCs in which the membrane has collapsed and fused pushing all the hemoglobin to one side creating a clear vacuole.
- Echinocytes: RBCs with multiple regular, uniform, evenly spaced spicules; in contrast to acanthocytes (Fig. 12-8c).
- Schistocytes: Small fragments of RBCs (Fig. 12-8d).
- Keratocytes: Blister cells or pre-keratocytes have an intact blister on the edge of the RBC (Fig. 12-9a). After rupture of the blister the RBC is known as a keratocyte (Fig. 12-9b).
- Rouleaux: RBCs that form like a stack of coins as opposed to agglutination (Fig. 12-10a); they may be observed in clinically normal cats. Confirm with a saline dilution/dispersion test (RBCs will disperse; see Fig. 12-6d).
- Agglutination: RBCs that form grape-like clusters as opposed to rouleaux (Fig. 12-10b). Confirm with a saline dilution/dispersion test (RBCs will not disperse; see Fig. 12-6c).
- Basophilic stippling: Multiple small blue dots in RBCs.
- Heinz bodies: Round to oval pale areas within the RBCs; these are difficult to identify until seen projecting from the RBC membrane

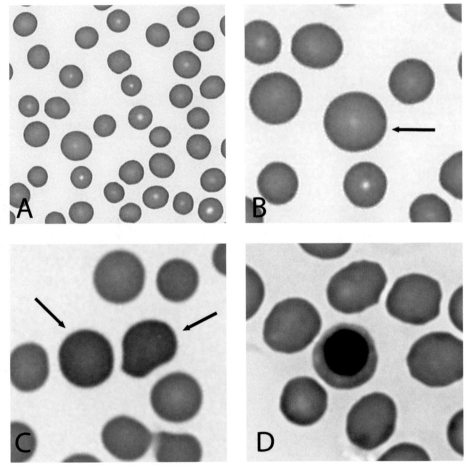

Figure 12-7 Feline erythrocytes. (a) Normal feline RBCs are round biconcave discs that stain orange-red with quick stains and often do not contain a pale center. (b) Anisocytosis or variation in size between cells is seen as a large RBC (arrow) surrounded by smaller RBCs. (c) Polychromasia is seen as a blue/gray hue in the two center cells (arrows). These are equivalent to aggregate reticulocytes on a NMBS and are used to evaluate bone marrow regeneration. (d) The nRBC or metarubricyte (center) has a circular dark nucleus with cytoplasm that is similar to the color of a mature RBC. Aqueous Romanowsky stain (a–d) original magnification 1000x. EDTA, ethylenediaminetetraacetic acid; NMBS, new methylene blue stain; nRBC, nucleated red blood cell; RBCs, red blood cells.

Courtesy of Dr. L. V. Lane.

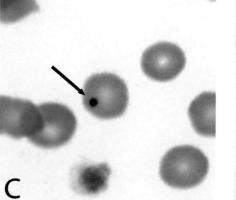

Figure 12-8 Feline erythrocytes. (a) Poikilocytes are abnormally shaped RBCs that should be further classified whenever possible. (b) Numerous acanthocytes with multiple, irregular, unevenly spaced spicules are present. (c) In contrast to acanthocytes, echinocytes *(arrows)* have multiple regular, uniform, evenly spaced spicules. (d) A schistocyte or RBC fragment (arrow) is surrounded by normal RBCs. Aqueous Romanowsky stain (a–d) original magnification 1000x. RBCs, red blood cells.

Courtesy of Dr. L. V. Lane.

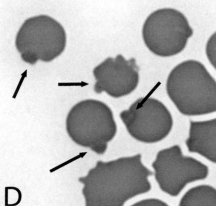

Figure 12-9 Feline erythrocytes. (a) A blister cell/prekeratocyte contains a blister on the edge of the RBC. (b) A keratocyte is a ruptured blister cell with the two ends projecting from the cell. (c) A Howell-Jolly body (retained nuclear chromatin, arrow) is seen in a RBC. (d) Heinz bodies projecting from the RBC membrane (arrows). NMBS will confirm their presence. Aqueous Romanowsky stain (a–d) original magnification 1000x. NMBS, new methylene blue stain; RBC, red blood cell.

Courtesy of Dr. L. V. Lane.

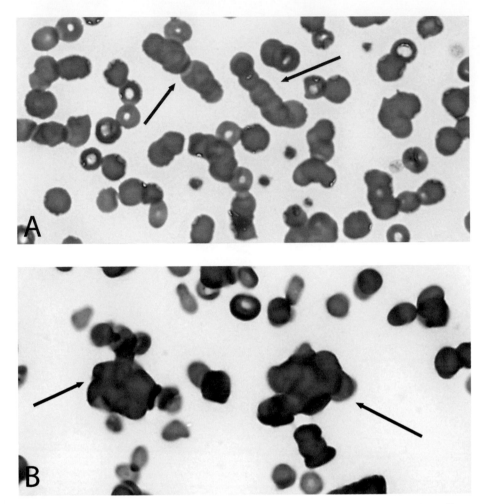

Figure 12-10 Feline erythrocytes. (a) Rouleaux is seen as a stacking of RBCs like coins (arrows). This may be seen in clinically normal cats. (b) In contrast, agglutination is seen as grape-like clusters of RBCs (arrows). A saline dilution/dispersion test is used to differentiate between the two. Aqueous Romanowsky stain (a–b) original magnification 1000x. RBCs, red blood cells.

Courtesy of Dr. L. V. Lane.

(Fig. 12-9d). Low numbers of small Heinz bodies may be seen in clinically normal cats. Confirm with a NMBS; the Heinz bodies will stain dark blue (see Fig. 12-5b).

- Howell-Jolly body: A single small dense round blue dot of nuclear chromatin in RBCs (see Fig. 12-9c). These must be differentiated from stain precipitate and infectious organisms.
- Hypochromasia: RBCs that have excessively pale centers.
- Nucleated RBC (nRBC): A RBC that has retained its nucleus (see Fig. 12-7d).
  ○ If the CBC analyzer reports total nucleated cell count (TNCC), the WBC count should be corrected for the nRBCs if they exceed 5/100 WBCs. Corrected WBC = TNCC x (100/100+nRBCs).
  ○ RBCs may be recorded separately while performing a WBC differential count and reported as number of nRBCs per 100 WBCs.
- Polychromasia: RBCs that have a blue/gray hue (see Fig. 12-7c). These cells are larger than normal RBCs and are used to evaluate bone marrow regeneration; they are equivalent to aggregate reticulocytes on a NMBS (see Fig. 12-5c). Polychromasia may be difficult to see with quick stains.

Parasites

- Cytauxzoon felis: Occasionally, large monocytes filled with hundreds of developing merozoites can be found on the feathered edge

(Fig. 12-11a). More commonly, small signet ring inclusions are seen in RBCs (Fig. 12-11b).
- *Mycoplasma hemofelis* (previously *Hemobartonella felis*): Small dot or rod-shaped blue bacteria on the surface of RBCs (Fig. 12-11c). They may be seen as ring forms and in chains. With prolonged storage in EDTA they will fall off the RBCs and may be seen in the background.

Leukocytes

Review Figures 12-12 to 12-16. There are five types of WBCs that must be categorized for a differential count on a CBC. These can be placed into two groups: the granulocytes that have a segmented nucleus and granules in their cytoplasm and the mononuclear cells that have a round nucleus and generally no granules in their cytoplasm.

- Neutrophils: These are the predominant granulocyte in health. The nucleus is blue, dense, and segmented. The cytoplasm is generally clear; occasionally pale pink granules may be seen (Figs. 12-12a-d).
- Eosinophils: These granulocytes are present in low numbers in health. They are slightly larger than neutrophils. The nucleus is blue, less dense, and less segmented than a neutrophil nucleus. The cytoplasm is filled with rod-shaped eosinophilic (orange) granules (Fig. 12-13a).
- Basophils: Only rarely are these granulocytes seen in health. They are slightly larger than neutrophils. The nucleus is blue, less dense, and less

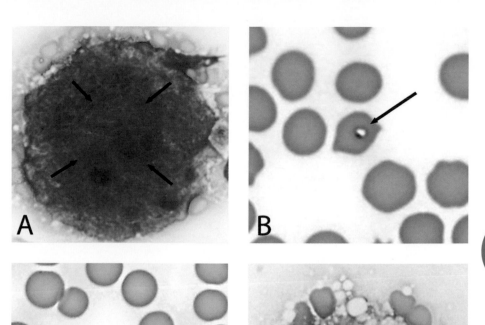

Figure 12-11 Parasites in peripheral blood. (a) *Cytauxzoon felis* schizont. A large monocyte is filled with hundreds of developing merozoites that often obscure the nucleus *(outlined by arrows)*. (b) The small signet ring inclusion in the RBC *(arrow)* is a *Cytauxzoon felis* piroplasm. (c) *Mycoplasma hemofelis* bacteria on the surface of the RBCs *(arrows)*. These may be seen in ring forms or in chains. (d) Numerous *Histoplasma capsulatum* organisms are present in a macrophage. These fungal organisms are round to oval with a crescent-shaped purple nucleus and a clear capsule. Aqueous Romanowsky stain (a–d) original magnification 1000x. RBCs, red blood cells.

Courtesy of Dr. L. V. Lane.

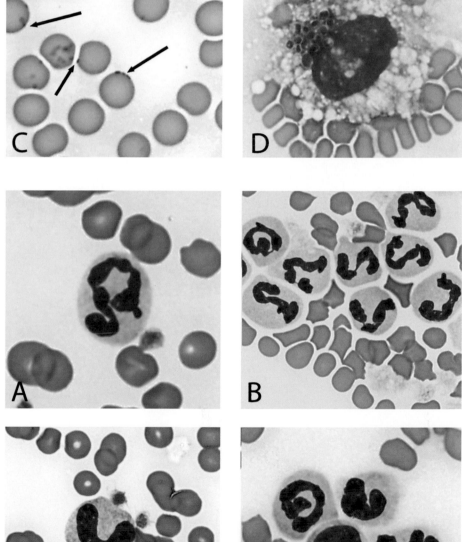

Figure 12-12 Feline leukocytes. (a) A mature segmented neutrophil. Note the blue, dense, and segmented nucleus and the clear cytoplasm. (b) Numerous segmented neutrophils. Note the variation in nuclear shape. (c) A band neutrophil has a horseshoe shaped nucleus that is not constricted and is not as dense as a mature neutrophil. The cytoplasm is lightly blue. (d) Four mature segmented neutrophils and a single band neutrophil are seen (arrow). Aqueous Romanowsky stain (a–d) original magnification 1000x.

Courtesy of Dr. L.V. Lane.

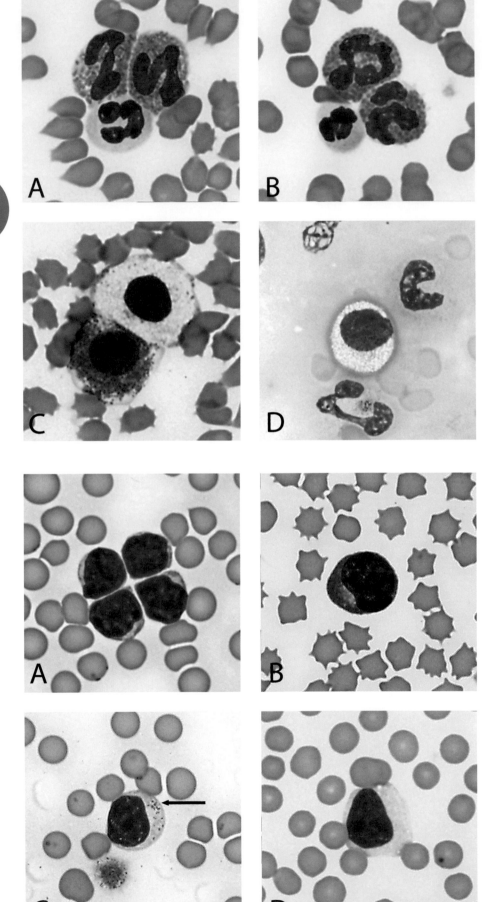

Figure 12-13 Feline leukocytes/mast cells. (a) Two eosinophils with segmented nuclei and rod-shaped eosinophilic (orange) granules in the cytoplasm are present. Note the neutrophil for comparison. (b) Two basophils with segmented nuclei and round lavender granules in the cytoplasm are seen. Note the neutrophil for comparison. (c) Two mast cells with round nuclei and abundant cytoplasm are present. The lower mast cell contains numerous purple granules, whereas the upper mast cell contains few purple granules. (d) A single mast cell with non-staining granules. Aqueous Romanowsky stain (a–d) original magnification 1000x.

Courtesy of Dr. L. V. Lane.

Figure 12-14 Feline leukocytes. (a) This field contains four small lymphocytes with round to cleaved, dense nuclei, and a thin rim of basophilic (blue) cytoplasm. (b) A reactive lymphocyte is present. It is slightly larger than a small lymphocyte with expanded and deeply basophilic cytoplasm. (c) A large granular lymphocyte is seen and is slightly larger than a small lymphocyte with expanded and clear cytoplasm that typically contains few variably sized pink granules (arrow) in the cytoplasm. (d) Large granular lymphocyte in which the granules have not stained is present. Aqueous Romanowsky stain (a–d) original magnification 1000x.

Courtesy of Dr. L. V. Lane.

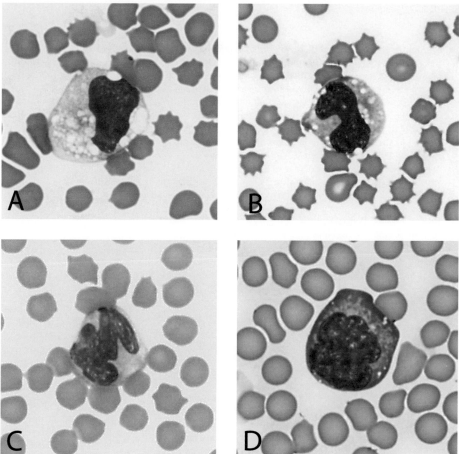

Figure 12-15 Feline leukocytes. (a–d) Monocytes are present with variable-shaped nuclei and variably abundant and vacuolated blue-gray cytoplasm. Aqueous Romanowsky stain (a–d) original magnification 1000x.

Courtesy of Dr. L. V. Lane.

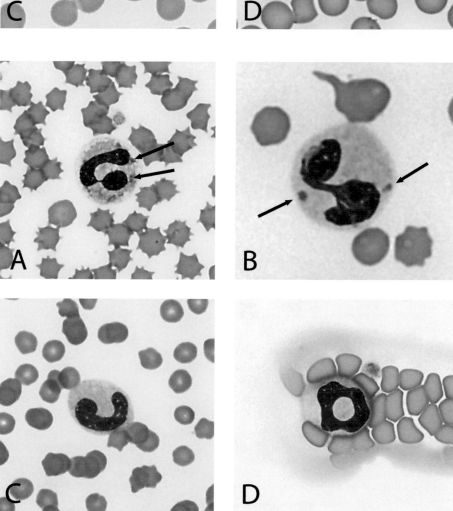

Figure 12-16 Toxic change in feline neutrophils. (a) A segmented neutrophil is seen with foamy vacuolated cytoplasm and numerous blue Döhle bodies (arrows) in the cytoplasm. (b) A segmented neutrophil is present with normal cytoplasm and two Döhle bodies (arrows). These may be seen in low numbers in clinically normal cats. (c) A band neutrophil with increased cytoplasmic basophilia (blueness) is seen. (d) A neutrophil with a ring-shaped nucleus is present. Aqueous Romanowsky stain (a-d) original magnification 1000x.

Courtesy of Dr. L. V. Lane.

segmented than a neutrophil. The cytoplasm is filled with round lavender granules (Fig. 12-13b). Eosinophils and basophils can sometimes be confused with mast cells because of the presence of granules; however, mast cells have a round nucleus and purple granules (Figs. 12-13c,d).

- Lymphocytes: These mononuclear cells are the second most abundant WBCs in health. They are slightly smaller than a neutrophil with a round to cleaved dense blue nucleus. The cytoplasm is seen as a thin blue rim (Fig. 12-14a). There are several variations of lymphocytes that may be seen. (Figs. 12-14b-d).
- Monocytes: These mononuclear cells are the largest WBC and are present in low numbers in health. The nucleus is variable in shape (round, oval, bean, and horseshoe) and is lighter and less dense than a neutrophil nucleus. The cytoplasm is abundant, blue-gray and often contains distinct vacuoles (Figs. 12-15a-d).
- Common changes that should be recognized and reported include:
  o WBC aging artifact may be the result of extended storage in EDTA. This is avoided by making a blood film soon after collection. Changes include deteriorated or shrunken pyknotic (condensed) nuclei, hypersegmentation (≥5 segments), and distinct holes in the cytoplasm (see Fig. 12-4c).
  o Toxic changes are seen in neutrophils as a result of accelerated bone marrow production. Döhle bodies are the most common mild change and may be seen in low numbers in clinically normal cats. These are small blue-green often multiple intra-cytoplasmic inclusions (Figs. 12-16a,b). Foamy cytoplasmic vacuolation (see Fig. 12-16a) and increased cytoplasmic basophilia (blueness; Fig. 12-16c) are commonly seen with moderate to severe inflammation while ring-shaped nuclei are observed only rarely and occur with severe toxic change (Fig. 12-16d).
  o Ruptured cells and bare nuclei should not be counted in the differential (see Fig. 12-4d). The differential is invalid if greater than 10% of the WBCs are ruptured.
  o A left shift refers to the presence of immature neutrophils most often consisting of band neutrophils (Fig. 12-12c,d). These are released prematurely from the bone marrow and should be counted separately from mature segmented neutrophils in the differential. See overview of the bone marrow for descriptions.
  o Neutrophils and monocytes are capable of phagocytosis (ingestion) of organisms. Although rare in peripheral blood, this may include bacteria or fungal organisms (e.g. *Histoplasma capsulatum*, see Fig. 12-11d).
  o Reactive lymphocytes: These are larger than the typical lymphocyte (slightly smaller than the size of a neutrophil) with more cytoplasm that is deeply basophilic (blue; Fig. 12-14b).
  o Large granular lymphocytes: These are larger than typical lymphocytes (slightly larger than a neutrophil) with abundant pale cytoplasm that typically contains a few variable sized pink granules in the cytoplasm (Fig. 12-14c). These granules do not always stain with quick stains (Fig. 12-14d).
  o Mast cells: These are large cells that tend to be pulled out to the feathered edge. They have large round deeply blue nuclei with variable numbers of round purple granules in the cytoplasm (Fig. 12-13c). These granules do not always stain with quick stains (Figs. 12-13c,d).
  o Leukemia/other neoplastic cells: If cells are seen that are not expected, contain nucleoli, or cannot be identified, review by a veterinary clinical pathologist is indicated.

Platelets

Platelets (Fig. 12-17) are cytoplasmic fragments of megakaryocytes that contain distinct purple granules. Feline platelets have a tendency to form clumps that can be seen on the feathered edge of a blood film (Fig. 12-17a) and are highly variable in size (Fig. 12-17b). These characteristics often cause an artifactual decrease in platelet counts from automated hematol-

ogy analyzers. Decreased platelet numbers must always be confirmed by microscopic evaluation of a blood film. If clumped/enlarged platelets are found the number generated by the analyzer should be viewed as a minimum number. Immature megakaryocytes (platelet precursors; Fig. 12-17c) and mature megakaryocytes (Fig. 12-17d) are present in the bone marrow and their numbers can be evaluated via bone marrow aspirate cytology.

Review Figures 12-17 to 12-19. Well-made bone marrow slides contain numerous particles composed of developing RBC, WBC, and platelet precursors along with fat, bone marrow stromal (supporting) cells, and minimal blood. The presence of other cells types not expected in the bone marrow is an indication for review by a veterinary clinical pathologist.

Stages of RBC (Erythroid) Maturation

- Rubriblast: The earliest identifiable stage; it is a large cell with a large round nucleus, a visible nucleolus, and moderately abundant deeply basophilic (blue) cytoplasm (Fig. 12-18a).
- Prorubricyte: This stage is similar in appearance to the rubriblast but does not contain a visible nucleolus (Fig. 12-18b).
- Rubricyte (aka nRBC): This stage is smaller; the nucleus is perfectly round and appears ropey. The cytoplasm is deeply basophilic (blue) (Fig. 12-18c).
- Metarubricyte (aka nRBC): This stage is smaller than rubricytes and may have orange or blue/gray cytoplasm. The nucleus is small and pyknotic (dense; see Figs. 12-7d, 12-18c).
- Polychromatophil: The final stage before mature RBCs. These cells do not have a nucleus, are slightly larger than mature RBCs, and have a blue-gray hue (see Figs. 12-7c, 12-18d). They are equivalent to aggregate reticulocytes on a NMBS (see Fig. 12-5c).

Stages of WBC (Myeloid) Maturation

- Myeloblast: The earliest identifiable stage; it is a large cell with a large round nucleus, a visible nucleolus and a moderate amount of basophilic (blue) cytoplasm (Fig. 12-19a).
- Promyelocyte: This stage is similar in appearance to the myeloblast but does not contain a visible nucleolus and has numerous small faint pink intra-cytoplasmic granules (Fig. 12-19b).
- Myelocyte: This stage is smaller with a round nucleus and clear cytoplasm (neutrophil; Fig. 12-19c, arrow). Orange granules (eosinophil; see Fig. 12-19a) or lavender granules (basophil) may be present.
- Metamyelocyte: similar to a myelocyte but with a bean-shaped nucleus and clear cytoplasm (neutrophil; Fig. 12-19d), orange granules (eosinophil), or lavender granules (basophil) may be present.
- Band cell: Slightly larger than a mature neutrophil with a horseshoe-shaped nucleus that is not constricted at any point and has parallel sides. The nucleus is not as dense as a mature neutrophil and the cytoplasm is lightly blue (neutrophil; see Figs. 12-12 c,d and 12-19e), with orange granules (eosinophil) or lavender granules (basophil).

Platelet Precursors

These are known as megakaryocytes and they are the largest cells in the bone marrow. As immature cells they have a round nucleus with scant deeply basophilic (blue) cytoplasm (see Fig. 12-17c). As they mature their nucleus starts to form many lobules, and the cytoplasm becomes more abundant, more purple, and appears granular (see Fig. 12-17d). The cytoplasm is sheared off in bone marrow sinusoids to form the platelets seen in peripheral blood.

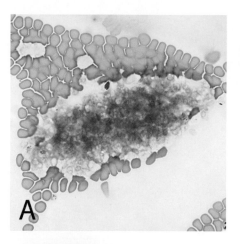

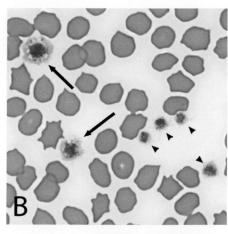

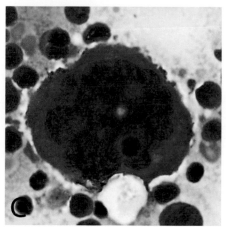

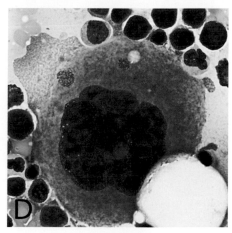

Figure 12-17 Feline platelets and megakaryocytes. (a) A platelet clump is seen on the feathered edge of a blood film. This may decrease the platelet count from automated analyzers. (b) Feline platelets are frequently seen varying in size from large (RBC size, arrows) to small (arrowheads). This may decrease the platelet count from automated analyzers. (c) An immature megakaryocyte (platelet precursor) is present in the bone marrow. Note the large size and deeply basophilic cytoplasm. (d) A mature megakaryocyte (platelet precursor) is prominent in the bone marrow. Note the large size, multi-lobulated nucleus and abundant granular purple cytoplasm. Aqueous Romanowsky stain original magnification 1000x. RBC, red blood cell.

Courtesy of Dr. L. V. Lane.

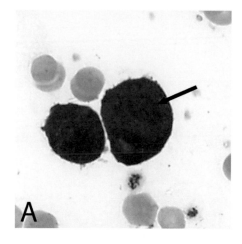

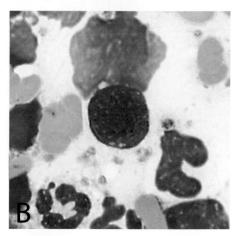

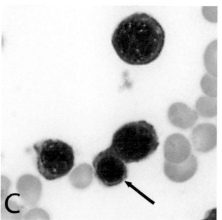

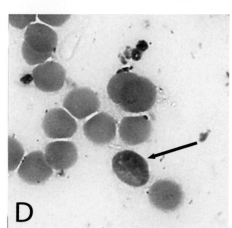

Figure 12-18 Feline bone marrow, erythroid maturation. (a) A rubriblast has a visible nucleolus (arrow). (b) Prorubricyte. (c) Three rubricytes and a metarubricyte (arrow). (d) A poly-chromatophilic cell (arrow) is surrounded by mature RBCs. Aqueous Romanowsky stain (a–d) original magnification 1000x. RBCs, red blood cells.

Courtesy of Dr. L. V. Lane.

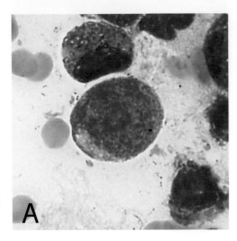
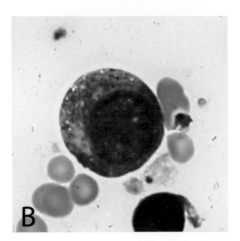
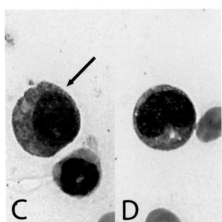
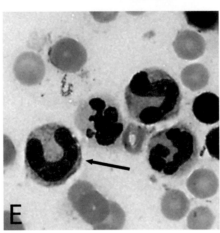

Figure 12-19 Feline bone marrow, myeloid maturation. (a) The myeloblast in the center has a visible nucleolus. A eosinophil myelocyte is located above. (b) A promyelocyte with faint-pink intracytoplasmic granulation, (c) a myelocyte with a round nucleus (arrow), and (d) a metamyelocyte with a bean-shaped nucleus are seen. (e) A band neutrophil (arrow) is noted with several segmented neutrophils. Aqueous Romanowsky stain (a–d) original magnification 1000x.

Courtesy of Dr. L. V. Lane.

Suggested Readings

Grindem CB, Tyler RD, Cowell RL. 2008. The Bone Marrow. In RL Cowell, RD Tyler, JH Meinkoth, et al., eds., *Diagnostic Cytology and Hematology of the Dog and Cat*, 3rd ed., pp. 422–50. St. Louis: Mosby Elsevier.

Reagan WJ, Irizarry Rovira AR, DeNicola DB. 2008. *Veterinary Hematology Atlas of Common Domestic and Non-Domestic Species*, 2nd ed. Ames: Wiley-Blackwell.

Thrall MA, ed. 2006. *Veterinary Hematology and Clinical Chemistry*. Ames: Blackwell Publishing.

Walker D. 2008. Peripheral Blood Smears. In RL Cowell, RD Tyler, JH Meinkoth, et al., eds., *Diagnostic Cytology and Hematology of the Dog and Cat*, 3rd ed., pp. 390–421. St. Louis: Mosby Elsevier.

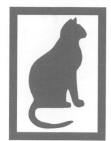

Surgery and Recovery

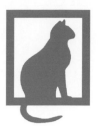

CHAPTER 13

Anesthesia: Sedation and General

Ludovic Pelligand

In a recent study on perioperative death in small animals, the risk of anesthesia- or sedation-related death was 0.24% in cats overall and 1.4% in sick cats. Although feline anesthesia appears increasingly safe, further reduction of mortality could be achieved with greater patient care and nursing during and after anesthesia.

A thorough clinical examination is necessary before sedation or general anesthesia. Even a healthy young cat subjected to "routine anesthesia" may hide subclinical congenital disease, which may become problematic during anesthesia. The proportion of the geriatric feline population is growing with the progresses of medicine; these animals may have chronic subclinical conditions.

Conditions and Drugs Affecting Anesthesia

- Respiratory: Pleural effusion, diaphragmatic hernia, and pneumothorax.
- Cardiovascular: Cardiomyopathy, systemic hypertension, hypovolemia, and distributive or septic shock.
- Renal: Chronic kidney disease, urinary obstruction, and electrolyte imbalance.
- Hepatic: Portosystemic shunt and hepatic lipidosis.
- Medications: Angiotensin-converting enzyme inhibitors, diuretics, beta blockers, and calcium channels blockers.

Further Preanesthetic Considerations

A stabilization period is beneficial to the outcome of anesthesia or sedation if a cat is presented in an unstable cardiorespiratory state. Laboratory analyses and diagnostic imaging are justified in an older or traumatized cat, particularly if the results might change the anesthesia protocol.

Some cats may not be amenable to minimal restraint for an examination so an educated guess must be made regarding their suitability for sedation or anesthesia based on their clinical history, age, and apparent symptoms. Sedation for better cooperation is usually preferred to a stressful restraint that can lead to sudden collapse.

Sedation

Sedation is required to facilitate a diagnostic procedure or placement of intravenous (IV) access. Sedation or premedication is also the first step of an anesthesia protocol that should include analgesics (opioids, alpha-2 agonists), hypnotic agents (induction agents, volatile anesthetic), and drugs that produce muscle relaxation (volatile agents, benzodiazepines and alpha-2 agonists). The choice of the most appropriate sedation protocol is influenced by the age and temperament of the patient, American Society of Anesthesiologists (ASA) status, and the degree of pain expected from the procedure.

Opioids are the cornerstone of intraoperative and postoperative analgesia. See Chapter 16. Nevertheless, opioids used alone do not generally provide good sedation in the cat. The pure mu agonists commonly used and their duration of action are: morphine (4–6 hours), methadone (4 hours), hydromorphone (4 hours), pethidine in Europe or meperidine in the United States (2 hours), and fentanyl (30 minutes). Their level of analgesia is dose related. Butorphanol (1.5 hours) is a kappa agonist and mu antagonist. It provides good sedation but only mild analgesia. Buprenorphine is a long-lasting partial mu agonist (6–8 hours) that may be included in a premedication protocol; however, its peak effect occurs 45 minutes after injection (Table 13-1).

Acepromazine in combination with opioids results in moderate to good sedation, which is often enough for catheter placement in calm conditions (*see* Table 13-1). This combination is frequently used as premedication prior to surgery. The action of acepromazine lasts 8 hours. This vasodilator should not be used in cats in shock because it may exacerbate hypotension.

An efficient and reversible immobilization is obtained with alpha-2 adrenoreceptor agonists alone or in combination with opioids (*see* Table 13-1). Nevertheless, they cause peripheral vasoconstriction and reflex bradycardia leading to reduction of cardiac output. Except in rare exceptions, they should only be administered to healthy cats that have a normal cardiac function.

Ketamine and midazolam are commonly combined in the same syringe to provide a profound sedation (*see* Table 13-1). This combination is preferred to the use of alpha-2 agonists when the cardiovascular function cannot be assessed prior to sedation. Recoveries are occasionally stormy with this protocol. A quiet, dark environment is essential for recovery after this protocol.

Insulin syringes or 1-cc syringes should be used for accurate volume measurement of medetomidine and acepromazine. The use of a diluted stock solution in saline (1:10 v:v) is also acceptable. Patients should be monitored following administration of sedation. Water bowls must be removed from the kennel. Sufficient time should be allowed for the drugs to reach their peak effect (5 minutes for medetomidine, at least 30 minutes for acepromazine).

General Anesthesia Procedure

Intravenous Access

Placement of a peripheral catheter is strongly recommended for general anesthesia. The cephalic vein or saphenous veins are usually catheterized with a 22-gauge catheter after clipping and preparation of the area. Initial skin perforation with the bevel of a needle prevents catheter tip damage when catheters are placed in male cats with thick skin. A T-connector filled with heparinized saline (1 unit per ml) is attached on the Luer-lock of the catheter and taped in place. Good handling by an experienced person and adequate chemical restraint make catheter placement easier and efficient. If IV access is required for more than 48 hours, placement of a central venous catheter under general anesthesia should be considered.

Placement of a temporary intraosseous catheter (spinal needle) in young kittens or dehydrated cats is another option. The best sites for their placement include the trochanteric fossa of the femur and the flat medial aspect of the proximal tibia.

Nursing the Feline Patient, First Edition. Edited by Linda E. Schmeltzer and Gary D. Norsworthy.
© 2012 John Wiley & Sons, Inc. Published 2012 by John Wiley & Sons, Inc.

TABLE 13-1: Combinations for sedation and premedication in the cat

Drug License Route		Dose	Butorphanol (Veterinary license) SC, IM	Buprenorphine (Veterinary license) SC, IM, IV	Pethidine (Veterinary license) SC, IM	Morphine or methadone IM, IV	Hydromorphone IM or IV	Comments
		Opioids alone	0.4 mg/kg	20 µg/kg	4–6 mg/kg	0.1–0.3 mg/kg	0.05–0.15 mg/kg	Possible hyperesthesia, increased sensitivity to stimulus and mydriasis
Ketamine IM (mg/kg) and midazolam IM (mg/kg)	Alone	3–10 + 0.2–0.3						Usually profound sedation
	with		0.2–0.4 mg/kg	10–20 µg/kg	3–5 mg/kg	0.1–0.2 mg/kg	0.05–0.15 mg/kg	Profound sedation, reduce dose if intravenous. Ideal to secure intravenous access on fractious cats
Acepromazine SC, IM (mg/kg)	Alone	0.025–0.05						Moderate sedation
	with	0.01–0.03	0.2–0.4 mg/kg	10–0 µg/kg	3–5 mg/kg	0.1–0.2 mg/kg	0.05–0.15 mg/kg	Moderate to good sedation. Reduce dose in elderly or in cardiovascularly unstable cats
Alpha₂-agonist Medetomidine IM (µg/kg)	Alone	20–40						Profound sedation
Normal cardiovascular function	with	10–20	0.2–0.4 mg/kg	10–20 µg/kg		0.1–0.2 mg/kg	0.1 mg/kg	Profound sedation; cat might be recumbent. Appropriate for diagnostic imaging and non painful procedures. Reversible
Dexmedetomidine IM (µg/kg)	Alone	10–20						Profound sedation
Normal cardiovascular function	with	5–10	0.2–0.4 mg/kg	10–20 µg/kg		0.1–0.2 mg/kg		Profound sedation; cat might be recumbent. Appropriate for diagnostic imaging and non painful procedures. Reversible
			Reduce dose if given IV		Pethidine *never* intravenous	Avoid intravenous (histamine release)		

IM, intramuscularly; IV, intravenously; SC, subcutaneously.

TABLE 13-2: Use of intravenous induction agents in the cat

	Veterinary license	Dose* depends on depth of sedation seen after premedication	Cardiovascular or respiratory depression	Analgesia	Accumulation	Recovery	Cost	Recommendation
Propofol	Yes	6–8 mg/kg (if mild sedation) 2–4 mg/kg (if deep sedation)	Marked	None	Yes if repeated or prolonged infusion	Good	Moderate	Low risk
Thiopental	No	10–12 mg/kg (if mild sedation) 5–10 mg/kg (if deep sedation)	Marked	None	Yes especially if young or liver disease	Good	Cheap	Low risk
Tiletamine and zolazepam	Depends on country	4–5 mg/kg (if mild sedation) 1–2 mg/kg (if deep sedation)	Mild, dose dependent	Some	Yes if kidney failure	Stormy	Moderate	Stable cat Avoid if cardiac
Ketamine with benzodiazepine	Yes for ketamine	5 mg/kg (if mild sedation) 1–3 mg/kg (if deep sedation)	Mild, dose dependent	Some	Yes if repeated administration	Stormy	Cheap	Moderate risk Avoid if cardiac
Etomidate	No	1–2 mg/kg (if mild sedation) 0.5–1.0 mg/kg (if deep sedation)	Almost none	None	None	Good	Expensive	High-risk cat
Fentanyl with benzodiazepine	No	Fentanyl: 5–10 mcg/kg Benzo.: 0.2–0.3 mg/kg	None for CV but severe for respiratory	Good	None	Good	Expensive	High-risk cat

* Slow IV injection to effect, as animal's requirement may be lower than the proposed dose. The proposed doses are reduced with deep sedation in comparison to mild sedation.
CV, cardiovascular.

Anesthesia Induction Agents

Healthy Cats

Propofol

This anesthetic agent is classically formulated in a white lipid emulsion. Open vials should be discarded within 24 hours because of the risk of bacterial contamination in the absence of preservative. The new "28-day" propofol contains the preservative benzyl alcohol. In the United States it is approved for dogs only. It is contraindicated in cats because benzyl alcohol is toxic to cats. The dose varies depending on animal status and premedication (Table 13-2). Propofol is given slowly to effect over 60 seconds (watch a clock). Propofol causes a marked respiratory and cardiovascular depression. Avoid repeated use of propofol in cats who are anesthetized on a daily basis due to the risk of developing Heinz body anemia and dyslipidemia.

Thiopental

Prepared as a 2.5% solution, thiopental is stable for 1 week. It should be given strictly intravenously; extravascular injection causes tissue necrosis. The induction dose depends on the effect of the premedication and the status of the cat (*see* Table 13-2). The dose should be further reduced in cats with acidosis. Half of the calculated dose is given as a bolus, and the rest is given to effect over 1 minute to reach the desired effect. Thiopental causes marked respiratory and cardiovascular depression. It also accumulates in fat, which delays recovery, especially after repeated administration.

Mask or Chamber Induction

Sevoflurane is preferred to isoflurane in this case because of the quicker uptake and the absence of the pungent smell. Initial excitement is commonly observed in early stages of the inhalant induction. Beware of pollution of the working place with such induction techniques. This induction technique may also expose the cats to high volatile anesthetic concentrations and may be dangerous for critical patients.

More Critical Patients

Ketamine + Benzodiazepine

Ketamine minimally depresses the cardiovascular system, but apnea can occur (*see* Table 13-2). Cranial nerves reflexes persist until the plane of anesthesia is deepened by other drugs. Ketamine provides good analgesia and has valuable properties for the management of chronic pain. Ketamine should be avoided in cats with cardiomyopathy or raised intraocular pressure. Similar effects but longer duration are obtained with the combination tiletamine and zolazepam.

Very Ill Cats

Etomidate given at 0.5–2 mg/kg intravenously or a combination of fentanyl (5–10 mcg/kg) and midazolam (0.2–0.3 mg/kg) can also be used in debilitated cats. The quality of induction with these protocols is poor.

Endotracheal Intubation

Endotracheal tubes should be placed in all cats undergoing general anesthesia. Laryngoscopy is advised to ensure laryngeal visualization and to limit laryngeal trauma. A short Miller laryngoscope blade should be used. Lidocaine may be applied to the arytenoids for intubation; it will also limit the risk of laryngospasm on recovery. If using a spray (not more than 2% concentration), apply only one squirt because cats are sensitive to lidocaine toxicity; allow at least 30 seconds for effect to occur. Preoxygenation is required (3–5 minutes) if a difficult intubation is anticipated to allow more time before hemoglobin saturation drops.

Cuffed endotracheal tubes are preferable (high volume, low pressure if possible). Disconnect the cat from the anesthesia machine when rolling it to its other side to avoid twisting the endotracheal tube and causing laryngeal or tracheal damage. Avoid excessive inflation of the endotracheal tube cuff, especially in dental patients. This can lead to mucosal damage or tracheal rupture. Place a pharyngeal pack to protect the airways during dental procedures.

Laryngeal mask airways can be used in some cases to deliver anesthetic agent and fresh gas. Because there is no tracheal intubation aspiration of gastric contents can occur. Positive-pressure ventilation may result in bloating.

Maintenance of General Anesthesia

The anesthesia machine and breathing apparatus should be checked at the beginning of each day (leaks, alarms, and oxygen supplies). In a normal setting, semi-open breathing systems such as the Bain, the "T-Piece," or the Mini Lack systems are used. Minute volume (MV) is calculated by multiplying the respiratory rate by the approximate tidal volume (10 ml/kg). MV is multiplied by a system coefficient (*2.5 for T-Piece or Bain and *1 for Mini Lack) to calculate the minimal flow to avoid rebreathing. Equipment dead space should be kept to the strict minimum in cats (short endotracheal tubes and connectors) to avoid rebreathing.

The drug given during premedication and induction may be enough to carry out a short procedure. In other cases maintenance of general anesthesia is achieved with repeated boluses or a continuous infusion of injectable agents (propofol). In both cases, the cat is connected to the anesthesia machine delivering at least 30% oxygen (the use of nitrous oxide will be discussed).

In most cases anesthesia is maintained with volatile anesthetic agents carried in an oxygen-rich mixture. All volatile agents cause a dose-dependent cardiovascular and respiratory depression.

The minimal alveolar concentration (MAC) of isoflurane in the cat is 1.6%. Changes in depth of anesthesia are faster than with previously used halothane because of lower solubility in blood. The respiratory depression is marked around MAC levels. Because isoflurane is a vasodilator, hypotension often occurs during anesthesia, but cardiac output will be better maintained.

The MAC of sevoflurane is 2.6%. The cardiovascular effects are similar to those of isoflurane, but sevoflurane is a lesser respiratory depressant. Because of its lower blood solubility, changes in anesthesia depth and recoveries are faster than with isoflurane.

Nitrous oxide may be used to facilitate gas uptake and possibly spare inhalant anesthetic. To reach the desired effect, it must represent at least 60% of the inhaled mixture (always keep at least 30% oxygen). Nitrous oxide is deleterious in case of gas-filed internal spaces (e.g. pneumothorax). It should be discontinued 10 minutes before disconnection from the breathing system.

The drug combination used during premedication and induction may reduce the requirement of the volatile agent of a given cat at sub-MAC levels, especially if alpha-2 agonists, ketamine, or fentanyl is used.

Maintenance of Homeostasis

Intravenous fluids should be administered for procedures exceeding 30 minutes unless contraindicated. Crystalloid solutions, such as lactated Ringer's solution or Hartmann's solution, are administered at a rate of 10 ml/kg/h during the first hour. The infusion rate can be reduced to 5 ml/kg/h thereafter if blood pressure is adequate. IV pumps or drip sets (normal or pediatric) are used. If an IV pump is not used, a burette drip set is recommended to allow precise monitoring of fluid administration and avoid overload. Protective or lubricant gel is applied to the cornea to avoid desiccation especially after ketamine administration. Because of their large surface volume ratio, cats are prone to heat loss during anesthesia. Hypothermia increases the risk of infection, delays recovery, and requires adjustment in anesthetic agents. Proactive temperature sparing strategies should be followed soon after induction because body temperature will drop initially following the use of vasodilatory agents. A heat and moisture exchanger should be attached between the endotracheal tube and the breathing system, and bubble wrap should be applied to the extremities to limit heat loss. Warm air blankets, perfusion warmers, and lavage of body cavities with warm saline contribute to warming the cat. Great caution must be exercised with electric heating blankets or gloves filled with hot water because of the concern of skin burns. However, the use of modern thermal-controlled heating blankets can be of great value.

Monitoring

The senses of an experienced anesthesia technician can be reliable for monitoring. The depth of anesthesia is assessed by looking at eye position and pupil size (from light to very deep: eye central with palpebral reflex present; ventrally rotated; back to central position with constricted pupil; central eye with dilated pupil). Serial assessment of jaw tone is useful to monitor muscle relaxation. Estimation of tidal volume can be obtained by observing chest excursions or movements of the rebreathing bag. Qualitative information on pulse may be obtained by palpating the femoral, metatarsal, or sublingual arteries. Peripheral perfusion is assessed by capillary refill time. An esophageal stethoscope permits cardiac and pulmonary auscultation.

Additional monitoring devices are useful to confirm clinical observations and to help to support vital physiological functions (Table 13-3). Their goal is to reduce the incidence of complication and accidents.

Pulse oximeters act as a pulse monitor and hemoglobin saturation monitor. The user must be aware of its technical artifacts (*see* Table 13-3). They are not sensitive for early detection of respiratory compromise when 100% oxygen is administered. Nevertheless, they will detect desaturation quickly if only 33% oxygen is administered (e.g. when nitrous oxide is used).

Capnography provides information on ventilation and gas exchange as well as cardiac output. Hypo- and hyperventilation must be addressed (*see* Table 13-3). A sudden drop of expired carbon dioxide (CO_2) with constant ventilation is a warning sign of a sudden drop in cardiac output. See Chapter 15.

A Doppler apparatus is a useful and affordable monitoring device to detect pulse and systolic blood pressure. It is a reliable noninvasive means of blood pressure monitoring in the cat. An ultrasound sensor is placed over a peripheral artery (metatarsal, palmar, or caudal). An

TABLE 13-3: Monitoring information and troubleshooting guide

Monitoring device	Reference range	Troubleshooting	Action
Pulse oxymetry (hemoglobin oxygen saturation)	More than 90%	1) Movements artefacts 2) Vasoconstriction 3) Interruption of flow 4) True hypoxemia	-> Stop movements -> Alpha-2 agonists, severe hypovolemia or hypothermia -> Move probe to another location -> Increase oxygen fraction, improve gas exchanges
Capnography (CO_2 partial pressure in expired gases and shape of the curve)	No more than 50 mm Hg	1) Increase CO_2 uptake	a) Rebreathing -> increase gas flow b) Check for faulty breathing system c) Excessive CO_2 inflation for laparoscopy?
		2) Hypoventilation	a) Assess anesthetic depth: reduce if possible b) Opioid or infusion related -> ventilate
	Not less than 30 mm Hg	1) Technical fault 2) Mixing with fresh gas 3) Hyperventilation 4) Imminent cardiac arrest	-> Check leak, obstruction, disconnection, dislodgement -> Reduce fresh gas or change breathing system -> Assess depth of anesthesia and analgesia -> Immediate cardiovascular status check
Doppler systolic blood pressure or oscillometric blood pressure monitor	No more than 160 mm Hg	1) Hypertension	a) Supply of anesthetic? (e.g. empty vaporizer) b) Lack of analgesia -> renew if due c) Check anesthesia depth -> deepen if too light d) Envisage endocrine or renal cause (clinical history)
	No less than 90 mm Hg	1) Technical fault	a) Disconnection; surgeon or instrument leaning on blood pressure device or Doppler probe b) Check cuff size and probe position
		2) Hypotension	a) Decreased venous return (bleeding, major vessel occlusion) b) Assess anesthetic depth: reduce if possible c) If bradycardia: anticholinergics d) Assess fluid status -> fluid load (crystalloids, colloids, blood) e) Use inotropes and pressors

audible signal is heard for each pulse. Contact gel is applied between the skin and the probe, which is taped in place. If hair is not shaved, alcohol then contact gel may result in sufficient contact. A cuff, with a width equal to about 40% of the limb circumference, is applied proximally to the probe. The pressure at which blood flow is heard again after cuff occlusion and gradual deflation is equal to the systolic blood pressure (*see* Table 13-3). Most oscillometric monitors tend to be less accurate at the extremes of the blood pressure range and fail to read during hypotension and vasoconstriction. Invasive arterial blood pressure monitoring via an arterial catheter placed in the dorsal metatarsal artery can be achieved in feline patients. If used it should not be left in place for postoperative monitoring, because in contrast to dogs, complications with blood supply to the paw can be seen.

Recovery

The cat should be taken to a quiet place where it can recover. Monitoring during the postanesthesia or postsedation period is paramount because many deaths happen during this phase. Brachycephalic cats should be monitored closely for airway obstruction following extubation.

Accidents and Complications

Respiratory

Most respiratory complications are detected with the use of pulse oxymetry and capnography. Respiratory obstructions are diagnosed by capnography and auscultation with a stethoscope. A mucus plug is frequently the cause of airway obstruction, especially endotracheal

tubes 3-French or less. Gentle suction or change of tube generally works in this case. Bronchoconstriction resulting from bronchospasm or anaphylactic reactions must be treated with bronchodilators (aminophylline or epinephrine respectively). Barotrauma is damage inflicted to the alveoli when excessive airway pressure is reached. The usual scenario is when the pop-off valve is accidentally left closed. Pneumothorax and cardiovascular collapse may occur if not detected immediately. Upper respiratory obstruction and pawing of the face (risking self-trauma) on recovery is frequent in the cat. Keep the neck extended, with the mouth slightly open and tongue out (if possible) until the cat is more awake.

Cardiovascular

The procedure for hypotension or hypertension is described in Table 13-3. Bradycardia may occur with large doses of opioids, hypothermia, intracranial lesions, or hyperkalemia. Hyperkalemia is frequent in cats with urinary obstruction and must be treated. See Chapter 30. The quantity of blood loss must be carefully monitored, and severe bleeding must be addressed intraoperatively. Depending on the volume lost, crystalloids, colloids, or whole blood (stored or fresh) should be used. The signs of impending arrest include: (1) weak or irregular pulse or loss of pulse signal, (2) sudden deepening of the anesthesia plane, (3) sudden drop of expired CO_2 level, or (4) grey mucous membranes or absent capillary refill time. Urgent assessment of the situation is needed. If cardiac arrest is confirmed, call for assistance, immediately discontinue anesthetic administration, give positive-pressure ventilation, antagonize cardiovascular depressants, and start cardiopulmonary resuscitation.

Miscellaneous

Excitement, dysphonia, or restlessness in recovery must be addressed. Express the bladder if necessary, and check the analgesic level. Sedation with small doses of acepromazine or medetomidine will be beneficial. Hypothermia and drug overload can lead to prolonged recoveries requiring active warming and support of elimination processes that include increasing diuresis and exhalation of volatiles. Partial or total reversal of opioids and alpha-2 agonists should be considered, but drug reversal should not result in insufficient analgesia. Marked postanesthetic hyperthermia can be seen in cats in association with the administration of hydromorphone or other opioids.

Suggested Readings

Brodbelt DC, Blissit KJ, Hammond RA, et al. 2008. The Risk of Death: The Confidential Enquiry into Perioperative Small Animal Fatalities. *Vet Anaesth Analg.* 35(5):365–73.

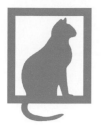

CHAPTER 14
Surgical Preparation

Eric Schmeltzer

Introduction

It was Alexander Graham Bell who said, "Before anything else, preparation is the key to success." Surgical preparation spans the time from which the patient fasts until the surgical drapes are placed and the surgeon begins. All the steps in between are crucial to a successful outcome.

Food Restriction

Restricting food prior to surgery prevents vomiting during the procedure and recovery, which can lead to aspiration pneumonia. Generally, food is withheld 8–12 hours prior to induction of anesthesia. In very young cats, restriction should be as little as 4–6 hours to prevent hypoglycemia. If the cat is admitted to the hospital on the day of surgery, question owners about anything ingested prior to surgery, including treats or snacks. It is also important to consider metabolic diseases that can affect anesthesia. One common protocol for diabetic cats is to give half of the normal dose of insulin the night before and none the morning of surgery because mild to moderate hyperglycemia is more desirable than hypoglycemia.

Patient Admission

Preparing a cat for surgery continues once it arrives at the hospital. Identification of the cat including, but not limited to, name and procedure type is critical. This information should be clearly stated on the cat's neckband, cage card, in the record, and on a surgical release form signed by the client. All of these should be double-checked for accuracy prior to proceeding. A complete physical examination including temperature, respiration rate, and pulse followed by a minimum laboratory work-up (complete blood count and serum chemistries) should always be done prior to any surgical procedure.

Preparation of Surgical Suite

All surgical supplies required for a given procedure should be gathered and in order prior to a patient's anesthetic induction. For routine surgeries, a checklist to include surgical pack, suture materials, surgical blade, surgical cap, gown, and gloves along with materials required to prepare the surgical site can be followed. For nonelective procedures it is important to consult with the surgeon for additional equipment and supplies that may be needed.

Patient Preparation

Preparation of the surgical site can be initiated prior to induction. If the patient has an accumulation of dirt, litter, or other debris in its coat, it is best to try to remove this prior to induction by combing, clipping, or bathing. This will shorten the time for surgical site preparation as well as the total length of anesthesia. Next, the placement of an intravenous (IV)

catheter can be done allowing for initiation of IV fluids and administration of IV anesthetic induction agents. Finally, the use of analgesics, as part of a complete pain management protocol, should always be addressed prior to surgery. See Chapter 16.

Preventing Hypothermia

Decline in body temperature begins as soon as an animal is placed under anesthesia. If a body cavity (thorax or abdomen) is opened and exposed to ambient temperature air, hypothermia develops more quickly. It is important to address these concerns prior to surgery with the use of a preheated circulating water blanket, surgical warming blanket (The ChillBuster® Vet Surgical Warming System), or forced air blanket (Bair Hugger®). Additional methods for limiting hypothermia include warmed towels, warmed IV fluid bags, and warm water-filled examination gloves. Electric heating pads and heat lamps are not recommended due to the possibility of thermal burns.

Preparation of Surgical Site

Numerous factors influence the ability to prevent postsurgical infections. The patient's ability to resist infection, the type and population of microorganisms present, and the interaction of the microorganisms with the host all play a role in determining postsurgical success. The size and location of the skin incision, alterations in blood supply around the incision, foreign materials (suture and surgical implants), age and physical condition of the patient along with, most importantly, the time taken for the surgical procedure all affect the likelihood of postoperative infections.

After anesthesia has been induced and surgical monitoring has begun, the patient's surgery site is clipped. This is ideally performed in a separate room from which the surgery will be performed. Procedure type, anatomical location, room for expanding the incision if necessary, and possible drain hole placements should all be considered when determining the size of area to be clipped. A number 40 clipper blade is used to first clip in the direction the hair lays, then as close to the skin as possible against the lay of the hair. Once the entire area has been clipped it is important to make sure the edges are as straight and smooth as possible. The appearance of the surgical site is often the client's first impression of their cat's surgery, so providers must take pride in making the clipped site look nice and neat. Clipped hair can be vacuumed away from the patient and an initial scrub (which will be described) can be performed prior to moving into the surgical suite.

There are a few anatomical locations that provide a challenge to surgical preparation. The clipping of hair around the paws, muzzle, and eyes can be difficult with a number 40 clipper blade alone. A disposable single blade razor can be used to remove hair in these areas if used carefully. Surgical scrub can be used to provide lubrication reducing the incidence of skin irritation in these areas. Hair from the scrotum can be plucked with fingers (widely thought to leave less irritation and a smoother surface) or removed with a number 40 clipper blade for the castration procedure.

The preparation of surgical sites involving the proximal portion of the limb also presents an added challenge. The lower extremities are frequently used as a handle by the surgeon during procedures of the upper limb, including femoral head and neck ostectomy, cranial cruciate

Nursing the Feline Patient, First Edition. Edited by Linda E. Schmeltzer and Gary D. Norsworthy.
© 2012 John Wiley & Sons, Inc. Published 2012 by John Wiley & Sons, Inc.

ligament repair, and fracture repairs. The use of a latex examination glove placed over the affected limb's distal extremity and attached with tape will keep the surgical field cleaner, and the surgeon will then be free to cover this with sterilized flexible cohesive bandage (Vetrap™ by 3M™) or aluminum foil after the final surgical scrub has been done.

There has been much discussion concerning the best antiseptic agent for surgical site preparation in feline patients. *Antisepsis* is defined as the inhibiting of the growth and multiplication of microorganisms. *Antiseptic* is defined as opposing sepsis, putrefaction, or decay, especially preventing or arresting the growth of microorganisms. It must be made clear that we are not sterilizing (destruction of all microorganisms) the skin surface when a surgical preparation is done.

One important aspect of the microorganism's interaction with the patient is the formation of a *biofilm* matrix. It was typically thought that free-moving bacteria were contributing to postoperative infections; however, new information suggests a bigger problem. The biofilm matrix is a layer of bacterial organisms and extracellular material capable of adhering to the patient's tissues, IV catheters, suture materials, and surgical implants. Although it cannot move on its own, it can be transferred to a new location on any object that touches it, such as a finger or a sterile surgical glove. It has been documented that bacteria in a biofilm matrix are 500–1500 times more resistant to antibiotics than are free-moving bacteria. Consequently, it is crucial that the veterinary staff be meticulous in every surgical site preparation.

The ideal surgical antiseptic would have specific characteristics: it would kill all forms of pathogenic (disease causing) microorganisms (bacteria, fungi, protozoa, viruses); it would not promote an allergic reaction or irritation at the skin surface; it would be nontoxic and not absorbed into the body; and it would have residual activity. There is no surgical antiseptic that has all of these characteristics, but some good choices are available. The two most commonly used antiseptic agents used in veterinary medicine are chlorhexidine gluconate and povidone-iodine. Both agents are available in a detergent (scrub) and a solution. Although not recommended for use by itself, isopropyl alcohol is often used in conjunction with the two previous agents for its ability to kill bacteria quickly and for its ability to break up fatty or oily material. There are also alcohol-based solutions containing a combination of antiseptics that improve its spectrum of activity.

Chlorhexidine gluconate is the fastest-acting antiseptic scrub with a consistent effect of more than 6 hours and residual activity for up to 2 days because of its attachment to the outer layers of the skin surface. The spectrum of activity for chlorhexidine covers gram-positive and some gram-negative bacteria, yeast, and some viruses. It also remains active in the presence of organic matter (blood or serum) and alcohol and is nonirritating to the skin surface. It is, however, ototoxic, neurotoxic, and toxic to the cornea, so it is not recommended for periocular procedures or surgeries within the ear canal. In addition, it has been proposed that chlorhexidine scrub, if ingested by the feline patient, can lead to glossitis (ulceration/inflammation of the tongue). This is prevented by thoroughly rinsing the surgical site with chlorhexidine solution, sterile saline, or alcohol.

Povidone-iodine is also a rapid-acting agent, although it is generally accepted that this antiseptic requires more than 5 minutes of contact time to be fully effective compared to about 2 minutes for chlorhexidine gluconate. It has persistent action of 4–6 hours but no residual activity. The spectrum of activity for povidone-iodine is broader than chlorhexidine, adding effectiveness against mycobacteria, more gram-negative bacteria, and bacterial spores with longer contact times. It is also the antiseptic of choice when preparing surgical sites close to the eye because of its lack of corneal toxicity. The effectiveness of povidone-iodine is diminished in the presence of organic matter and alcohol. It has also been found to be more irritating to skin.

No matter which surgical antiseptic agent is chosen, the technique used for the final sterile surgical preparation is of utmost importance. The final surgical prep is done in the surgical suite after the patient has been properly positioned for the given procedure. It is common practice to use a sterile wash bowl filled with the antiseptic agent of choice, sterile gauze squares, and sterile gloves for this procedure. Air-tight canisters filled with antiseptic soaked gauze squares and isopropyl alcohol soaked gauze squares can also be used.

The final surgical scrub is started at the incision site closest to the center of the clipped area. Use a circular motion to move from the center to the periphery of the clipped area. Once the gauze has touched the haired margin, it is discarded and must not be returned to the center of the clipped area. If using alcohol between povidone-iodine scrubs, it is important to remember that alcohol inactivates this detergent and will affect its total contact time. A recent study has shown that rinsing chlorhexidine gluconate with alcohol after the final scrub can increase the likelihood of postoperative infections. Either a dilute chlorhexidine solution or saline can be used to rinse the final scrub without decreasing its effectiveness. This type of rinse is also used for laser and electrosurgical procedures when alcohol must be avoided.

There have been several new developments in the field of surgical site preparation and prevention of postsurgical infections. New, one-step solutions (DuraPrep™ by 3M™, ChloraPrep® by CareFusion, and ACTIPREP® by Healthpoint Biotherapeutics) have been formulated to contain multiple antiseptic agents applied in a single layer. After a 2- to 3-minute drying time, the surgical site is ready and has been shown to provide equal effectiveness to older conventional techniques. Another area of interest has been the use of an antimicrobial incise drape (Ioban™ by 3M™) that is applied over the surgical site and seals off bacteria through a barrier film technique. More recently, the development of a cyanoacrylate barrier preparation (InteguSeal™ by Kimberly-Clark™) that is painted onto the surgical site and helps to lock pathogens in place has been promising.

No matter how skilled the surgeon, if the cat is not properly and thoroughly prepared for surgery the outcome may not be optimum. All of the fine details from the time of admittance to the hospital until the patient has recovered from surgery have to be undertaken precisely. Attention to detail and a thorough knowledge of the procedures required for obtaining surgical site asepsis are crucial to a successful surgery.

Suggested Readings

Cockshutt J. 2002. Principles of Surgical Asepsis. In DH Slatter, ed., *Textbook of Small Animal Surgery*, 3rd ed., pp. 149–54. Philadelphia: Elsevier Saunders.

Davidson JR, Burba DJ. 2006. Surgical Instruments and Aseptic Technique. In DM McCurnin, JM Bassert, eds., *Clinical Textbook for Veterinary Technicians*, 6th ed., pp. 701–5. St. Louis: Elsevier Saunders.

Fossum TW. 2007. Preparation of the Operative Site. In TW Fossum, ed., *Small Animal Surgery*, 3rd ed., pp. 32–37. St. Louis: Elsevier Mosby.

Osuna DJ, DeYoung DJ, Walker RL. 1990. Comparison of Three Skin Preparation Techniques. II. Clinical Trial in 100 Dogs. *Vet Surg.* 19:20–23.

Paulson DS. 2005. Efficacy of Preoperative Antimicrobial Skin Preparation Solutions on Biofilm Bacteria. *AORN Journal.* 81:491–501.

Phillips MF, Vasseur PB, Gregory CR. 1991. Chlorhexidine Diacetate Versus Povidone-Iodine for Preoperative Preparation of the Skin: A Prospective Randomized Comparison in Dogs and Cats. *J AHAA.* 27:105–8.

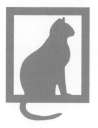

Anesthetic Monitoring of the Feline Patient

Susan Bryant

Introduction

The purpose of anesthetic monitoring is to ensure a safe anesthetic experience and outcome. Because most, if not all, of the anesthetic drugs used in veterinary medicine affect body systems in some way, it is the anesthetist's responsibility to monitor those systems and reduce or eliminate the side effects of the anesthetics before they cause irreversible crises. The astute and knowledgeable anesthetist will be able to anticipate potential complications and to intervene accordingly through diligent monitoring of patient parameters. Parameters to be monitored on any patient under anesthesia include cardiovascular (heart rate and rhythm) and blood pressure. Respiratory function should be assessed by monitoring the rate and character of respirations. Patient temperature should always be monitored because any patient placed under anesthesia loses the ability to thermoregulate.

Measurement of the patient's parameters should take place at regular intervals, usually every 5 minutes, and the results tracked on an anesthetic record. This record should become part of the patient's permanent record, and it also becomes a legal document. By regularly monitoring and recording physiologic parameters, trends can be monitored and easily tracked. The record provides a visual aid in which even slight but steady decreases or increases in parameters can be tracked. Monitoring trends means watching parameters and taking note of any subtle changes that result. For instance if the anesthetist has been monitoring blood pressure every 5 minutes and the results have been a systolic reading in the range of 100–120 mm Hg for the first half hour of the procedure, that is a trend. If at 35 minutes the reading begins to decrease to a systolic below 100 mm Hg and does not rebound, that is a change in the trend, or norm, and this information should be a flag to the anesthetist that a crisis could be looming. Now would be the time to investigate the reasons for the change, begin troubleshooting the cause, and begin treatment for it before it progresses or becomes a life-threatening emergency.

Mechanical monitors are useful and desirable, but there is no replacement for the diligent and observant anesthetist. Monitors need to be monitored for accuracy because several extrinsic factors can alter reliability, such as electrical interference from cautery devices and movement or occlusion of the instrumented area by the surgical team. The skilled anesthetist will use all of the senses to successfully monitor the anesthetized patient especially concerning the physical signs of anesthetic depth. The anesthetist must be able to get access to the patient during the procedure so that anesthetic depth can be assessed and monitor issues can be addressed. Anesthetic depth can be assessed by judging the amount of jaw tone when trying to open the mouth, measuring the withdrawal reflex by using a toe pinch, and by assessing palpebral reflex. (The latter can be affected by the use of ketamine; the palpebral reflex may never disappear.) The loss of reflexes corresponds with increasing anesthetic depth, as does a relaxed jaw. The anesthetist should be able to assess pulse strength on the patient. If the patient is in sternal or lateral recumbency, eye position can be used to assess depth. A cat in a medium plane of surgical anesthesia will have an eyeball that is rotated ventromedially (except with use of ketamine where it does not rotate). The anesthetist will use his or her eyes to visualize spontaneous movement in the patient. Even the sense of smell can be used to detect a leak in the anesthetic circuit, or it can tip off the anesthetist to sepsis or infection. Monitors may need to be readjusted during the procedure. The use of a surgical halo can be extremely useful for allowing access to feline patients during anesthesia so that the surgical drape does not occlude view and access to the patient.

Temperature

Body temperature should be monitored regularly throughout any anesthetic procedure. The anesthetic drugs used can cause vasodilation that can exacerbate heat loss through the skin. When patients are anesthetized they lose their ability to thermoregulate. During surgery, open body cavities will be exposed to the cool ambient temperatures of the surgery suite.

Hypothermia or decreased body temperature can result in a number of complications including prolonged recovery, reduced metabolism of anesthetic drugs, impaired platelet function, and even death. Hypothermia reduces anesthetic drug requirements and without careful monitoring, can result in anesthetic overdose. Heat supplementation for feline patients can be supplied by circulating warm water blankets, forced warm air blowers or an electric thermal pad such as the Hot Dog Patient Warmer (Augustine Temperature Management, Eden Prairie, MN) or the ChillBuster Blanket (ThermoGear, Inc., Tualatin, OR). These thermal pads can be folded over the patient for procedures involving the head, such as ophthalmic procedures or dental procedures. Warmed lavage fluids should be used intraoperatively, especially for abdominal flushing. Fluid warmers can be helpful as long as they are placed as close to the patient as possible. Drip rates for feline patients are low and fluids will likely recool before reaching the patient if the warmer is placed further away from the patient. Warm fluid bags or hot water-filled gloves must be used with great care, if at all. Cats have thin skin that is easily burned and these warming tools must be covered well with a towel so that they do not rest directly against the skin to prevent burns.

Heat retention can be further accomplished by wrapping the feet with plastic wrap or bubble wrap or applying baby socks for the duration of the procedure and into recovery. Many multiparameter monitors come with an esophageal temperature probe that provides continuous temperature readings. Every effort should be made to maintain body temperature to at least 99°F.

Blood Pressure

Blood pressure is the measurement of the force applied to the walls of the arteries as blood is pumped by the heart through the body. Blood pressure is determined by the force with which the heart pumps (contractility) and the volume of blood pumped. It is also determined by the size and flexibility of the arteries.

Ideally, any cat under anesthesia should have regular blood pressure monitoring because most of the anesthetic drugs used affect blood pressure in some way. Prolonged hypotension (more than 15–30 minutes) can lead to nephron damage. Although the effects may not be immediately apparent because 65%–75% of nephrons need to be damaged before renal disease becomes clinically observable, the effects could certainly play a role in the onset of renal disease later in a cat's life. Consider that this means untreated or unrecognized hypotension during the cat's spay surgery at 6 months of age or even during a dental prophylaxis in midlife

Nursing the Feline Patient, First Edition. Edited by Linda E. Schmeltzer and Gary D. Norsworthy.
© 2012 John Wiley & Sons, Inc. Published 2012 by John Wiley & Sons, Inc.

could be a contributing factor to renal disease a cat develops later in its life. Severe untreated hypotension can lead to cardiac and respiratory arrest. Hypertension, or excessively high blood pressure, can lead to problems as well. A mean arterial pressure (MAP) of at least 60 mm Hg is needed to properly perfuse the heart, brain, and kidneys. Mean arterial blood pressures consistently below 60 mm Hg can lead to renal failure, decreased hepatic metabolism of drugs, worsening of hypoxemia, delayed recovery from anesthesia, neuromuscular complications, and central nervous system abnormalities, including blindness after anesthesia.

Methods of Measuring Blood Pressure

Pulse Palpation

If no monitor is available, manual palpation of an arterial pulse can give some indication of the state of the blood pressure. A palpable pulse pressure is the difference between the systolic and diastolic pressures. A difference of at least 30 mm Hg is necessary to palpate a strong pulse. Peripheral pulse palpation sites in the cat include the lingual, dorsal metatarsal, carpal, and coccygeal arteries. It is best to monitor the peripheral arteries because these pulses are lost at a much higher mean pressure than the central (femoral) arteries.

Potential cardiovascular abnormalities may be detected by regular palpation. Pulses should be assessed for strength, rate, and regularity, and palpation should begin prior to induction so that any differences in them can be tracked (monitor trends) from the onset of anesthesia through recovery. Certainly pulse palpation should be done prior to induction so that any abnormalities caused by premedications can be detected and dealt with if necessary prior to the administration of induction drugs.

Capillary Refill Time

Blanching the mucous membranes with direct pressure should result in a refill time of less than 2 seconds. Delays in refill time can indicate intense vasoconstriction (potentially from anesthetic drugs, such as alpha-2 agonists) or hypotension.

Indirect Blood Pressure Monitoring

Oscillometric devices work by picking up pulsation under an occlusion cuff placed over an artery. The cuff is connected to a monitor that can be programmed to measure blood pressure at specific intervals of time. These devices deliver systolic, mean, and diastolic readings, as well as the heart rate. Most have alarms that can be set to alert when readings are out of the accepted range. Unfortunately many of these devices do not work well or at all on the feline patient. Many of the blood pressure machines used in veterinary practice are actually designed for human use and, therefore, designed for much larger patients. There are, however, some veterinary specific monitors available (Cardell Blood Pressure Monitor, SurgiVet, Smiths Medical, Dublin, OH; PetMap, Ramsey Medical, Inc., Tampa, FL; HDO, DVM Solutions, San Antonio, TX; VetGard+, VMed Technology, Mill Creek, WA) that are designed specifically to work on smaller veterinary patients. These are much more reliable on cats because the settings and calibration are set for smaller patients (Fig. 15-1).

The cuff size for any blood pressure monitor should be approximately 40% of the circumference of the limb around which it will be placed. Cuffs that are too large will lead to artificially low readings, and cuffs that are too small will give false high readings. For average-sized cats this usually means a size 2 cuff. Kittens may need a size 1 cuff. Ideally, cuffs should be placed on a limb that is in the same horizontal plane as the heart when the patient is in position for the procedure taking place. (The level of the right atrium is the zero mark for blood pressure.) Limbs well above the heart may give artificially low readings. Legs hanging well below the heart will give false highs. The cuffs are usually marked

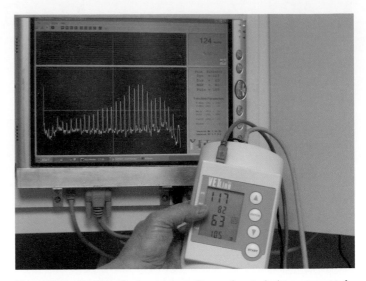

Figure 15-1 The HDO blood pressure monitor can be attached to a computer for computerized analysis of the quality of the reading. A bell-shaped curve indicates a reliable reading.

with the proper placement over the artery. They must not be applied too tightly because this may occlude flow and cause inaccurate readings as well as swelling distal to the cuff. Poor pulse signals from poor flow or any movement of the limb during a reading will interfere with the device and may cause it to fail or deliver an inaccurate reading.

Doppler Ultrasonic Flow Detector

Doppler ultrasonic blood pressure monitors are useful for feline patients. They are relatively inexpensive and easy to use once the anesthetist is properly trained on placement and use (Fig. 15-2).

Doppler flow detectors involve the placement of an ultrasonic probe (crystal) over an artery. The frequency of the sound reflected from the moving arterial blood differs from that of the sound from the crystal and the shift in frequency is converted into an audible sound. Doppler probes may be placed over any artery, but the most useful for measuring blood pressure in cats are the palmer arterial arches of the forelimb and hindlimb (Fig. 15-3).

Consideration of patient recumbency and accessibility of the crystal should determine the choice of artery because these monitors occasionally need to be troubleshot during the procedure. The crystal may need to be readjusted or relubricated. Trying to troubleshoot the monitor by blindly reaching under a surgical drape to find it adds stress and frustration for all involved in the procedure. The area should be shaved and a generous amount of ultrasonic or lubricating gel applied to the area or to the concave side (the side toward the body) of the crystal. The crystal is secured in place snuggly (but not too tightly) with tape. The device can then be turned on to make sure it is properly placed over the artery. There should be an audible "whooshing" sound that corresponds with the pulse rate. If no sound is heard, the crystal should be repositioned until the sound is heard. A properly sized occlusion cuff is placed above the crystal. The cuff is inflated using a sphygmomanometer until the sound of the pulse is eliminated. The cuff is allowed to deflate slowly until the sound of the flow returns. The first audible sound heard is said to correspond with the systolic blood pressure. There are some controversies over what the first audible sound heard in cats is. Some suggest that the first audible sound heard correlates most closely with MAP in feline patients. In some patients it may be possible to detect a second sound, this is said to be the diastolic pressure. With the Doppler and in the absence of a MAP, systolic pressure, or the first sound heard, should

(a)

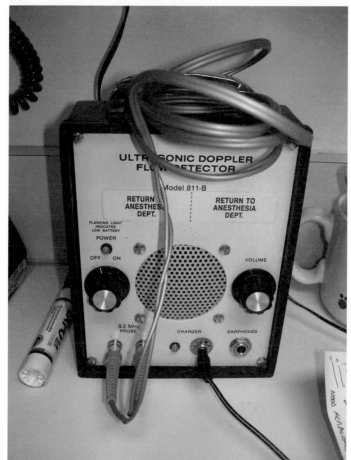

(b)

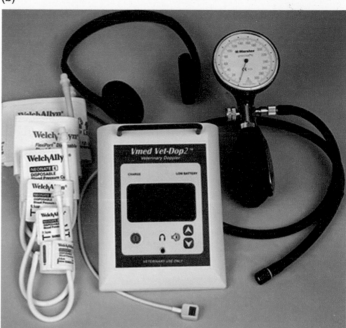

(c)

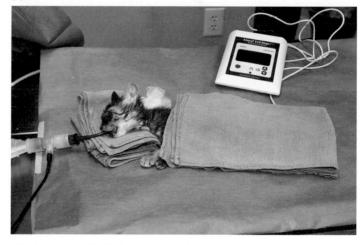

Figure 15-2   The Doppler ultrasonic flow detector monitor is a reliable means of measuring blood pressure. (a) The Parks Medical Doppler (Model 811-B, Parks Medical Electronic Sales, Inc., Las Vegas, NV, www.parksmed.com) has been used successfully in cats although it is designed for neonatal human use. (b) The Vet-Dop2 (Vet-Dop2, VMed Technology, Mill Creek, WA, www.vmedtech.com) is a newer unit made specifically for feline and canine patients. (c) Due to its sensor, the Vet-Dop2 can be used on kittens weighing less than 0.5 kg (1 pound). It was attached to a rear leg on his 0.4 kg (12 ounces) kitten during surgery for enucleation of the left eye.

be maintained above 80–90 mm Hg. Doppler flow detectors are useful monitors, with one of the biggest advantages being the audible sound of blood flow. Changes in flow, especially a reduction, can be heard as well as changes in the regularity of the pulse. Doppler probes are sensitive to movement or bumping by the surgical team, and they are also sensitive to air flow such as that caused by a warm air blower. To prevent interference a Doppler "guard" can be easily constructed from a small plastic bottle (such as a saline bottle). Cut the bottle lengthwise in half and cut a small half-circle on one end that can fit over the instrumented limb. This structure provides protection from bumping or occlusion from the surgeon inadvertently leaning on the limb, and it also provides a barrier from excessive air flow from the warm air blower/blanket.

Direct Method

Direct blood pressure measuring is the gold standard for blood pressure measurements. It involves placing a catheter into an artery and attaching the catheter to a transducer. The transducer (placed at heart level) is connected to an oscilloscope that gives systolic, mean, and diastolic readings continuously. In addition, most monitors also display a wave form that corresponds with the pulse. This provides important information about the patient and the blood pressure. The arterial wave form should match the electrocardiogram complexes. Arterial catheters can be difficult to place in feline patients, but if the anesthetist has experience catheters may be placed in many arteries. The most common sites are the same as listed previously. The possible complications of arterial catheter

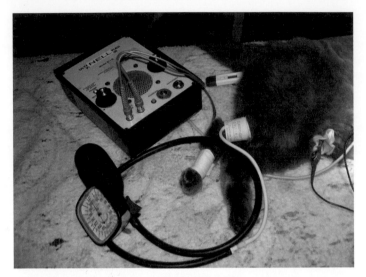

Figure 15-3 This image shows the proper placement of a Doppler ultrasonic flow detector probe and cuff on the hindlimb of a feline patient undergoing endoscopy. The cuff can also be placed on the forelimb or the base of the tail.

placement should be considered when deciding whether direct measurement is necessary and when choosing a site to catheterize. Hematomas, air embolism, thrombosis, and infection are the most common, yet rare, complications. Sterile technique should be considered when placing these catheters to reduce complications. Arterial catheters should be clearly marked so that nothing but heparinized saline is ever injected into them. The catheter needs to be flushed at regular intervals with heparinized saline to prevent clotting. Drugs should never be given through an arterial catheter. Unfortunately, direct arterial blood pressure measuring technology can add $1,000 or more to the price of a monitor making cost a big factor when choosing blood pressure measuring components on a monitor.

Troubleshooting Abnormal Blood Pressure Readings

Hypotension is classified as a MAP of less than 60 mm Hg. When using a Doppler device, which is common with feline patients, the systolic reading should be greater than 80–90 mm Hg. It is important to be able to identify the cause of a blood pressure abnormality to know how to begin treatment for it. There are generally three things to consider when looking for causes of hypotension. Look for drugs or physiological or pathological factors that may reduce systemic vascular resistance (SVR), which is the amount of resistance to flow through the vessels. Some vessels may be dilated and, therefore, allow more flow at less resistance. Constriction of vessels may limit blood flow and require more pressure to get blood through. Look at heart rate, and look for things that affect stroke volume (preload/contractility). As mentioned previously, many of the drugs used in anesthesia cause some degree of hypotension, and less often, hypertension. Knowing the side effects of these drugs and how they work will help in determining treatment. Drugs that decrease SVR (and cause vasodilation) in a dose-dependent manner include acepromazine, propofol, isoflurane, and sevoflurane. Other physiologic factors that may cause a decrease in blood volume or vascular tone include hemorrhage, inadequate volume administration or replacement, dehydration, shock, sepsis, anaphylaxis or severe hypercapnia (high carbon dioxide). Patients with acid-base abnormalities should be stabilized prior to anesthesia if possible to help reduce the possibility of hypotension. Drugs that can decrease heart rate include opioids (although not that commonly in cats), alpha-2 agonists, and the inhalant drugs isoflurane and sevoflurane. Patients with intracranial disease or that are hypothermic may have low

heart rates (bradycardia). Anesthetic drugs affecting the contractility of the heart include the inhalants, propofol, and alpha-2 agonists. The inhalant drugs are potent vasodilators and are often major contributors to hypotension. For this reason a balanced anesthesia technique is recommended. Alpha-2 agonists cause vasoconstriction of blood vessels that result in hypertension. The effects of hypertension from the alpha-2 agonists is transient, lasting only a few minutes before the vessels relax and then hypotension can result. The dissociative drugs, ketamine and tiletamine/zolazepam (Telazol, Pfizer Animal Health, New York) have indirect positive effects on the cardiovascular system and thus, increase heart rate, but this can cause a reduction in stroke volume. Patient positioning can affect blood pressure. Patients that are obese, bloated, or pregnant or patients with large abdominal masses placed in dorsal recumbency may be hypotensive because of excessive pressure on the caudal vena cava. This pressure may compromise venous return and result in hypotension. The same can happen when positive-pressure ventilation is used.

Certain disease states common in feline patients that can contribute to hypertension include renal disease and hyperthyroidism. Ideally these patients will have their hypertension well controlled before surgery. If a patient develops hypertension under anesthesia that is not related to a disease state, the cause is most likely related to inadequate anesthetic depth or inadequate analgesic administration. Adjusting anesthetic depth and providing additional pain medications should result in normotension.

The first step in developing a plan for treatment of hypotension is determining the cause. If the patient is otherwise normal and healthy, the anesthetic drugs are most likely the cause of hypotension. The effects of these drugs are dose related, and therefore, the best first treatment always involves reducing the dose of the drug or reducing anesthetic depth by turning down the vaporizer. Anesthetic protocols that include appropriate analgesics, preoperatively and perioperatively, will allow lower doses of all anesthetic drugs to be used, lowering the side effects of each drug as well. Any patient anesthetized with inhalant drugs or premedicated with acepromazine will have some degree of vasodilation. Intravenous fluid administration of crystalloids at a rate of 10 ml/kg/hr is recommended in patients under anesthesia to help "fill the space" caused by vasodilation and to replace normal ongoing losses that occur for patients under anesthesia with normal cardiovascular and renal function; patients with certain cardiac and renal diseases may not be able to handle excessive fluid overload. Fluid therapy is best begun before hypotension exists. For suspected hypovolemia in a cat with normal cardiac and renal function a fluid bolus of "one hour's worth" the patient's maintenance rate may be given (i.e. 6-kg cat = 60-ml bolus, along with maintenance fluids). Reassess following the bolus. If the patient is instrumented with a Doppler monitor you may be able to hear the improvement and "stronger" flow. Blood loss should be replaced with two to three times the suspected amount of loss (i.e. 1 ml of blood loss should be replaced with 2–3 ml of crystalloid). Excessive hemorrhage may require replacement with colloids such as hetastarch and blood products.

If blood pressure fails to respond to these therapies, and surgical stimulation does not fix the problem, then pharmacologic intervention may be necessary. Pharmacologic agents stimulate the cardiovascular system through two primary mechanisms. Vasopressor effects increase MAP through changes in heart rate, myocardial contractility, or affecting the tone of the vasculature through vasoconstriction. Inotropic effects increase the contractility of the heart muscle and cardiac output. The most common drug used for increasing blood pressure in cats is dopamine. Less commonly, ephedrine, phenylephrine, and vasopressin can be used. In extreme circumstances, epinephrine and norepinephrine may be indicated. Before beginning dopamine therapy it is important to ensure proper vascular volume. Side effects of this drug include tachycardia and possible arrhythmias. Tachycardia is more prevalent in hypovolemic patients or with overdose. Electrocardiograms should be monitored for potential arrhythmias when beginning therapy. Therapy should be reduced or discontinued at any sign of side effects. The half-life of dopamine is relatively short and side effects should diminish with

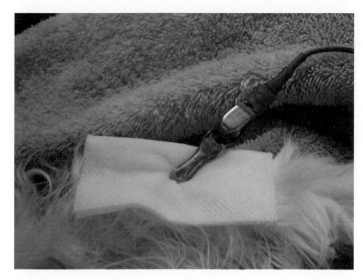

Figure 15-4 Alligator clips can be traumatic to the thin skin of feline patients. Even with the teeth flattened, a "buffer," such as a gauze square, is recommended between the clip and the skin.

the discontinuation of therapy. Dopamine is given as a constant rate infusion with the dose varying from 2 to 10 mcg/kg/min. Infusions should be started slowly and increased to the desired effect while the heart rate and rhythm are monitored closely.

Blood pressure should be routinely measured on any feline undergoing general anesthesia. The best way to prevent hypotension is to detect changes in blood pressure as soon as they begin.

Electrocardiogram

As the heart undergoes depolarization and repolarization, the electrical currents that are generated spread not only within the heart but also throughout the body. This electrical activity generated by the heart can be measured by electrodes placed on the body surface. The recorded tracing of this activity is called an electrocardiogram (ECG). The different waves that comprise the ECG represent the sequence of depolarization and repolarization of the atria and ventricles. The complete cardiac cycle that is portrayed on the ECG is represented by waves that are identified as P wave, QRS complex, and T wave.

It is important to note that the ECG measures only the electrical activity of the heart. It does not measure the function or effectiveness of the heart muscle as a means to pump blood around the body. The ECG may be a useful adjunct to other monitors in determining and recording heart rate but, as with all monitors, results should be verified by simultaneously feeling and counting pulses. ECG machines for veterinary patients usually use the alligator clip type leads. For cats and other small patients that can suffer a skin injury from the alligator "teeth" a buffer is recommended. Usually a small gauze pad in between the teeth and the skin helps protect it (Fig. 15-4). The gauze can be moistened with conductive gel along with the lead to prevent drying out (like alcohol) under the drape from the warm air blower or other heating device. Normal heart rates in cats under anesthesia range from 100 to 180 beats per minute.

Bradycardia, or a slow heart rate, that develops under anesthesia may be caused by anesthetic depth that is too deep, hypothermia, vagal stimulation, or opioid administration. As always when dealing with complications try and lighten the anesthesia first. If the heart rate does not rebound after troubleshooting these potential causes and the blood pressure is reduced as well, treatment with an anticholinergic is likely indicated. Note that anticholinergic drugs such as atropine and glycopyrrolate do not work well in hypothermic patients.

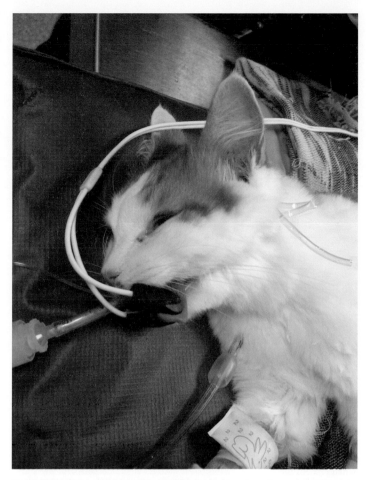

Figure 15-5 The pulse oximeter probe is usually placed on the tongue. The probe should be adjusted occasionally to ensure perfusion to the tissue beds underneath it. On this light-skinned cat the probe would likely work on a toe, the tail, flank, or ear.

Tachycardia, or a fast heart rate, that develops in a cat under anesthesia can be the result of an anesthetic plane that is too light, pain, hypercarbia, blood loss, or hypovolemia. Investigate the cause and treat for it.

The ECG is useful for recording and identifying cardiac arrhythmias. Cardiac arrhythmias are not prevalent in cats with a healthy heart. If it is only occasional and not affecting blood pressure no action need be taken. It is always a good idea to try and identify the cause and eliminate or rectify it if possible. Some causes of potential arrhythmias in cats under anesthesia include pain, hypercarbia, and electrolyte disturbances, such as high potassium in a cat with urethral obstruction.

Pulse Oximetry

Pulse oximetry is a simple, noninvasive method of monitoring the percentage of hemoglobin that is saturated with oxygen. The pulse oximeter does not directly measure ventilation adequacy. The pulse oximeter consists of a probe attached to the patient. Usually in cats the tongue is a common site for measurement, although for dental patients, the probes can work equally well on the tail, a toe, or even the flank skin of a light-colored nonpigmented cat (Fig. 15-5). The probe is connected to a computerized unit that displays the percentage of hemoglobin saturated with oxygen together with an audible signal for each pulse beat, a calculated heart rate, and in some models, a graphical display of the blood flow past the probe. A pulse oximeter can detect hypoxia (low oxygen content) before the patient becomes clinically cyanotic. The

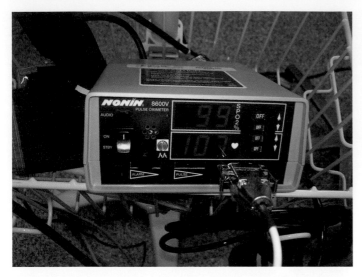

Figure 15-6 This pulse oximeter is light and mobile. The top number represents the oxygen saturation; the lower number represents the heart rate.

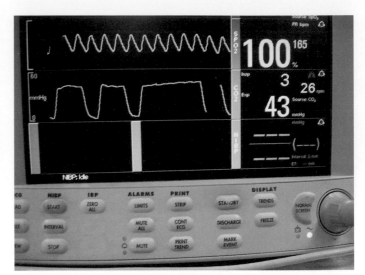

Figure 15-7 A multiparameter monitor displaying the plethysmograph or SpO$_2$ wave form on top beside the oxygen saturation reading. The smaller number to the right of the 100 is the calculated heart rate. Below the plethysmograph is the capnograph displaying the classic shape universal to all animals on a scale where the high limit is 60 mm Hg. To the right of the capnograph is the ETCO$_2$ number, 43 mm Hg. Note the number 3 above the ETCO$_2$ that represents the inspired CO$_2$. Ideally this number should be 0. The 3 represents a small amount of rebreathing of expired gas containing CO$_2$. The monitor also displays respirations per minute. CO$_2$, carbon dioxide; ETCO$_2$, end-tidal carbon dioxide; SpO$_2$, oxygen saturation of blood.

oximeter is dependent on a pulsatile flow and produces a graph of the quality of the flow. Any reduction in pulsatile flow produced by vasoconstriction, hypovolemia, severe hypotension, hypothermia, and some cardiac arrhythmias will result in an inadequate signal for analysis. Sometimes moving the probe to a new location will work. The probe can cause constriction of the vessels beneath it over time, so repositioning it occasionally is a good idea. Wetting the tongue, a popular myth among technicians, does not improve the signal. It is likely the repositioning, and therefore reperfusion, of the area that helps. Bright ambient light can affect the signal as well. Movement artifact is a problem for the pulse oximeter. This comes mostly into play during recovery when patients begin shivering or gaining control of their tongues. The oxygen saturation should always be above 95% (Fig. 15-6). Slight changes over time may just mean the probe needs to be repositioned, but the overall patient should be assessed for desaturation. Sudden steady decreases, especially during thoracic surgery or in the critical patient, should be investigated immediately and supportive measures taken. Usually this means instituting positive-pressure ventilation and improving oxygen delivery immediately while the cause is determined and rectified.

Ventilation

Observations

Monitoring ventilation on feline patients under anesthesia can be done a number of ways. Respirations should be assessed in terms of rate, rhythm, and tidal volume. Initially, careful observation of the patient's chest excursions prior to induction should be done to evaluate for quality and effort. Auscultation of the lungs should be performed prior to sedating or anesthetizing any patient. Normal lung sounds should be heard on both sides of the chest. Any abnormal sounds should be investigated prior to moving forward with anesthesia because anesthetic drugs can depress respiration and ventilation and may worsen existing problems.

Mucous membrane color should be assessed regularly during anesthesia. The tongue and gums should be pink. Any change in color, especially blue or purple tingeing, can indicate hypoxemia.

Apnea Monitors

Apnea or respiratory monitors detect the movement of gas through the proximal end of the endotracheal tube. They provide no information on

tidal volume or the physiologic state of the patient. These monitors can add dead space to the anesthesia circuit causing a rebreathing of expired carbon dioxide, so care should be taken to monitor for this especially in feline patients whose tidal volumes are normally low. They can also be falsely activated by pressure on the chest or abdomen of the patient or by cardiac oscillations that cause gas movement in the trachea.

Capnography

Capnography measures the carbon dioxide concentration in expired gas. It provides a noninvasive means of measuring arterial carbon dioxide pressure (PaCO$_2$). At the end of expiration, assuming there is no rebreathing, the airway and the lungs are filled with carbon dioxide free gases. Carbon dioxide diffuses into the alveoli and equilibrates with the end-alveolar capillary blood. As the patient exhales a carbon dioxide sensor at the end of the endotracheal tube will detect no carbon dioxide as the initial gas sampled will be the dead space gas. As exhalation continues carbon dioxide concentration rises gradually and reaches a peak as the carbon dioxide-rich gas from the alveoli makes its way to the sensor. At the end of exhalation the carbon dioxide concentration decreases to 0 (base line) as the patient commences inhalation of the carbon dioxide free gases. The number given on the capnograph is called the end-tidal carbon dioxide(ETCO$_2$). The ETCO$_2$ value is approximately 5–10 mm Hg less than the PaCO$_2$ of the patient with normal pulmonary function. The evolution of the carbon dioxide from the alveoli to the sensor during exhalation and inhalation of carbon dioxide free gases during inspiration gives the characteristic shape to the carbon dioxide curve on the capnograph. It is identical in every animal (Fig. 15-7). Any deviation from this identical shape should be investigated to determine a physiological or pathological cause producing the abnormality. A report of inspired carbon dioxide (graph not returning to baseline 0) on the monitor means rebreathing of carbon dioxide is occurring and can indicate equipment problems such as expired soda sorb or a malfunction in the valves of the anesthetic machine. Excessive dead space can also be a cause and can be

The Capnograph

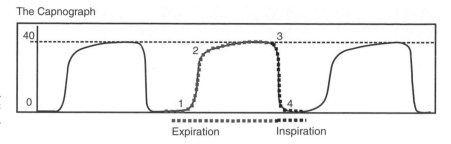

Figure 15-8 The capnograph representing a normal breath pattern. The upswing, (numbers 1–2) represents expiration, numbers 2–3 represent the alveolar plateau, and numbers 3–4 represent inspiration. Drawing courtesy Kristen Cooley.

seen in feline patients when additional equipment (the respiratory monitor and even the carbon dioxide sensor) is added to the patient's endotracheal tube. Abnormal shapes on the capnograph can be caused by a number of things and can be interpreted if normal wave physiology is understood. The beginning of exhalation should be the baseline. The upswing represents the variable emptying of alveoli; however, airway disease will flatten out the slope. The plateau reflects alveolar gas. The down slope represents inspiration (Fig. 15-8). Rebreathing will make the down slope less steep. If there is no waveform, it means the patient is apneic for some reason. If the baseline is increased it represents rebreathing malfunction. An increased plateau is representative of hypoventilation or increased rate of carbon dioxide production. A decreased plateau to a new stable level indicates hyperventilation, hypothermia, airway leaks, tachypnea, or a calibration error. An abrupt drop to 0 means an airway obstruction, disconnect, apnea, or cardiac arrest. An unstable, fluctuating plateau represents patient "bucking" the ventilator.

Normal carbon dioxide is 35–45 mm Hg. Low carbon dioxide can indicate overventilation or poor perfusion. High carbon dioxide (hypercarbia) can indicate hypoventilation, airway disease or obstruction, or anesthetic machine malfunction.

Capnography is easy to use and noninvasive. It provides a continuous measurement of end-tidal carbon dioxide. It provides information on the adequacy of ventilation, airway obstruction, disconnection from the breathing system, and severe circulatory problems. It is also a useful tool in an arrest situation to help determine the adequacy of cardiopulmonary resuscitation. Expense may limit its use in practice, but smaller handheld capnographs are available that are significantly less expensive than one of the multiparameter monitors with the technology included.

Blood Gas Interpretation

Blood gases are the gold standard method of monitoring ventilation. The analysis of carbon dioxide and oxygen tensions in an arterial blood sample provides useful information on pulmonary function. Most analyzers also provide acid-base status and some electrolyte values. There are now many different bedside portable blood gas units available, although expense will limit their availability in general practice.

Blood gas samples are drawn from an artery, either directly or through an arterial catheter, into a heparinized syringe. Care must be taken to make sure that the sample is not exposed to room air or drawn into a syringe with excessive heparin in it because this can affect results. Most blood gas analyzers will measure or calculate partial pressure of oxygen in arterial blood (PaO_2), partial pressure of carbon dioxide in arterial blood ($PaCO_2$), pH, base excess (BE), bicarbonate (HCO_3-), potassium (k+), sodium (Na+), and perhaps other electrolytes (Table 15-1).

In cats breathing room air and with normal lung function PaO_2 should be 80–85 mm Hg. Numbers below this can indicate hypoxemia. Increases in inspired oxygen lead to increases in PaO_2. As a general rule PaO_2 should be five times the inspired oxygen concentration. Therefore, a cat on 100% oxygen should have a PaO_2 of greater than 500 mm Hg. To evaluate blood gas results for ventilation effectiveness first look at the pH to determine acid-base status. Normal pH should be 7.35–7.45. Results are

TABLE 15-1: The iStat* is a cage-side analyzer that is capable of performing blood gas analysis using three cartridges

CG4+	CG8+	EC8+
pH	pH	pH
PCO_2	PCO_2	PCO_2
HCO_3	HCO_3	HCO_3
TCO_2	TCO_2	TCO_2
Base Excess	Base Excess	Base Excess
PO_2	PO_2	Anion Gap
sO_2	sO_2	Hct
Lactate	Hct	Hgb
	Hgb	Glu
	Glu	BUN
	iCa	Na+, K+
	Na+, K+	Cl-

ACT, activated clotting; AnGap, anion gap; BE, base excess; BUN, blood urea nitrogen; Cl-, chloride; Glu, glucose; Hb, hemoglobin; HCO, bicarbonate; Hct, hematocrit; iCa, ionized calcium; K+, potassium; Na+, Sodium; PCO₂, partial pressure of carbon dioxide; PO₂, partial pressure of oxygen; SO₂, oxygen saturation; TCO₂, total carbon dioxide concentration.
*VetScan i-Stat 1, Abaxis North America, Union City, CA, www.abaxis.com.

considered acidotic if the pH is less than 7.35 or alkalotic if the pH is greater than 7.45. Next look at the $PaCO_2$. Remember normal is considered to be 35–45 mmHg. If pH is less than 7.35 and $PaCO_2$ is greater than 45–50 mm Hg it is indicative of a respiratory acidosis, and the patient is underventilating or not being ventilated adequately. If the pH is alkalotic and the $PaCO_2$ is low, it is indicative of a respiratory alkalosis, and the patient is hyper- or overventilating. It can help to think of carbon dioxide as an acid. Therefore, if there is a lot of it (result is high) then the pH should indicate acidosis, and vice versa.

Positive-Pressure Ventilation

Positive-pressure ventilation (PPV) is indicated when a cat cannot ventilate adequately on its own. This indication may be defined as one or more of the following: hypercarbia (increased CO_2, >60 mm Hg), desaturation (SpO_2 < 95%) despite oxygen therapy, hypoxemia (PaO_2 of less than 100 mm Hg on oxygen), or a low observed or measured minute volume. PPV is always indicated in any surgery requiring an open chest, whenever paralytic neuromuscular blocking drugs are to be used, neuromuscular diseases, chest wall problems, abdominal enlargements, or pulmonary parenchymal disease. Any patient that is to be anesthetized with potentially increased intracranial pressure should be mechanically ventilated. PPV is of great benefit to many patients, but it is not without

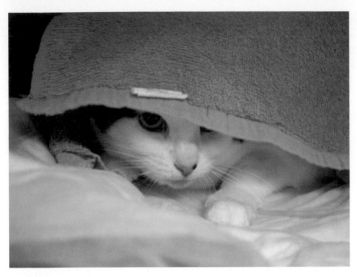

Figure 15-9 Patients should be continuously monitored throughout anesthetic recovery until they are alert and able to maintain their airways unassisted. Some feline patients feel more comfortable if they are able to hide, but care should be taken to make sure they easily viewed in early recovery.

potential complications. These can be avoided with careful monitoring, attention to detail, and a good understanding of the underlying physiological processes. A major contraindication for PPV is a closed pneumothorax because PPV will make it worse. PPV can decrease arterial blood pressure and reduce cardiac output, especially if airway pressures are consistently more than 10 mm Hg or if circulating blood volume is low. Artificial ventilation decreases pulmonary blood flow, and, therefore, may lead to ventilation-perfusion abnormalities. Circulatory changes during PPV are caused by prolonged increases in mean airway pressures and decreases in carbon dioxide.

Tidal volumes are generally calculated as 10–20 ml/kg of lean body weight. Smaller patients like cats will most often do well with the lower volumes. Usually in small animals the peak inspiratory pressure should not exceed 20 cm H_2O to prevent damage to the tissues from excessive pressure, but in cats with large abdominal masses, bloating, respiratory disease, or compliance issues, and in

dorsal recumbency, higher pressures may be needed. Overall, whatever it takes to deliver the needed minute volume and adequately ventilate the patient should be done. Ideally, ventilation assessment and adequacy will be determined by monitoring $ETCO_2$ and blood gases. In the absence of these monitors it is possible to successfully use PPV as long as close attention is paid to peak inspiratory pressure, chest excursions, pulse oximetry, mucous membrane color, and blood pressure. Hypotension can be indicative of hypocarbia (low CO_2) and overventilation because carbon dioxide causes sympathetic stimulation and a subsequent rise in arterial blood pressure. Brick red (injected) mucous membranes can be indicative of hypercarbia.

Monitoring the cardiovascular system function, respiratory system function, and temperature of patients under anesthesia should be a routine part of the overall monitoring plan for each and every patient. Monitoring should continue well into recovery. More critical patients that have had surgery may need ongoing support throughout recovery and beyond. Many times the recovery period is crucial. Patients may have had high levels of physiologic support (100% oxygen, blood pressure support, fluid therapy, temperature support) throughout the anesthetic period; to take it all away suddenly can cause a crisis. Most patients will recover smoothly if they have been monitored closely throughout the procedure and complications have not been allowed to develop. Nonetheless, until the patient recovers enough that it can maintain its own airway, is alert, and can right itself from lateral recumbency (if feasible), it should continue to be closely monitored. Some patients may need ongoing physiologic support, and any patient recovering from a surgical procedure will need pain assessment and management. These patients will benefit from recovering in the intensive care unit or where one person is designated to recovery so they can be continuously monitored. Overall, a warm, quiet, darkened room will help facilitate a calm, stress free recovery for the patient (Fig. 15-9).

Suggested Readings

Haskins SC. 2007. Monitoring Anesthetized Patients. In W Tranquilli, J Thurmon, K Grimm, eds., *Lumb and Jones' Veterinary Anesthesia and Analgesia*, 4th ed., p. 537. Ames: Blackwell Publishing.

Smith LJ. 2002. Hypotension. In SA Greene, ed. *Veterinary Anesthesia and Pain Management Secrets*, pp. 135–40. Philadelphia: Hanley & Belfus, Inc.

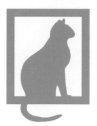

CHAPTER 16

Pain Assessment and Management

Susan Bryant

Introduction

Pain is a difficult sensation to characterize and assess despite the frequency of situations in which it is encountered. Managing pain in felines involves acquiring knowledge of the basic physiology and types of pain, understanding the pharmacology of the different drugs used today to treat pain, and learning and practicing methods of assessing pain in cats. Veterinary technicians provide the bulk of nursing care to the hospitalized patients and are, therefore, better able to detect changes in behavior of the patient and alert the veterinarian that the patient seems painful.

Pain Assessment

In humans, pain management is based largely on verbal communications between the patient and the physician. This is not possible in the feline patient. Feline patients present special challenges because their instincts and survival techniques often prevent them from showing visible signs of pain and distress. In general, if there is difficulty in interpreting the behavioral characteristics of a patient, the anthropomorphic approach should be used. If the cat has undergone surgery or is suffering from a disease that is known to be painful in humans or if there is a history of trauma, the cat is likely to have some level of discomfort and should be treated as such. An appropriate dose of analgesic should be given to treat the anticipated level of pain, and the response to therapy should be evaluated. Inflammation, which occurs to some extent after any surgical intervention, is known to be a major cause of pain. Inflammation is likely to intensify following surgery and can amplify pain. It is known that untreated pain can lead to any number of deleterious physiological changes, delayed healing, and even death. Pain is an individualized experience, for humans and animals, and patients undergoing the same procedure may recover quite differently. Assessment of pain intensity in animals varies greatly between caregivers. Because of this and because pain management is best tailored to each individual patient, it is important to develop and use a pain assessment plan that can be routinely and consistently used by all members of the practice who provide patient care. When an effort is made to routinely study and observe the behavior of the patients before and after surgery changes in "normal" behavior can be detected more readily. For patients with chronic pain or those nonsurgical patients coming into the clinic because "they are not quite right," it may be necessary to rely on the owner's insight regarding the pet's behavior changes at home in a nonstressful situation. The ultimate goal of any pain management plan should be to assist the patient in returning to normalcy as soon as possible.

Things to consider when assessing pain in cats include age, personality, and normal feline behavior. Potential prey species, like felines, are more likely to hide signs of pain. Some cats can act dramatically when they are in the hospital by hissing and yowling when approached, even before surgery. It is important not to ignore these behaviors and dismiss them as exaggerated postoperatively without properly assessing the individual. For these patients and others who show signs of anxiety and stress an anxiolytic or tranquilizer added to the analgesic therapy can often provide optimal relief.

Hyperalgesia, or an exaggerated sensitivity response, can be potentiated in anxious and stressed animals. The stoic or fearful cat can be difficult to assess, but if close attention is paid to its behavior, subtle changes can often be noted; it should be treated with analgesics according to assessment results and anticipated levels of pain. Many older patients may have arthritic pain that can worsen if they are anesthetized and not carefully positioned. They may recover with pain from more than one area. Younger patients, especially kittens, are usually less stoic, but they can be more fragile as well and less able to handle intense pain and illness (Fig. 16-1).

Sometimes the size of these patients makes the idea of administering analgesics a frightening one, but pain medications can be diluted and titrated to effect in tiny kittens. Fear of side effects from analgesics is noted to be one of the biggest excuses veterinarians give for not treating pain. Knowledge, experience, and education can help to eliminate these fears. Many analgesics can be given to effect, and many (pure opioids) can be reversed if absolutely necessary. Reversing the drug completely will also reduce or eliminate the analgesic effects, so alternative therapies should to be used. If caregivers understand the potential side effects of the analgesics used then the patient can be monitored for these side effects and dosages adjusted accordingly. Ethically and otherwise there are no valid excuses for not treating pain.

There are many pain scales available designed to help with pain assessment. Although use of pain scales can help ensure that every patient is evaluated for pain, they all have their limitations especially when assessing a prey species like the feline. Many are subjective and are prone to observer variability to some degree. There has not been a perfect scale developed yet. The ideal scale would be highly specific to detect a patient's pain level and would not produce any false-positives. It would be highly reproducible so identical, or at least similar, results would be obtained by any observer. To base a patient's pain level on one number does not take into consideration the variability of pain perception from patient to patient and observer to observer and may lead to under or overestimating pain levels in patients. Pain scales that have mainly been

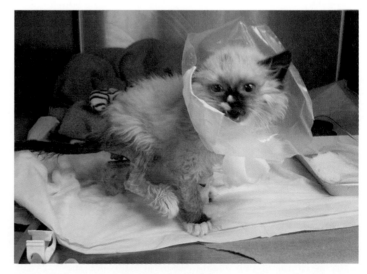

Figure 16-1 Young or neonatal patients are less able to cope with pain and stress.

Nursing the Feline Patient, First Edition. Edited by Linda E. Schmeltzer and Gary D. Norsworthy.

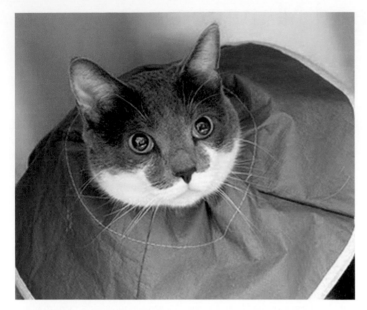

Figure 16-2 Softer, more flexible Elizabethan-collars are better tolerated by patients than the traditional plastic collars.

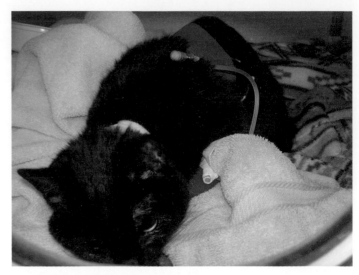

Figure 16-3 This cat demonstrates many of the signs that can be attributed to pain in the feline patient. The cat is lying in an awkward position and appears very uncomfortable. Perhaps it is unable or unwilling to reposition itself. The patient is staring aimlessly and has wide, dilated pupils. The cat never acknowledged the picture taker opening the cage door.

used to assess acute postoperative pain may not be effective for assessment of pain that is chronic in nature or that is caused by disease states such as pancreatitis, sepsis, or even cancer pain. Pain scales are generally used to help guide analgesic therapies and to help track the recovery process. Monitoring physiological parameters (e.g. heart rate, respiration rate) alone can be a helpful tool in determining whether a patient is in pain when under general anesthesia, but in postoperative patients the results can be variable and typical signs (elevated heart rate, respiration rate) can be the result of factors other than pain. If a high heart rate exists after appropriate analgesic treatment the patient may be hypotensive or hypovolemic, and alternative physiologic causes should be identified. Patients should be evaluated for pain on a regular, predetermined basis through the recuperative phase and the response to analgesic therapy should be evaluated as well.

Observation of behaviors should be measured by noninteractive methods (observation of the patient from outside of the cage) and also by interactive methods. Patients may behave differently when they know they are being watched. Some patients are comforted by human contact and may seem more relaxed when someone is with them. This does not mean that they are not in pain, perhaps just less anxious than when alone. Remember, anxiety and distress can intensify pain. Other patients are reluctant to show any pain behaviors in strange and often stressful environments. It is important to note that good nursing care can help to alleviate some pain and anxiety. Full bladders can cause discomfort and distress, and many patients are more relaxed with clean, dry bedding if they have soiled their current beds and are unable to move away from the mess. Many cats are social eaters and will not eat unless someone sits with them and encourages them. Many cats will not eat with an Elizabethan collar on. There are soft, more flexible Elizabethan collars available, and these may be better tolerated by feline patients (Fig. 16-2).

If patients are immobile following surgery, be sure food and water bowls are within reach. Patients that are unable to change positions themselves may need to be turned and repositioned to prevent pressure soreness. An important tool for pain and analgesic therapy assessment involves the patient's response to gentle palpation of the incision or injury. A nonpainful area should be assessed first to determine the particular cat's response to being touched in general. Without risking injury (to clinician) apply slight pressure to the wound and watch the patient's response. Reactions may include vocalization, attempts to get

away, hissing, growling, swatting, and biting. These responses require additional analgesics depending on the intensity of the response and depending on the observation of other behaviors.

Behaviors to consider when assessing pain include posture, facial expression, ability/willingness to walk or move around, ability and willingness to use the litter box, ability to lie down and sleep, position in cage, appetite, demeanor or mental status, greeting behavior, attention to wound, and vocalization. For posture, consider whether the cat is lying in a normal position or lying continuously in one position. Is the cat sleeping sitting up? Most relaxed and pain-free cats sleep laterally recumbent with the spine curved. Is the cat sitting with its front legs stiffly in front of it? Is the cat lying in lateral recumbency with its front legs stiffly extended or leaning a hind leg up on the cage wall so that the abdomen is not under pressure from the limb? Is the head hung low; is the cat reluctant to move its head? It is possible to assess the facial expression in cat. Is there a noticeable "grimace" to the face? Are the brows furrowed? Is the cat squinting? Are the pupils dilated? Are the ears flattened and to the side or up at alert? Is the tongue in the mouth or hanging out? Does the patient get up and change position frequently or has it been in the same position for an extended period of time seemingly unwilling to move around (Fig. 16-3)? Has the cat defecated or urinated where it lies? Normal cats not in pain will usually show some reaction to passersby. Painful or sick cats often face the rear and are oblivious to what is going on outside their area. Some frightened cats may hide in the back of the cage but will usually keep an eye on what is happening outside (Fig. 16-4). Has the patient returned to eating and drinking? Look at the general demeanor of the patient. Has the cat stopped normal grooming? Does it have an unkempt appearance? Was the cat happy and excited to greet you at the front of the cage presurgically and now barely acknowledges company? Does the cat flick its tail or does the tail remain still? Most healthy cats will use their tails to convey how they are feeling. Has the friendly cat suddenly become aggressive? Does it growl or flinch when touched? Is the patient trembling or shaking? Is the patient actively chewing or biting at the wound or bandage? Catheter wraps are a frequent irritation to the meticulous cat. Be sure that the wrap is not too tight or irritating the skin (Figs. 16-5 and 16-6). Is there growling or yowling? Does the patient scream or howl when approached or touched? Note that cats in pain may purr. It is thought that purring releases endorphins that can help to alleviate pain. Some patients may develop an

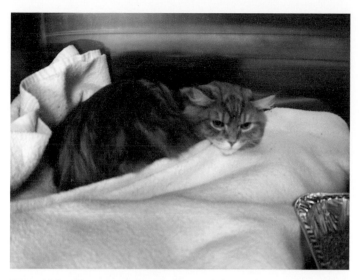

Figure 16-4 This orange cat demonstrates some behaviors that may warrant further pain assessment. The cat is hunched, the ears are slightly flattened, and he is trying to hide. The cat also refuses to make eye contact. In this instance pain cannot be determined by observation alone. More information is needed to determine whether this cat is in pain or just fearful.

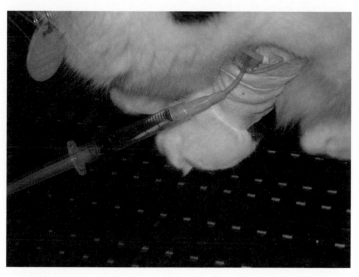

Figure 16-6 This catheter wrap is too tight and has resulted in a swollen foot, likely a source of pain for this cat.

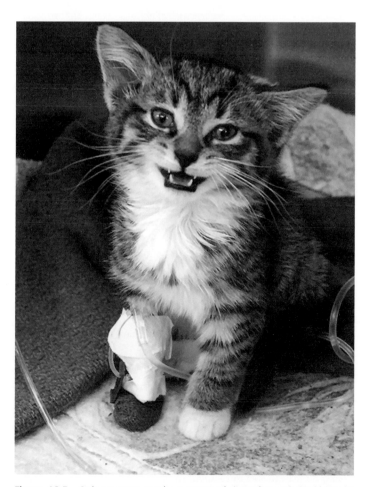

Figure 16-5 Catheter wraps can be a source of discomfort and should not be overlooked as a potential source of pain.

abdominal breathing pattern or excessive respiratory effort in response to pain so watch for these respiratory signs.

As mentioned previously, the goal of good pain management should be to help restore the animal to normalcy as soon as possible while minimizing pain and discomfort. Using appropriate analgesic techniques preoperatively, perioperatively, and postoperatively helps patients to recover more quickly, with less stress on them, their caregivers, and their owners, and it helps them to return to their normal routines sooner than patients left untreated. Learning how to accurately assess and treat pain in cats takes practice, but the results can be rewarding and well worth the effort (Table 16-1).

Anticipating Pain Levels

Some of the surgical procedures, injuries, or illnesses associated with severe to excruciating pain include neuropathic pain, extensive inflammation, crush injuries, large ulcerated fibrosarcomas, and fractures with soft-tissue injury. Moderate to severe pain is expected from osteoarthritis, intra-articular surgery, limb amputation, onychectomy (declaw), traumatic diaphragmatic hernia, urethral obstruction, total ear canal ablation, queening, and corneal ulcers. Procedures or injuries causing moderate pain include some dental procedures, some laparotomies (with minimal tissue manipulation), castration, and ovariohysterectomy in older patients (or done by inexperienced veterinarians), some mass removals, and enucleation. Mild to moderate pain is expected from uncomplicated ovariohysterectomy and castration in younger patients, lump removals, some dental procedures, some ophthalmic surgical procedures, lacerations, cystitis, and otitis.

In general it is better to treat pain before it happens if possible. Pain is known to be more difficult to treat after the insult. Treating pain preemptively can help prevent some of the pain transmissions from traveling along the pain pathway and can dull or eliminate its perception. It can also help prevent the phenomenon known as "wind-up." Wind-up involves the hypersensitivity of neurons and leads to hyperalgesia and allodynia. Cats that develop wind-up are more difficult to treat. Premedication with an analgesic drug is recommended.

Multimodal Analgesia

Another proven technique in managing pain in cats is called multimodal analgesia or balanced analgesia. The theory behind this technique involves understanding that certain drugs work differently along the

TABLE 16-1: Signs of pain or discomfort

Posture: not lying in normal position; lying continuously in one position; sitting with front legs stiffly in front of the cat; lying in lateral recumbency with front legs extended; leaning a hind leg up on the cage wall; head hung low; reluctance to move head

Facial expression: grimace; furrowed brow; squinting; dilated pupils; ears flattened; tongue hanging out of mouth

Increased heart rate

Increased respiratory rate

Withdrawal or aggression from palpation of the incision or injury

Lying in urine or stool

Nonresponse to passersby

Facing the rear of the cage

Hiding in the back of the cage

Lack of eating or drinking

Lack of grooming

Flicking of the tail

Aggression

Growling

Flinching when touched

Trembling or shaking

Chewing or biting a wound or bandage

Growling or yowling

Abdominal breathing

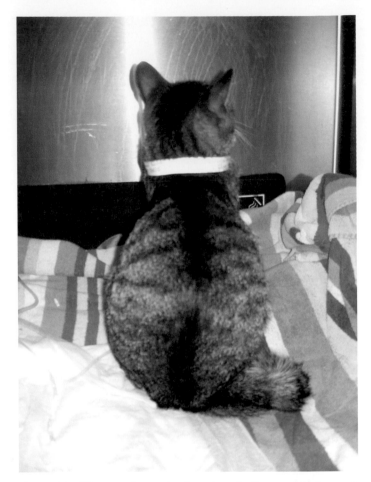

Figure 16-7 This cat was discovered staring at the walls of her cage following a postoperative dose of oxymorphone. She was not uncomfortable, just a little dysphoric.

pain pathway. Also using the balanced technique, or more than one analgesic drug, usually reduces the therapeutic doses needed, and therefore, reduces the potential side effects of all drugs used. An example of this for a cat undergoing anesthesia is the use of an opioid and tranquilizer as a premedication and then adding a nonsteroidal anti-inflammatory drug and perhaps more opioid postoperatively for a moderately painful procedure. A protocol such as this should allow for less induction drug and lower vaporizer settings for maintenance.

Opioids

Opioids, which characteristically produce analgesia without loss of proprioception or consciousness, are currently the most efficacious systemic means of controlling acute or postoperative pain. Pure agonist opioids used in veterinary medicine include morphine, oxymorphone, hydromorphone, and fentanyl. These drugs can be used in a variety of ways to alleviate pain, including as premedications, intra- or postoperatively as small boluses or as a constant rate infusion (CRI), intra-articular, and epidurally. Fentanyl is also available as a transdermal patch although plasma fentanyl concentrations are variable in the cat and may not reach effective, steady doses. If used, cats must be assessed regularly for effectiveness. Using them as premedication drugs allows for lower doses of induction and inhalant drugs to be used. When opioids are given as part of the premedication plan prior to surgery, the patient's blood pressure and heart rate tend to remain stable because they are not influenced by noxious stimuli. These drugs are potent analgesics, and

they are not without side effects. Many cats non-painful given a dose of an opioid preoperatively respond with sedation and euphoric behavior. This can manifest as extremely friendly behavior, where the cat will become interactive, rubs up along the handler or the cage sides, purrs, and kneads with the front paws. Opioids can cause dysphoria in some feline patients where they seem "high," staring at imaginary things on the wall, rolling around in their cages, and even vocalizing randomly (Figs. 16-7 and 16-8). If excessive and self-destructive dysphoria results, it can often be treated with a low dose of acepromazine, with a tranquilizer, or sometimes with the addition of a low dose of an alpha-2 agonist such as dexmedetomidine. Adverse side effects with opioid administration are usually dose related and may include excessive sedation, respiratory depression, bradycardia, and nausea and vomiting. Patients non-painful seem more susceptible to vomiting when given an opioid preoperatively and more often with morphine and hydromorphone given by subcutaneous or intramuscular routes. Opioid-induced bradycardia and respiratory depression are not as prevalent in cats as in other small animal species when used at clinically effective doses. Opioid-induced hyperthermia is a common side effect in cats, especially with the use of hydromorphone. Although its use does not produce hyperthermia in all cats, in one report 60% of cats that received the drug had elevations in temperature to greater than 40°C (104°F). It is something that should be monitored for throughout recovery. If hyperthermia results it can be treated by removing heat sources and bedding so that the cat lies directly on the cool cage floor, administration of alcohol to the foot pads, fans, and the administration of cool subcutaneous or

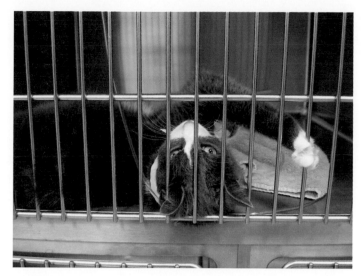

Figure 16-8 This cat is demonstrating euphoric behavior following premedication with an opioid.

intravenous fluids. In some cases giving a dose of acepromazine will promote vasodilation and further cooling. In extreme cases the drug can be reversed through the use of the antagonist naloxone. Be aware that fully reversing the opioid will also eliminate the analgesic effects so alternative therapies should be used for pain management.

Cats seem to respond well with the fewest side effects to oxymorphone. Oxymorphone can be expensive, and its availability has been intermittent in recent years, but it can be a good analgesic option for cats with moderate to severe pain. Morphine should be given very slowly if given intravenously because it can cause histamine release that can cause a severe drop in blood pressure and potential cardiovascular collapse. Fentanyl given intravenously is a potent synthetic opioid with a short half-life so its duration of action is brief. For this reason it is often a good drug to use on more critical patients as a constant rate infusion (CRI) during surgery or with a tranquilizer for induction of critical patients. Using an opioid CRI during surgery allows for less inhalant anesthesia to be used because it lowers minimum alveolar concentration (MAC) significantly. And using CRIs can eliminate the peaks and valleys in plasma concentrations associated with a bolus of drug. If an opioid was not included in the premedication, a loading dose will need to be given before starting the CRI so that therapeutic levels of the drug may be achieved and then maintained. The pure agonist opioids have the advantage of being reversible with the antagonist naloxone. However, as mentioned previously, reversing the negative side effects (excessive sedation, hyperthermia, respiratory depression) also reverses the analgesic effects, and the results may be sudden and dramatic. It is best to titrate the reversal to effect unless it is an emergency situation. Butorphanol, an agonist-antagonist, can be used to partially reverse the effects of an opioid while retaining some of the analgesic effects. To do this, calculate a dose of 0.05–0.1 mg/kg, dilute to desired volume, and give in incremental doses until desired effect is achieved.

Butorphanol

Because it is an agonist-antagonist butorphanol does not induce the profound analgesia that the full agonists do. Butorphanol should only be used to treat mild pain; thus, it is not an effective analgesic for orthopedic procedures or other invasive procedures. It does appear to be more effective in treating visceral pain, such as that associated with interstitial cystitis. Butorphanol does tend to provide good sedation in cats and can be a good choice for premedication or sedation for noninvasive

diagnostic procedures, such as ultrasounds or radiographs. It might also be a good choice for a patient receiving a dental prophylaxis without extractions.

Buprenorphine

Buprenorphine is a partial mu-agonist opioid, so it does not induce the same effects as a full agonist nor the degree of side effects that full agonist opioids can induce. Buprenorphine is a popular and effective drug for treating pain in cats. Research over the past few years has proven that buprenorphine is effective at providing moderate analgesia in cats and can be administered by a variety of routes. It can be given intramuscularly and intravenously, but it is also highly effective when given transmucosally, which is thought to occur because of the cat's highly alkaline saliva. Doses of 0.02 mg/kg given by the transmucosal route have proven to be equally as effective as the intravenous route at the same dose. This allows buprenorphine premeasured doses to be sent home with owners for continued analgesia after leaving the hospital. Buprenorphine has strong affinity for mu receptors, but this effect can be slow in onset. Peak effects of buprenorphine take 30–45 minutes; therefore, it is not a titratable drug. Its analgesic effects can last 6–8 hours. Buprenorphine is difficult to reverse, but reversal is rarely indicated as the side effects tend to be minimal compared with those of the pure agonist opioids. This drug is acceptable to use in patients with mild to moderate pain.

Nonsteroidal Anti-Inflammatory Drugs

Drugs in this class can be used to relieve pain in feline patients. They can be used to help control moderate to severe acute and chronic pain. They are usually given postoperatively rather than preoperatively because of their potential for harm and the inability to reverse their effects; their mechanism is to inhibit COX-1 and COX-2 enzymes. Because they work differently along the pain pathway from opioids, nonsteroidal anti-inflammatory drugs (NSAIDs) can be used synergistically with opioids. There are definite contraindications for the use of NSAIDs, and the overall health of the patient needs to be determined before administering these drugs. NSAIDs should only be given to well-hydrated, normotensive patients with normal renal and hepatic function, with no hemostatic abnormalities, not receiving corticosteroids, and with no evidence or concern of gastric ulceration. When used judiciously, they can be a useful tool in a multimodal technique and can be used routinely in normal healthy cats undergoing routine surgeries such as ovariohysterectomy and castration and for routine dental procedures requiring extractions.

Currently, meloxicam and robenacoxib are frequently used in cats. Both are used in many countries; however, the oral use of meloxicam is not approved in the United States. Robenacoxib is approved in the United States for three-day use although long-term use of this drug for arthritic pain is common.

Ketamine

Ketamine has traditionally been used as a dissociative anesthetic in cats for induction purposes. More recently ketamine has been identified as an N-methyl-D-aspartate (NMDA) receptor antagonist. Stimulation of these receptors causes central nervous system sensitization. Blocking these receptors provides a degree of analgesia. Subanesthetic doses (microdoses) of ketamine can provide analgesia and may help to reduce opioid doses. Ketamine is used in conjunction with other analgesics and is ideally given as a CRI. An initial dose of 0.5 mg/kg intravenously before surgical stimulation can be given (unless ketamine was used for induction) followed by a CRI of 0.1–0.6 mg/kg/hr. This is an effective adjunct analgesic technique for cats. It is usually recommended to discontinue the CRI 20–30 minutes prior to recovery, but for painful

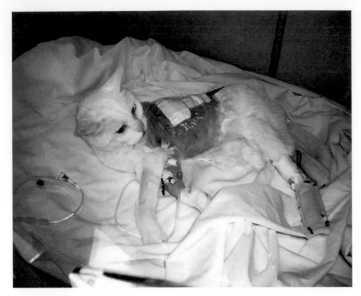

Figure 16-9 This cat had a lateral thoracotomy. She has a diffusion catheter. Note her half flattened ears and the way she is looking at her wound. Gentle palpation can tell us if she is reactive to the bandages covering her incision and diffusion catheter or if she needs additional analgesics.

procedures it may be continued into recovery as part of a multimodal analgesic plan.

Alpha-2 Agonists

Alpha-2 agonists are powerful analgesics that are effective as part of a multimodal approach in young healthy cats. They can also potentiate the analgesia provided by other drugs such as opioids and NMDA antagonists. Alpha-2 agonists can provide sedation and act as anxiolytics, as well as provide analgesia. They can reduce anesthetic requirements significantly. Dexmedetomidine is probably most commonly used in small animals today. It can be used as an adjunct to other anesthetic and analgesic drugs at a dose of 0.0001–0.0005 mg/kg intravenously or intramuscularly. It can also be used as a CRI at 1 μg/kg/hr. The dose can be adjusted accordingly if the patient seems too sedate. The alpha-2 agonists are not without side effects, and these drugs are not recommended for use on any patient that is shocky or has renal, kidney, or cardiovascular disease. Overall their use should be limited to otherwise healthy and cardiovascularly stable patients only. Alpha-2 agonists can be reversed with the antagonists yohimbine and antipamazole, if necessary.

Local Anesthetics

Local blocks are a great addition to an analgesic protocol. Local anesthetics can be used as "splash blocks," injected into joints and nerves, and infiltrated through the dermis and subcuticular to facilitate minor procedures such as laceration repair. A commonly used block in cats is the digital nerve block for declaw. Epidural anesthesia can be a good choice for cats having urethral surgeries. Brachial plexus blocks can provide analgesia for amputations of the forelimb or elbow surgery. Cats are more sensitive to toxicity by local anesthetics so doses should be carefully calculated, and a dose of 6 mg/kg should be considered the maximum dose. In general doses much below the potential toxic dose can be effective at blocking pain impulses during surgery.

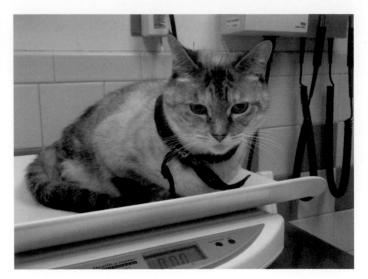

Figure 16-10 Many cats are tolerant of acupuncture treatments. Note the acupuncture needles in this cat's head.

Wound Soaker Catheters

A wound soaker or diffusion catheter is a variable length (2–10 inches long) catheter that has small holes incorporated into it at one end (like a soaker hose) that are used to infuse local anesthetic into a wound bed for an extended period of time (Fig. 16-9). The surgeon buries the catheter into the deepest part of the wound bed possible and the end of the catheter remains exposed and capped with an injection cap. Local anesthetic can be infused at certain intervals or the device can be attached to a syringe pump for continuous infusion. Because cats are so sensitive to local anesthetics, doses at 4- to 6-hour intervals are recommended over the syringe pump method. Soaker catheters are proven effective at reducing postoperative opioid doses in cats with limb amputations. They are also a good choice for postoperative thoracotomy patients. These soaker catheters can be "homemade" out of a red rubber catheter and sterilized or they are now commercially available (Diffusion/Wound Catheter, Mila International, Inc., Erlanger, KY).

Alternative Methods of Pain Control

Other alternative methods of pain control can and should be added to drug therapy. Ice packing wounds or surgical sites can dramatically help reduce inflammation, which is known to be painful. Acupuncture can be chosen as adjunctive therapy to other analgesics, or it can be effective used alone for chronic pain. Acupuncture is said to have some value in assisting painful, nonappetent cats to eating again (Fig. 16-10).

Good nursing care is an important part of a patient's recovery and includes attending to full bladders, hungry stomachs, and the overall comfort of the patient. Stress and anxiety can add to the level of pain a patient experiences. Adding an anxiolytic to an analgesic protocol is often helpful, allowing the patient to relax and rest. Giving the cat a place to hide, such as a box, can help them to feel more comfortable, but cats needing close monitoring postoperatively still need to be carefully watched.

Summary

Pain management in cats can be a challenge, especially because they cannot verbally communicate and to say what is effective. Experience with particular protocols and the willingness to "try it and see" when additional therapies are needed will help to aid in succeeding at treating pain in the feline patient. In general, pain medications should be tapered down slowly over time instead of discontinuing them abruptly.

Suggested Readings

Grimm K. 2002. Recognition of Pain in Small Animals. In SA Greene, ed., *Veterinary Anesthesia and Pain Management Secrets*. Philadelphia: Hanley & Belfus, Inc.

Mathews K. 2000. Management of Pain. In *The Veterinary Clinics of North America, Small Animal Practice*. Philadelphia: WB Saunders.

Robertson S. 2009. Pain Management in the Cat. In R Gaynor, W Muir, eds., *Handbook of Veterinary Pain Management*, 2nd ed., pp. 415–36. St. Louis: Mosby, Inc.

Skarda RT, Tranquilli WJ. 2007. Local Anesthetics. In RT Skarda, WJ Tranquilli, eds., *Lumb and Jones' Veterinary Anesthesia and Analgesia*, 4th ed., p. 408. Ames: Blackwell.

CHAPTER 17

Postoperative Care

Linda E. Schmeltzer

Introduction

The care a cat receives after the surgeon has finished the procedure is paramount to the success of the procedure. Lack of postoperative care can result in injury, infection, or even death. Being as prepared as possible for every step of the recovery process can prevent life-threatening complications.

Transport to Recovery Area

Every cat should have a designated area setup for recovery before it is transferred from the surgery suite. The ideal recovery area is clean, dry, warm, and quiet while allowing for easy observation and access by the staff. The cat should be confined to a safe area large enough for the cat to lay comfortably outstretched. A kennel containing a large bath towel is usually sufficient.

When carrying the cat from surgery to recovery, use caution to avoid restriction of the airway. If the endotracheal tube is still in place, hold the head to prevent the tube from prematurely slipping out of place.

The surgical technician should verbally communicate any pertinent information to the recovery technician when the cat is transferred. The verbal information should include any complications that occurred during the procedure, medications given, the last recorded body temperature, heart rate, and respiration rate. Special care instructions from the surgeon that deviate from normal postoperative guidelines must be discussed. All of the instructions should also be recorded in the patient chart as a reference.

Extubation

To decrease the possibility of choking or suffocating extubation should not occur until the cat's swallowing reflex is present. In some cats jaw tone will return before the swallowing reflex returns creating a risk that the cat may chew or bite through the endotracheal tube, therefore making it necessary to extubate the cat immediately. For cats that have had a procedure causing blood or other secretions to collect in the mouth or upper airway keep the cuff inflated to prevent aspiration. Ensure the cuff is deflated before pulling the endotracheal tube. Recovering these cats at a slight incline (head tilted down) can decrease the risk of aspiration. Care should be taken not to tear the cuff with the teeth when the tube is removed.

It is always a good idea to keep the supplies needed to reintubate a cat in the event of an airway obstruction after extubation.

Temperature Regulation

The majority of postanesthetic cats will have some degree of hypothermia. Providing cats with supplemental heat in the form of a warmed towel, warming cage mat (Chillbuster®), forced warm air blanket (Bair Hugger®), warm water bottle, warm bean or rice bag, or circulating water blanket will help them to retain body heat. To prevent hyperther-

Nursing the Feline Patient, First Edition. Edited by Linda E. Schmeltzer and Gary D. Norsworthy.
© 2012 John Wiley & Sons, Inc. Published 2012 by John Wiley & Sons, Inc.

mia, remove the supplemental heat as soon as the cat's body temperature is within the normal range.

Pulse, Heart Rate and Respiration

Pulse quality, heart rate, and respiration rate should be checked at regular intervals throughout the recovery period. Elevations in any of these parameters can be an indication of pain and should be addressed. See Chapter 16. An elevated heart rate accompanied by weak pulses, pale mucous membranes, and slow capillary refill time may be an indication of internal hemorrhage. Auscultation of the chest gives the technician an opportunity to access heart rate and rhythm as well as the lungs. Lung sounds in the cat are quieter than in the dog. Wheezes or short popping noises (crackles) heard during lung auscultation are abnormal and should be brought to the attention of a veterinarian.

Fluid Therapy

Intravenous fluid therapy should be continued as prescribed by a veterinarian. Whenever possible continue to use warmed fluids until the cat's body temperature is within the normal range. Intravenous infusion of room temperature fluids will slow the body-warming process and prolong recovery.

Care of Surgical Incision Site

The area around the incision site should be kept as clean as possible. Initial cleaning typically occurs in the surgical suite. Postoperatively it is important to prevent the incision site from being soiled by stool or feces. It is ideal to place cats that are not able to posture to properly use a litter pan on a rack that allows the urine and stool to fall away from them. If the cat becomes heavily soiled a bath may be necessary. Be gentle when washing around the incision site to avoid breaking sutures loose. Use a mild shampoo to prevent irritation to the skin. Dry the cat as quickly as possible, using towels or a warm cage dryer to prevent hypothermia. In some cases cleanup of minor blood soiling may best be left to the cat following anesthetic recovery.

Feeding

Check the chart or ask the veterinarian if special diet or feeding instructions need to be followed. Unless otherwise indicated, small amounts and food and water may be offered to the cat as soon as it is fully awake and able to stand. Offering small amounts at frequent intervals can help prevent vomiting from overeating. If the cat does not eat consult a veterinarian for further instructions to administer needed nutritional support.

Preparing for Discharge from the Hospital

On the day the cat is scheduled to be released to the owner it should be examined by the veterinarian. Make sure that intravenous catheters, identification collars, and nonessential bandages have been removed. The cat should be as clean as possible when it is transferred back to the owner. The technician should ensure that all home care instructions are clearly written down for the owner. Gather all medications, food and personal belongings in one place before the owner arrives.

Discharge from the Hospital

The technician should review all home care instructions and medications with the owner before discharging the cat. Having the instructions clearly written down for the owner will allow them to reference the instructions at home and prevent call backs from owners who did not retain verbal instructions.

Postdischarge Call

A staff member should call the client within 24 hours of discharge to check on the cat's progress at home. This will be an opportunity for the owner to ask questions or express concerns as well as for the technician to reiterate important home care instructions. Concerns or complications should be addressed by the veterinarian.

Suggested Readings

Looney A, Bohling M, Bushby P, et al. 2008. The Association of Shelter Veterinarians Veterinary Medical Care Guidelines for Spay-Neuter Programs. *J Amer Veter Med Assoc.* 233(1):814–83.

Pattengale P. 2009. The Postoperative Period. In *Tasks for the Veterinary Assistant*, 2nd ed., pp. 489–93. Ames: Wiley-Blackwell.

Willard MD, Seim HB. 2002. Postoperative Care of the Surgical Patient. In TW Fossum, ed., *Small Animal Surgery*, 3rd ed., pp. 90–93. St. Louis: Mosby Elsevier.

CHAPTER 18

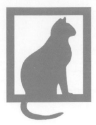
Physical Therapy and Rehabilitation

Barbara Bockstahler and David Levine

Overview

Physical therapy and rehabilitation is a rapidly growing field in veterinary medicine. To help ensure optimal treatment adequate knowledge should be obtained not only about the different types of treatments utilized, but also about the pathophysiology and treatment of the underlying disease, the anatomy and physiology of the tissues and their healing processes, and the timing of introducing rehabilitative techniques to the tissues based on their strength. In this chapter a short overview of common physical therapy interventions are given. For more detailed information, several recent textbooks on physical therapy for small animals are available.

In contrast to dogs, the feline patient is underrepresented in veterinary physical therapy and rehabilitation. This might be a consequence of the (false) belief that cats are not treatable with traditional methods of physical therapy because of their behavior. Although the species-related behavior of cats makes it somewhat more difficult to handle the patient, cats have some unique characteristics that can be used in the development of a rehabilitation program.

Examination

Before starting a physical therapy program a thorough clinical examination has to be performed by the veterinarian. Never start a rehabilitation program without a clinical diagnosis and recommendations or prescriptions from the veterinarian on the scope of the rehabilitation program. In addition to the physical examination special attention should be given to:

- The general muscle condition, symmetry, and tone. Older cats or cats that have undergone a prolonged period of immobilization, such as cage rest, often show a loss of muscle (muscle atrophy) and decreased muscle strength. The muscle mass of the limbs can be easily measured using a tape measure, but it is crucial to always measure the limb circumference in the same location. In cases of neurological disorders, such as a disc rupture, the muscle tone can be diminished or increased based on where the injury has occurred. Painful muscle spasms that often occur secondary to orthopedic and neurological disorders can also be detected.
- The passive range of motion of joints. This means the full comfortable motion that a joint can be moved through without resistance or signs of discomfort. The passive range of motion can be measured with a goniometer. The joint is flexed and extended through its range of motion and the values are read from the goniometer (Figs. 18-1 and 18-2). Jaegger reported range of motion values in normal cats for the carpal joint 22 degrees (flexion)/198 degrees (extension), elbow 22 degrees/163 degrees, shoulder 32 degrees/163 degrees, tarsal 21 degrees/167 degrees, stifle 24 degrees/164 degrees, and hip 33 degrees/164 degrees.

Special Recommendations

- In general cats are less tolerant than dogs; therefore, it is more difficult to perform exercises with them.
- Cats are relatively impatient and quickly bored. Therefore, the time of the session should be as short as possible and offer a variety of different activities.
- Behavioral characteristics of cats such as playing and hunting can be used to design active exercise.
- Not all treatments are tolerated by all cats. Some cats enjoy electrotherapy or ultrasound treatment, and some do not. Therefore, each therapy should be introduced carefully to avoid injuries of the patient and the therapist.
- Some cats will tolerate being in the water as a treatment (hydrotherapy). However, for the majority of the cats this causes high stress and should be only used as a last option.

Techniques

Massage

Massage has been proven as an effective treatment modality in several conditions such as low back pain in humans and is often recommended for rehabilitation of small animals.

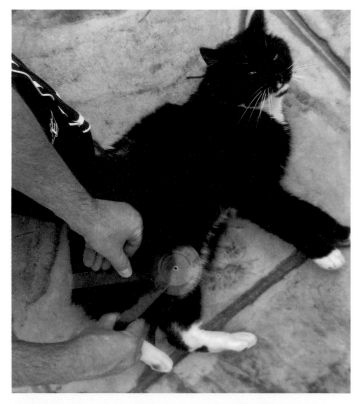

Figure 18-1 Measuring knee flexion range of motion with a goniometer.

Nursing the Feline Patient, First Edition. Edited by Linda E. Schmeltzer and Gary D. Norsworthy.
© 2012 John Wiley & Sons, Inc. Published 2012 by John Wiley & Sons, Inc.

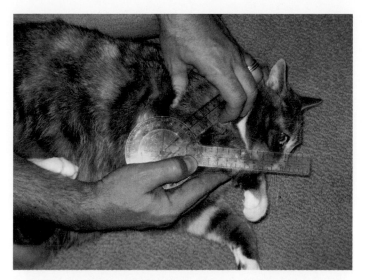

Figure 18-2 Measuring elbow flexion range of motion with a goniometer.

Biological Effects

There are many beneficial therapeutic effects of massage such as the increase of blood flow, increasing oxygen supply to the area, and the release of endogenous endorphins (the bodies natural painkillers), which can be used effectively in the rehabilitation.

Methods

A lot of different massage techniques are described in the literature; the most commons classic or "Swedish" ones are:

- Effleurage, which means gliding, is a superficial technique to increase blood flow and make the cat comfortable with the treatment.
- Petrissage is a kneading type of massage and is effective at increasing blood supply and the mobility and length of connective tissues.
- Friction is a deep form of massage that can help to restore the mobility between tissue interfaces.

Indications and Precautions/Contraindications

The indications are the improvement of muscle spasms secondary to musculoskeletal disorders, increasing the blood flow, increasing the elasticity of tendons and ligaments, improving the joint and muscle function, and to prevent tissue adhesions after surgery. Massage should not be used in case of tumors, infections, cardiac decompression, fever, and bleeding disorders.

Use of Heat

Biological Effects

Heat can be applied to increase the blood flow and the metabolic rate of tissues, relax muscles, relieve pain, and increase the extensibility of connective tissues.

Methods

Commercially available hot packs can be used to heat tissues up to a depth of 2 cm. They are applied to the affected body part for about 15–20 minutes, one to three times daily, commonly before an activity such as range of motion (ROM) and stretching or to decrease pain.

Indications and Precautions/Contraindications

It is useful in cases of osteoarthritis, back pain resulting from conditions such as spondylarthrosis or disc lesions, muscle spasms, and to prepare tissues such as muscles and tendons for exercise. Contraindications include acute inflammation, tumors, open wounds, severe cardiac insufficiency, and decreased sensation in the treatment area.

Use of Cold

Biological Effects

The application of cold (or cryotherapy) causes vasoconstriction and therefore, reduces bleeding in the area after injury or surgery. Cold also decreases the metabolism of cells, decreases nerve conduction velocity, and helps to alleviate pain.

Indications and Precautions/Contraindications

Cold is used to decrease swelling, pain, and the overall inflammatory process after surgery and exercise, and to reduce swelling and pain in acute stages of osteoarthritis, for example. Cold should not be used in case of paresthesia and circulatory disorders.

Methods

To cool tissues commercial available cold packs or ice packs can be used. They are typically wrapped in a towel and placed directly on the affected body part for 10–15 minutes, one to three times daily.

Therapeutic Ultrasound

In physical therapy therapeutic ultrasound is commonly used for deep tissue heating to improve the extensibility of connective tissues, to decrease pain and muscle spasms, and to promote tissue healing and improve the quality of scar tissue.

Two frequencies are used, 1.0 MHz and 3.3 MHz; 1 MHz is absorbed at a depth of 2–5 cm, and 3.3 MHz acts more superficially at a depth of 0–3 cm. Two modes of ultrasound are used; continuous (100%) and pulsed (typically 20%).

Biological Effects

Depending on the mode the biological effects of ultrasound differ:

- Continuous mode: The thermal effects are higher, and it is primarily used for tissue heating prior to stretching.
- Pulsed mode: The thermal effects are minimal, but a variety of effects may occur based on the phase of tissue repair. These include an acceleration of the inflammatory process, increased fibroblast proliferation, increasing tensile strength of healing tissues, and numerous other effects.

Indications and Precautions/Contraindications

Common indications include increasing tissue temperature prior to stretching, decreasing pain, treatment of calcifying tendinitis, and acceleration of the wound healing process. It should not be used over the heart or in animals with pacemakers, in areas at risk for embolism, over tumors or infections, over the epiphyseal area of immature physis, and over the spinal cord after laminectomy.

Methods

- The choice of the mode (continuous/pulsed) depends on the desired effects. The thermal effects are pronounced with a continuous mode, the tissue healing effects if a pulsed mode is used.

- The choice of the frequency depends on the depth of the target tissue.
- The intensity for ultrasound is generally between 0.5 (little soft tissue) and 1.5 (large amount of soft tissue) W/cm². For pulsed treatments with the goal of wound healing, specific guidelines have been developed.
- The treatment time depends on the size of the area and of the sound head. Generally four minutes for each sound head that fits into the treatment area (e.g. sound head size 5 cm², treatment area 10 cm²: 8 minutes).
- The treatment area must be shaved and a suitable contact gel must be used. Hair must be clipped for effective transmission and to avoid burns.
- The sound head must be slowly moved during the treatment to avoid overheating the skin.

Electrotherapy

Electrical stimulation is a useful therapeutic modality and is often possible to use in cats; in fact many cats like this modality. The two most common uses for electrical stimulation are for muscle strengthening and pain control.

Biological Effects

For muscle strengthening the motor nerve is stimulated, which causes a muscle contraction. For pain control, analgesia occurs as a result of several mechanisms such as the Gate Control Theory and the release of endogenous endorphins.

Indications and Precautions/Contraindications

Electrical stimulation is often used for pain management, improvement of muscle spasms, prevention of muscle atrophy, and muscle strengthening.

Precautions/contraindications include anesthetized areas of skin, acute inflammation, infection, and tumors.

Electrodes

A variety of electrodes are available (rubber, gel, bristle). With exception of bristle electrodes (Fig. 18-3) the skin must be clipped before treatment, and a suitable contact medium such as ultrasound gel must be applied.

Electrodes can be placed directly on the painful area, segmentally via the nerve innervating the target tissue, over acupuncture/trigger points, and to stimulate muscle over the motor point and the muscle-tendon junction.

Therapeutic exercises

Therapeutic exercises are one of the most important parts of the rehabilitation process. The design of the therapy program depends strongly on the needs of the individual patient and should ensure that the exercises can be performed safely without the risk to worsen the symptoms. The exercises should be selected based on the stage of tissue repair; therefore, the therapist should understand the underlying pathology, the expected recovery progress and biomechanical considerations. Exercises are performed to achieve many goals including improving ROM, increasing muscle mass, strength, conditioning and endurance, active pain-free ROM and joint function, use of the limbs, coordination and proprioception, and performance and daily function.

Indications and Precautions/Contraindications

Therapeutic exercises are contraindicated if the desired movement could worsen the state of the disorders (e.g. high impact exercises in acute cases of osteoarthritis or directly after fracture stabilization).

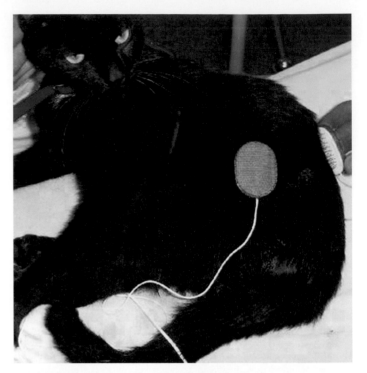

Figure 18-3 Electrotherapy using needle electrodes (PT2000, S+BmedVet) on the back.

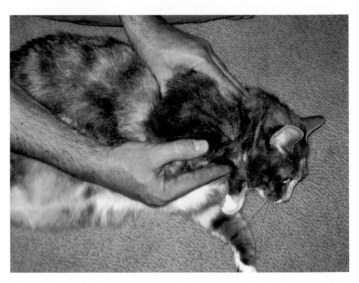

Figure 18-4 Performing passive range of motion to increase flexion of the elbow joint.

Passive Range of Motion

Passive range of motion (PROM) occurs when a joint is moved without an active muscle contraction of the patient within the available range of motion (Figs. 18-4 and 18-5). Adding and holding additional pressure to increase the ROM is termed stretching. PROM exercises are therefore performed to maintain the flexibility of joints, not to increase the flexibility, muscle strength, or endurance.

Usually all joints in the affected limb are treated, starting distally and 10–30 repetitions can be performed two to three times daily.

Bicycling

Bicycling movements are a type of PROM that involves moving all the joints in a limb through their ROM in a bicycling type of motion. It can be

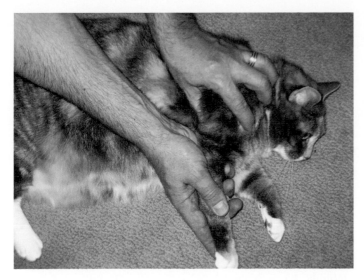

Figure 18-5 Performing passive range of motion to increase extension of the elbow joint.

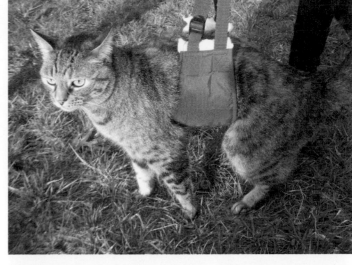

Figure 18-6 Cat with a neurological injury needed a sling support (Four Flags Over Aspen, Inc., P.O. Box 190, St. Clair, Minnesota 56080).

performed in lateral recumbency or in the standing position. The exercise is performed to train the passive ROM of the joints and gait patterns. The tarsal or carpal region is grasped gently and the limb is moved smooth circular in caudal to dorsal to cranial movements. If the animal is in a standing position it should be assisted to prevent falling.

Stretching

Whereas PROM exercises are performed to maintain joint mobility, stretching is performed to increase the flexibility of joints and periarticular tissues such as the joint capsule, tendons, and muscles. The joint is flexed until a restriction is detected and the muscles and connective tissues are stretched. The stretch is held for 20–30 seconds. The same procedure is repeated in the extended direction. Repeat for two to five repetitions, one to three times daily.

Assisted Standing

This is a valuable exercise especially after orthopedic and neurological surgery. It is useful to strengthen the patient, to train the neuromuscular function, and improve proprioception. Usually body slings or harnesses are used to support the cat (Fig. 18-6). The limbs should be placed squarely underneath the body. The cat should be allowed to bear as much weight as possible for several seconds. As soon as the cat shows signs of weakness it is lifted back into a standing position. As the cat becomes stronger, less support is provided by the therapist. Repeat for 5–15 repetitions, one to three times daily.

Weight Shifting

If the cat is able to stand safely this exercise is useful to improve balance, proprioception, and the use of a limb the cat does not want to put down. The therapist tries to disturb the balance by gently pushing the animal on the shoulder or the pelvis momentarily causing as loss of stability for the cat. Repeat for 5–15 repetitions, one to three times daily.

Playing with Laser Lights, Toys, and Treats

Cats may be difficult to motivate, but some of their playing and hunting behaviors can be used to design active exercises. The use of laser lights

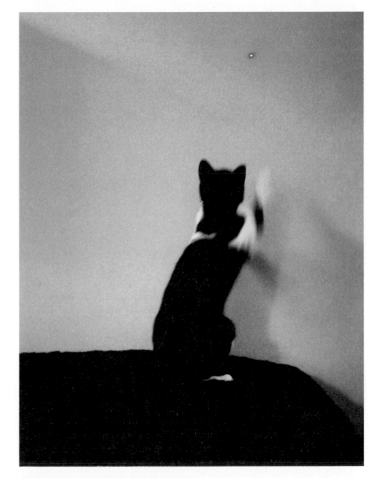

Figure 18-7 Cat playing with a laser light.

(Fig. 18-7), toys, and treats can help to motivate the cat to perform the desired exercise. For example moving the light along the wall can motivate the cat to stretch the legs to reach the light. Other possibilities involve playing with toys or treats.

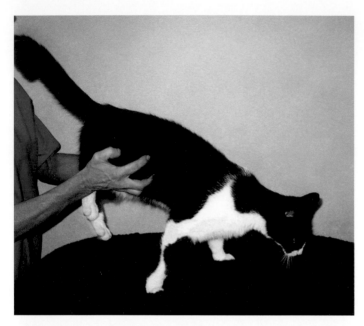

Figure 18-8 Cat in a wheelbarrowing exercise.

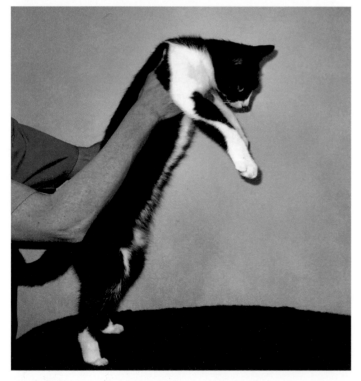

Figure 18-9 Cat in a dancing exercise.

Wheelbarrowing and Dancing

The wheelbarrowing exercise (Fig. 18-8) is designed to improve the use of the forelimbs and to strengthen or stretch the forelimb muscles. The rear legs are lifted off the ground and the cat is moved forward. Dancing is performed to improve use and muscle strength or ROM of the hind legs (Fig. 18-9). The forelimbs are lifted off and the cat is encouraged to move several steps forward or backward.

Osteoarthritis

Osteoarthritis (OA) in cats is underdiagnosed. This might be caused by the fact that cats do not articulate pain as clearly as dogs. Often they do not show lameness but only changes in their behavior such as aggression, house soiling, and difficulty with activities such as stair climbing and jumping onto a bed. Nevertheless, OA in cats is a common problem.

Clinical Signs

The clinical diagnosis might be difficult, but affected animals can show pain during manipulation, limited ROM, or joint effusion.

Goals of Physical Therapy

Pain treatment (in addition to the conservative pain medication) and improvement of the ROM are the goals.

Methods

- Acute stage: Cold (two to three times/day, 15 min), therapeutic ultrasound (20% pulsed) daily, 0.3–0.5 W/cm², gentle PROM exercises two times/daily.
- Chronic stage: Massage, heat (hot pack or therapeutic ultrasound continuous, 0.5–0.75 W/cm²) before therapeutic exercises (PROM and stretching), electrical stimulation (usually transcutaneous electrical nerve stimulation (TENS), two to three times/week, therapeutic exercises for muscle strengthening.

Pelvic Fractures

Pelvic fractures frequently occur as a result of a high-rise syndrome (fall from a height) or if the cat was hit by car.

Clinical Signs

Clinical signs depend on the location and severity of the fracture. The cat might show lameness up to the inability to move. The kind of therapy (conservative, surgically) depends on the specific fracture.

Goals of Physical Therapy

Pain treatment (in addition to the conservative pain medication), maintain or improve ROM, prevent or improve muscle atrophy, and improve lameness are the goals.

Methods

Start during cage rest with cold packs on the fracture side. As soon the swelling is improved start PROM exercises (carefully), bicycling in standing, or lateral recumbency. Active-assisted exercises can be introduced as soon as the cat can bear some weight. Increase to more active exercises if the fracture is stable.

Be gentle. Conservatively treated cats (longer cage rest) must be treated carefully!

Brachial Plexus Lesions

These injuries usually occur as a result of an accident. They are often extremely difficult to heal, and it is necessary to make a thorough diagnosis (e.g. using electromyography) before start of the treatment. If the prognosis is poor, the owner must be clearly informed accordingly.

Clinical Signs

The clinical signs depend on the extent of the nerve damage. Neurogenic muscle atrophy can develop very quickly.

Goals of Physical Therapy

Physical therapy is important to maintain the ROM of the joints and to decrease the amount of muscle atrophy. Physical therapy will be only successful if the injury is reversible. In cases in which partial weight bearing is present, active exercises like weight shifting can be performed.

Methods

Thermotherapy (hot packs or therapeutic ultrasound continuous, 0.5–0.7 W/cm²) before PROM exercises and stretching. Massage might be useful to prevent muscle tensions. Electrical stimulation of denervated muscle can be useful to prevent muscle atrophy provided the nerve is intact and can recover with time.

Cruciate Ligament Rupture

Cruciate ruptures in cats are often traumatic and often involve more ligaments than only the cruciate.

Clinical Signs

Cats show mild to severe lameness, pain during manipulation, and joint effusion. The management can be conservative (cage rest) or surgical.

Goals of Physical Therapy

Pain treatment (in addition to the conservative pain medication), maintenance or improvement of ROM, prevention or improvement of muscle atrophy, and improvement of lameness are the goals.

Conservatively Treated Cats

Start with cold packs to reduce swelling on the affected stifles during the cage rest. As soon the swelling is improved start PROM exercises (carefully) and bicycling in standing or lateral recumbency. Transcutaneous electrical stimulation can be applied during the acute phase segmentally and during later stages locally. Active-assisted exercises can be introduced as soon as the cat can bear some weight. Increase to more active exercises during the following weeks, but avoid exercise that can lead to high degrees of extension (like dancing) during the first weeks. If a restricted ROM is present stretching after warming up of the joint should be performed (hot packs or therapeutic ultrasound). Remember that heat should be not used during the acute stage of the wound healing.

Surgically Treated Cats

Start with cold packs and careful PROM exercises at the day after surgery. If the cat is able to bear weight on the operated leg start with assisted active exercises like weight shifting. If the weight bearing improves, increase to active exercises, but avoid any exercise that could damage the surgical stabilization. Transcutaneous electrical stimulation can be applied during the acute phase segmentally and during later stages locally. In case of a restricted ROM apply heat before stretching exercises (not in the acute stage).

Fractures of the Spine

Fractures of the spine are frequently seen and usually caused by a high-rise syndrome or car accidents.

Clinical Signs

Cats show pain, kyphosis, or neurological symptoms and vary depending on the location of lesion.

Goals of Physical Therapy

In the first days after injury the goals are the improvement of the neurological function and the maintenance of the joint's ROM. As soon the fracture is stable, more effort can be placed on the improvement of muscle mass and strength.

Methods

In general these patients must be treated carefully to avoid any aggravation of the symptoms. During the first days start with PROM exercises of the joints of the legs and bicycle movements. If the fracture is stable, introduce assisted standing exercises and weight shifting. These patients can profit from underwater treadmills exercises, but this type of training should only used if the cat tolerates the water well. Further useful exercises like laser light playing can be introduced if the cat is pain free and able to walk safely.

Obesity and Weight Management in Physical Therapy

Weight management is an important aspect of physical therapy in cats with orthopedic and neurological problems. Excess weight contributes to the development of musculoskeletal diseases and places excessive strain on joints, muscles, tendons, and ligaments, thus aggravating existing health problems. Numerous body condition scoring systems are used to evaluate for obesity in cats.

Possible consequences of obesity in cats include:

- Cardiovascular disease, heart failure, and high blood pressure.
- Diabetes mellitus.
- Gastrointestinal problems such as constipation and flatulence.
- Loss of liver function.
- Reproductive disorders such as decreased breeding performance and dystocia.
- Increased risk of complications during anesthesia.
- Higher frequency of skin problems.
- Susceptibility to infection due to decreased immune defense.
- Shorter life expectancy.

Cats with long-term exercise restrictions because of medical reasons may have decreased energy requirements. It is therefore important to devise a weight maintenance plan for these patients and to switch them to low-calorie foods if needed. The decision as to which food the cat receives lies mainly in the hands of the cat owner. Clients who have problems restricting their cat's food intake as prescribed should be encouraged to use low-calorie cat foods. Because premium diet cat foods contain high-quality ingredients with a balanced mixture of all essential nutrients, they facilitate dietary management considerably. When low-calorie cat foods are used, the owner must simply follow the feeding recommendations printed on the product label.

Home Modifications

The home environment (for indoor cats) may need to be modified for a patient to meet their needs. Nonslip flooring for cats with neurological deficits or osteoarthritis may improve their stability during walking. Sleeping areas should be padded and warm to help minimize pain from conditions such as arthritis. Raised feeding and water bowls are available for cats that have neck disorders. Ramps can be used when a cat can no longer ambulate on stairs. Cats that were predominantly living outside may need to transition to an indoor life if their injuries are serious or if being outside poses a potential risk of exacerbating their problems (such as a spinal cord lesion resulting in paralysis). Paralyzed cats require tremendous effort and commitment on the part of the owner, especially if the cat is incontinent.

Suggested Readings

Bockstahler B, Levine D, Millis D, eds. 2004. *Essential Facts of Physiotherapy in Dogs and Cats*. Babenhausen, Germany: BE VetVerlag.

Furlan AD, Imamura M, Dryden T, et al. 2009. Massage for Low Back Pain: An Updated Systematic Review Within the Framework of the Cochrane Back Review Group. *Spine (Phila Pa 1976)*. 34(16):1669–84.

Jaegger G. 2007. Validity of Goniometric Joint Measurements in Cats. *Amer J Vet Res*. 68(8):822–26.

Levine D, Millis DL, Marcellin-Little DJ. 2005. Introduction to Veterinary Physical Rehabilitation. *Vet Clin North Am Small Anim Pract*. 35(6):1247–54.

Millis LM, Levine D, Taylor RA., eds. 2004. *Canine Rehabilitation and Physical Therapy*, St. Louis: Saunders.

Saunders DG. 2007. Therapeutic Exercise. *Clin Tech Small Anim Pract*. 22(4):155–59.

Saunders DG, Walker JR, Levine D. 2005. Joint Mobilization. *Vet Clin North Am Small Anim Pract*. 35(6):1287–1316.

Steiss JE, Levine D. 2005. Physical Agent Modalities. *Vet Clin North Am Small Anim Pract*. 35(6):1317–33.

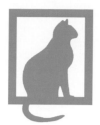

Dentistry and Dental Radiography

Diana Eubanks

Overview

In decades past, the importance of veterinary dentistry has been underemphasized. Largely due to the increasing awareness of animal pain and the strengthening of the human-animal bond, dentistry has emerged as a vital and important area of veterinary medicine. Owners are becoming more educated about the value of dental services and the problems associated with neglecting oral health care.

Dental diseases are among the most common ailments affecting felines; most may be alleviated and some even prevented with proper oral health care. The role of the technician is paramount in the evaluation of dental disease, its prevention and treatment on a professional level, and the education of pet owners concerning home care. The technician can perform a variety of the tasks associated with dental cleanings, dental radiology, charting, and pain management. Additionally, the educated technician is an invaluable source of information for the client.

Normal Anatomy and the Oral Examination

The oral examination is the first, and arguably the most important, step in overall oral evaluation of a patient. Head symmetry, oral or facial swellings, and nasal discharge can be evaluated without touching the cat. Especially cooperative cats may allow a full intraoral examination including evaluation of the gingiva, teeth, mucous membranes, palate, tongue, and caudal mouth to be conducted without the aid of anesthesia. "Lifting the lip" can be performed as part of petting and generally "loving on" many cats. If a cat yawns (or hisses), that can be an advantageous time to sneak a peek at the caudal mouth. Still, many cats will require sedation or general anesthesia to allow a thorough oral assessment.

To identify disease, the veterinary technician must be familiar with the normal anatomy of the feline mouth. The incisive and maxillary bones hold the teeth of the upper arcade. Collectively these structures are referred to as the maxilla, or upper jaw. Likewise, two mandibles, a left and right, are fused at midline by a fibrous symphysis and serve to hold the teeth of the lower arcade.

Occlusion refers to the manner in which the upper and lower portions of the mouth "meet" one another. The normal occlusion in the feline is termed the "scissors bite." In a proper scissors bite, the upper incisors should rest immediately rostral to ("in front of") their lower counterparts. The lower canine tooth on each side should fit in the space between the upper lateral incisor and the upper canine tooth. Premolars should interdigitate, like a pair of pinking shear scissors. Finally, because the upper arcade is slightly wider than the lower arcade, the fourth upper premolar should be located just outside (or buccal to) the lower first molar (Fig. 19-1).

Some cats may exhibit variations of the scissors bite. These variations may be normal for a particular breed (especially seen in brachycephalics) or they may be an abnormal finding. Misaligned teeth may be more prone to trauma or can themselves traumatize surrounding tissues.

The Unique Feline Mouth

The feline mouth differs somewhat from other species. One of the most remarkable differences stems from the fact that cats are true carnivores, having sharp cusps on nearly all cheek teeth (molars and premolars) and having no flat occlusal surfaces like those found in most other species.

Many a beginning veterinary or technician student has mistaken the membranous molar pad, a fleshy protrusion of tissue located bilaterally caudal to the lower molars, as an abnormal structure. This pad is a normal finding and it envelops a small salivary gland (Fig. 19-2).

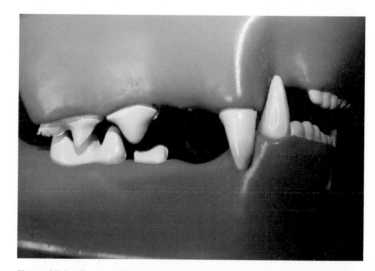

Figure 19-1 The normal occlusion for a cat is termed a "scissors bite." The lower canine tooth should fit in the space between the most lateral incisor and the upper canine tooth.

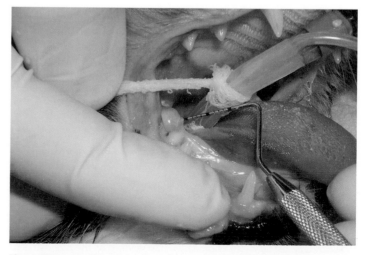

Figure 19-2 A membranous molar pad is located just behind the lower molar on each side and should not be mistaken for an abnormal finding.

Nursing the Feline Patient, First Edition. Edited by Linda E. Schmeltzer and Gary D. Norsworthy.
© 2012 John Wiley & Sons, Inc. Published 2012 by John Wiley & Sons, Inc.

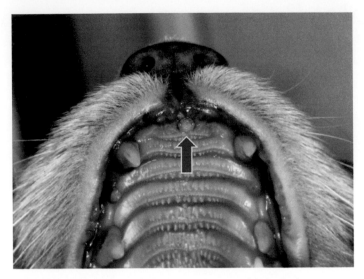

Figure 19-3 The incisive papilla *(arrow)* and the rugae of the hard palate.

Likewise, the incisive papilla is located on the hard palate immediately behind the upper incisors and can appear quite large in some cats. Tiny openings on either side of this structure lead to the vomeronasal organ, which responds to pheromones. Caudal to the incisive papilla, the hard palate is traversed by a series or ridges called rugae (Fig. 19-3).

Kitten Eruption Times and Normal Adult Feline Dentition

Kittens have 26 teeth, deciduous predecessors of all the adult teeth except for the four molars, which erupt only as part of the permanent dentition. Primary (deciduous) canine teeth erupt at approximately 3–4 weeks of age in the kitten. Primary incisors are visible 1 week prior and premolars generally follow in 1–3 weeks, though some premolars may erupt at the same time as the canine teeth. Permanent incisors, canine teeth, and premolars erupt at 3–4 months, 4–5 months, and 4–6 months, respectively. The molars erupt at 4–5 months of age.

The adult cat has 30 teeth, a number far fewer than many other domestic species. When considering the mouth in four separate quadrants (upper, lower, right, and left), each quadrant has three incisors and a canine tooth. The upper arcade has three premolars (designated second, third, and fourth because there is not a tooth in the space that would normally be occupied by the first premolar in many other similar species such as the dog). The large (and sharp) fourth upper premolar is followed caudally by a single smaller molar that may be difficult to see on cursory examination.

The lower arcade has only two premolars (designated third and fourth premolar) but has a rather large, sharp molar tooth on each side.

In the cat, the incisors, canines, and second upper premolar have one root each. The upper fourth premolar is the only tooth with three roots. The remainder of the teeth have two roots, with the possible exception of the upper molar which can have one to three, usually fused, roots.

Periodontal Disease and Staging

The *periodontium* is composed of the following four tissues: alveolar bone, cementum on the root surface of a tooth, a network of collagen fibers termed the *periodontal ligament*, and the gingiva. Periodontal disease is simply inflammation and infection of these tissues. Periodontal disease is the result of bacterial colonization within the mouth that leads to secondary tissue destruction as well as seeding of the bloodstream. Organs with the highest blood flow, such as the heart and kidneys, may be most prone to bacterial infections secondary to periodontal disease.

TABLE 19-1: The stages of periodontal disease.

Stage 1	Gingivitis only. No attachment loss.
Stage 2	Early periodontal disease. Attachment loss <25%.
Stage 3	Moderate periodontal disease. Attachment loss 25%–50%.
Stage 4	Advanced periodontal disease. Attachment loss >50%.

Although definitive links have been established in humans between periodontal disease and systemic diseases, research in veterinary medicine is ongoing.

Despite the best oral health care, a layer of glycoproteins begins to develop on the tooth surface only minutes after cleaning. This layer, termed the *pellicle*, traps bacteria on the surface of the tooth giving rise to plaque. Initially plaque bacteria is composed of mostly gram-positive organisms, but if left undisturbed, the organisms yield to the more pathogenic gram-negative bacteria as well as anaerobes and spirochetes. The latter can lead to a great deal of tissue destruction. As the patient's immune system attempts to fight the infection, tissue destruction may worsen.

Periodontal disease is one of the most common findings in cats. Healthy gingiva should be pink (or in some cases pigmented) with knifelike margins. Gingivitis represents the least pathogenic level of periodontal disease (Stage 1), and with proper cleaning and treatment the gingiva can return to normal. True periodontal disease can be classified as stages 2, 3, and 4 and is based on increased periodontal probing depths and radiographic bone loss (Table 19-1).

Prevention of periodontal disease through a combination of professional and home care can be rewarding and provide many health benefits for a cat including a longer life and decreased pain. Treatment of existing periodontal disease may be a more frustrating undertaking as the patient tends to require lifelong treatment once the destructive process begins.

The Periodontal Probe and Dental Explorer

Periodontal probes come with a variety of markings and are used for measuring the depth of the gingival sulcus. This instrument should be carefully inserted into the space between the tooth and the free gingiva. The depth of the sulcus in a cat should measure not greater than 0.5mm. Increased probing depths are found in cases of periodontal disease and result from the loss of soft-tissue attachment to the tooth. Any measurement greater than 0.5mm should be noted on the patient's chart (Fig. 19-4). Many periodontal probes have an explorer on the opposite end of the handle. This instrument can be used to carefully probe broken teeth and assess pulp exposure. The explorer is sharp and should not be introduced into the gingival sulcus.

Common Abnormalities of Cats

Tooth Resorption

Formerly known as feline odontoclastic resorptive lesions (FORL), among other names, tooth resorption is not entirely unique to the feline. Other species have demonstrated resorptive lesions though none are as frequently affected. Tooth resorption is the most common pathological condition associated with the hard substance of the tooth. Lesions can appear anywhere along the tooth surface and on any tooth but may first be identified immediately above the gum line on the mandibular premolars. A crater-like defect occurs on the tooth and inflamed gingiva may cover the affected area of the tooth surface in an attempt to "patch"

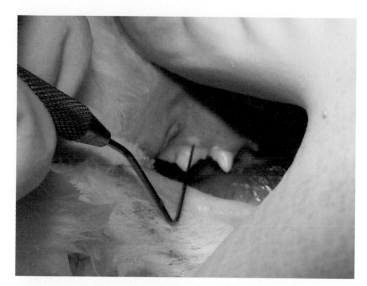

Figure 19-4 Use of a periodontal probe.

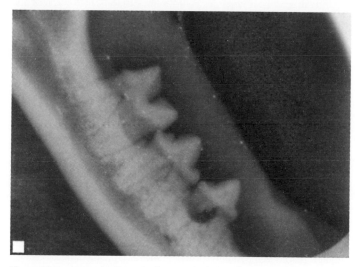

Figure 19-5 Intraoral radiograph of a resorptive lesion affecting 407 (lower right third premolar) in a cat. 408 and 409 appear normal.

the defect. Affected cats are quite painful and may drop food when they eat. An almost certain sign of tooth resorption is that the cat will "chatter" when the painful area is touched with a cotton-tipped swab, thumbnail, or periodontal probe. The chattering response can still be elicited even under anesthesia because there is direct nerve stimulation.

Intraoral radiographs are needed to assess the full extent of the pathology and most of these teeth require extraction. The cause of tooth resorption is still not fully understood and affected cats are likely to continue to develop more lesions as they age (Fig. 19-5).

Stomatitis

Although stomatitis may affect any species, cats are particularly prone to lymphocytic plasmacytic gingivostomatitis. This immune-mediated disease can result in severe pain and a remarkable decrease in the quality of life for a cat. Clinical signs include decreased appetite, dropping food, and excessive salivation. Painful cats may be reluctant to groom, and thus, their hair coat may be unkempt. Stomatitis is characterized by

severe inflammation in the caudal portion of the mouth, affecting primarily the palatoglossal arches. Treatment can be challenging and may include immunosuppressive medications, tooth extraction, and more recently, carbon dioxide laser therapy. A small portion of cats are unresponsive to all modes of treatment.

Persistent Primary Teeth

Other terms used for persistent primary teeth include retain teeth, deciduous teeth, or "baby" teeth. Besides the obvious problems associated with periodontal disease (trapping of debris and tartar by these teeth), persistent primary teeth may be associated with certain orthodontic abnormalities, and therefore, should be removed shortly after the adult tooth begins to erupt. Veterinary dentists adhere to the general rule that "no two teeth should try to occupy the same space at the same time."

Lance Canines

Rostroversion of the upper canine teeth, sometimes called lance canines, often results from persistent primary canine teeth in the maxilla. The adult maxillary canines erupt mesial to (in front of) the primary (or baby) canines. A persistent primary tooth can force the adult to incline rostrally, resembling a knight's lance as the cusp of the tooth aims forward in the animal. Extraction of the primary canine teeth may correct the problem if discovered early. Otherwise, orthodontic correction may be necessary.

Base Narrow

Base narrow canines are frequently the result of persistent primary mandibular canines. In the lower arcade, adult canines erupt lingual to (toward the tongue) their normal position. Persistent primary canine teeth in the mandible can prohibit the normal eruption and lateral "tilting" of these teeth as they emerge. Extraction of the primary canine teeth may correct the problem if discovered early. Otherwise, orthodontic correction may be necessary.

Missing Teeth

Termed *anodontia*, the absence of teeth can affect the entire mouth or simply a single tooth. Causes include teeth that never formed, are slow to erupt, or were present but were lost. A radiograph should be taken to determine if there is any underlying pathology associated with the area, such as a cystic structure or imbedded tooth.

Extra Teeth

The term *supernumerary* is used to describe extra teeth in the mouth. In most cases, supernumerary teeth do not cause a problem.

Periapical Abscess

The area around the root of a tooth (the apex) may become infected, usually as a result of pathology located within the pulp canal. Infectious debris leaks from the pulp canal into the surrounding soft tissues resulting in an abscess or granuloma, which can usually be detected by a halo surrounding the apex on radiographs. These teeth must be treated either with extraction, or in some cases, root canal (endodontic) therapy.

Stains

Enamel normally resists staining though exposed dentin is porous and may stain easily. Staining does not usually result in pathology.

Hypoplasia

Enamel is formed during a specific phase of development of the tooth. Trauma or an infection resulting in a high fever can negatively affect enamel development. Immediately after eruption, teeth many appear normal but begin to show signs of excessive wear only weeks later. Sometimes termed enamel hypoplasia, this condition is more correctly referred to as enamel hypocalcification.

Luxations and Avulsions

A tooth that is dislocated from its socket, either partially or entirely, has probably had its blood supply disrupted, which will result in subsequent death of the pulp. A tooth that is completely out of the socket should be transported to the clinic in milk and reimplanted immediately for best results. A reimplanted tooth will need to have root canal therapy at a later time.

Oronasal Fistulas

A fistula may be associated with any of the maxillary teeth but especially the canines. Nasal discharge is often noted as the fistula allows direct communication between the oral and nasal cavities. Oral secretions and food may leak into the nasal cavity causing odorous infections.

Discolored Teeth

Teeth should normally be white and transilluminate when a light is shone on them. Any dullness may indicate a dead or diseased pulp. A pink or purple hue indicates pulpitis, which often leads to a dead pulp.

Oral Masses

Because many oral masses can be malignant, any questionable mass should be evaluated by a veterinarian. The most common malignant neoplasm of the oral cavity in the feline is squamous cell carcinoma (SCC). SCC tends to be locally aggressive and often difficult to cure. Other oral malignancies include fibrosarcoma, malignant melanoma, and lymphosarcoma. Careful evaluation and possible biopsy or imaging is warranted in any suspect case.

Charting

Any abnormality noted on the oral examination should be noted on the patient's dental chart. The chart becomes a part of the patient's medical record as well as an excellent means for monitoring progression of disease and response to treatment. Knowing the correct dental formulas and eruption times is important. There are a number of systems for identifying teeth. The following abbreviation may be used: I, incisor; C, canine; P or PM, premolar; and M, molar. Writing the formula as a fraction represents teeth in the upper and lower arcades. The total number is arrived at by multiplying by 2 to account for left and right sides of the mouth.

Deciduous: I = 3/3; C = 1/1; P = 3/2; Total = 26 teeth
Permanent: I = 3/3; C = 1/1; P = 3/2; M = 1/1; Total = 30 teeth

The Triadan tooth numbering system assigns a three-digit number to each tooth. The first number corresponds to the quadrant of the mouth: 1, upper right quadrant; 2, the upper left quadrant; 3, the lower left quadrant; and 4, the lower right quadrant. The second and third numbers correspond to the tooth itself with the incisors being numbered 01–03 starting with the most central one. Canine teeth are assigned 04. Hence, an upper right canine tooth would be number 104 and a left lower central (middle) incisor would be designated 301. Cats do not have first premolars as do many other species. As such, they do not have a 105, 205, etc. The first tooth encountered behind the upper canine is termed the 06, or upper second premolar. The system requires some practice to become proficient, but once the veterinary technician masters the language, its benefits become apparent. Deciduous teeth are numbered in much the same way except that the quadrants are numbered as follows: 5, upper right quadrant; 6, the upper left quadrant; 7, the lower left quadrant; and 8, the lower right quadrant. A lower left primary canine tooth would therefore be labeled as 704.

A sort of shorthand for charting is often used to indicate abnormalities found on examination. A list of commonly used charting terms and symbols can be found at www.avdc.org/dental-charts. Many veterinary dental textbooks also contain charting information.

Dental Radiography

The importance of intraoral radiographs cannot be underestimated. Many common conditions affecting oral structures cannot be visualized during the oral examination. Conditions such as tooth resorption, broken roots, and periapical abscesses are often unapparent. Intraoral radiographs illuminate the area beneath the gum line and allow for accurate diagnosis of what lies beneath the surface. The tooth root and surrounding structure are the most important area to capture in a radiograph since the crown can be visualized.

The veterinary technician can perform all aspects of positioning and producing dental radiographs. Although positioning may be a bit frustrating at first, quality radiographs are easy to produce with a little practice. Traditional intraoral films require developing in a dark room (many practices utilize a "chairside darkroom" [Fig. 19-6]). Newer digital imaging systems reduce the amount of time required to produce a quality image. Both systems use the same positioning techniques as both the traditional film packet and the digital probe are used similarly.

Although areas of the mouth, such as the mandibular premolars, may have enough room to position a probe for a parallel technique similar to that utilized in radiographing extremities such as the paw, many areas are not amenable to this technique (Figs. 19-7 and 19-8).

Because of the presence of the hard palate, a probe cannot be positioned in such as way as to acquire a parallel radiograph of the upper premolars. The bisecting angle technique must be used. This technique relies on visualizing angles, much like that used in a game of billiards. A film or probe is placed in the mouth parallel to the hard palate. If one considers a line drawn down the longitudinal axis of the tooth to be radiographed, the line and the film will make approximately a 90-degree angle with each other. The bisecting angle technique then splits the angle (bisects it),

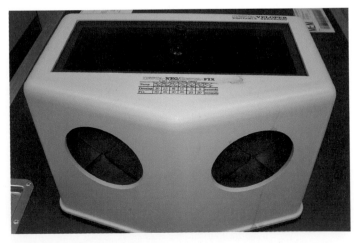

Figure 19-6 A chairside darkroom.

and the x-ray tube head is then aimed perpendicular to the bisecting angle (Figs. 19-9 and 19-10).

Another way to look at it is that the x-ray tube head is the sun shining. The tooth to be radiographed can be thought of as a tree. To produce a shadow that is neither too long (such as occurs late in the afternoon) or too short (at noontime), picture the sun at mid-afternoon. The x-ray tube head (the sun) should be positioned at about a 45-degree angle to the tree (the tooth). The resulting shadow is our radiographic image as captured on the probe or film. Obvious adjustment will need to be made depending on the individual tooth, interference with other oral structures, such as the zygomatic arch, and other considerations. Patience and practice will pay off in learning to produce quality images.

At times oral structures may overlap one another such as often occurs with the mesial roots of the fourth upper premolar. Simply shifting the tube head more rostral (toward the front of the mouth) or caudally (toward the back of the mouth) will separate superimposed structures and allow better diagnosis.

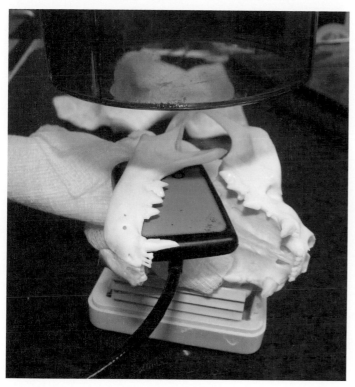

Figure 19-7 Positioning for the parallel technique.

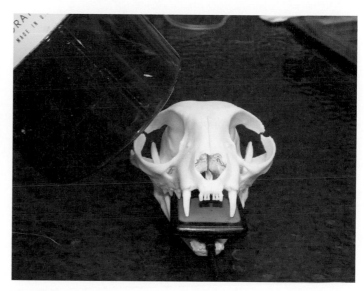

Figure 19-9 Positioning for the bisecting angle technique.

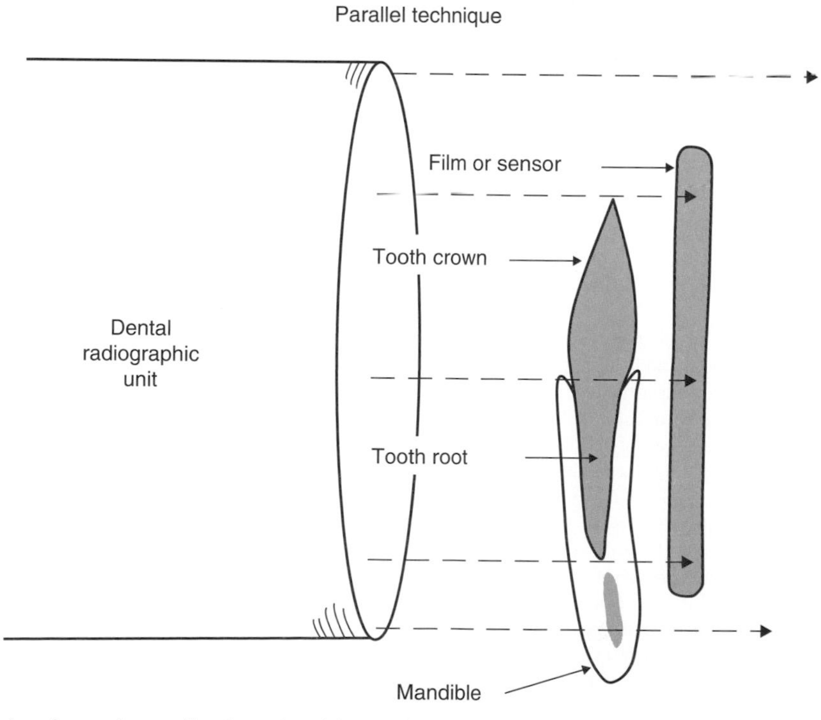

Parallel technique

Film or sensor

Tooth crown

Dental
radiographic
unit

Tooth root

Mandible

Figure 19-8 Using the parallel technique the x-ray beam strikes the tooth and the x-ray film at 90 degrees to their long axis.

149

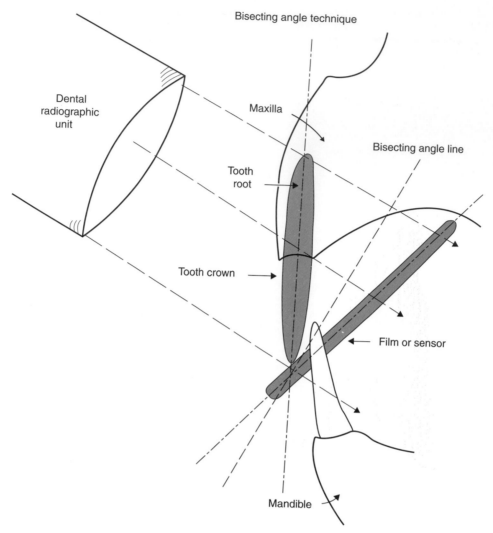

Bisecting angle technique

Dental radiographic unit

Maxilla

Bisecting angle line

Tooth root

Tooth crown

Film or sensor

Mandible

Figure 19-10 Using the bisecting angle technique the film is placed in as close proximity as possible to the desired object. The angle formed between the tooth's long axis and the film is then bisected, and the primary beam is directed perpendicular to this bisecting angle.

Home Care

Many clients may ask the question: "Why isn't professional cleaning enough; why do I need to worry about homecare?" As discussed previously, within minutes to hours of a thorough professional teeth cleaning, a layer of salivary glycoprotein begins to form on the surface of the tooth. This layer (the pellicle) gives rise to plaque that is primarily composed of bacteria. If left undisturbed, more pathogenic bacteria begin to colonize the tooth surface as well as the surrounding structures. Within a period of about 10 days, salivary minerals initiate the formation of tartar or calculus. Once calculus has formed, a professional scaling will be necessary to remove the build up. Thus, the results of a professional cleaning begin to be lost within days following the procedure. Disrupting the pellicle before it has time to mature is the goal of home therapy. With proper homecare, the interval between professional cleanings can be greatly extended.

The best time for an owner to begin oral homecare is when a kitten has deciduous teeth, building up to proper brushing technique and frequency (daily) by the time the adult teeth erupt. Early treatment of plaque and tartar build up allows an owner to start with a comfortable mouth rather than trying to treat a mouth that has already become uncomfortable from periodontal disease. Additionally, kittens are naturally curious and more adaptable to a new procedure than are many older cats.

Tooth brushing is considered the gold standard in veterinary oral health care. It is the single most effective means of removing plaque, significantly outpacing other dental products. Though some cats may be reluctant to accept this procedure, many will willingly participate if the owner has patience. It is important to emphasize the need for veterinary toothpastes because human toothpastes contain detergents and fluoride that should not be swallowed. The tuna flavoring is also more acceptable to the feline palate. Finger brushes may be used for the initial training period, but a brush with traditional bristles should eventually replace the finger brush.

The veterinary technician can provide a helpful client service by demonstrating proper brushing technique using a model or a clinic cat. Although it is beneficial to brush the incisors and the inner surfaces of all teeth, these areas usually have less tartar and plaque build up. The areas of primary concern are the outside surfaces of the cheek teeth and the canines. The toothbrush should be held at a 45-degree angle to the long axis of the tooth and small circular motions should be made on the tooth surface. Brushing should take approximately 30–60 seconds on each side of the mouth.

A vast array of additional products is on the market for reducing plaque, calculus, and gingivitis. These include water additives, waxy polymers, rinses, chew toys, and dental diets. Although most of these are not as effective as brushing, they can augment the effects of brushing or replace brushing in those pets that do not tolerate the procedure. It should be emphasized to the owner that oral healthcare begins in the veterinary clinic and continues at home.

The Veterinary Oral Health Council (VOHC) is an independent body that reviews research on the effectiveness of veterinary dental products. The VOHC exists to recognize products that meet preset standards of plaque and calculus (tartar) retardation in dogs and cats. Products are awarded the VOHC Seal of Acceptance following review of data from trials conducted according to VOHC protocols. The VOHC's most current list of products can be found at www.vohc.org.

Suggested Readings

Holmstrom SE. 2000. *Veterinary Dentistry for the Technician and Office Staff.* Philadelphia: Saunders.

Lobprise HB, Wiggs RB. 1999. *The Veterinary Companion to Common Dental Procedures*. Denver: AAHA Press.

Wiggs RB, Bloom BC, Ruth SL. 2010. Oral and Dental Radiography. In GD Norsworthy, ed., *The Feline Patient*, 4th ed., pp. 610–13. Ames: Wiley-Blackwell.

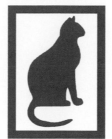
Major Diseases of the Cat

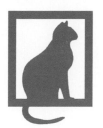

CHAPTER 20

Cardiology

Gary D. Norsworthy

Introduction

About 40 years ago it was believed that cats did not have significant heart disease. However, major increases in awareness and diagnostics have shown that feline cardiac disease is common and a frequent cause of severe illness and death.

Cardiac Anatomy and Function

The heart is a hollow organ with muscular walls and four chambers separated by valves. An electrical system generates electrical impulses that stimulate the two upper chambers – the atria – to contract simultaneously followed by simultaneous contraction of the two lower chambers – the ventricles.

In a simplistic way, the heart has two major purposes. The first is to move blood from the organs that use oxygen to the lungs for oxygen acquisition and then back to the oxygen-consuming organs. The second is to collect nutrients from the gastrointestinal tract, move them to the liver for further processing, and then move the nutrients to the various organs. If either of those functions is impaired as a result of poor cardiac function, the cat cannot sustain life.

The heart is the body's pump. It receives oxygen-depleted blood from the body into the right atrium, moves it through the tricuspid valve into the right ventricle, and then pumps it to the lungs. Following oxygenation, the blood moves into the left atrium then goes through the mitral valve to the left ventricle from which it is pumped vigorously to the distant part of the body (Fig. 20-1).

Diagnostics

Diagnosis of cardiac disease is based on several modalities. The findings will vary considerably between asymptomatic cats and cats in heart failure.

Asymptomatic Cats

Clinical Signs

These cats typically show no obvious clinical signs of heart disease. However, upon close questioning owners may report slow growth of kittens compared to their littermates and reduced activity or reduced stamina following exertion that may include short periods of panting.

Murmurs

The most common finding on a physical examination is the presence of a murmur (abnormal sound heart sound). Murmurs in cats are usually not detected in the same locations as dogs; rather, they are usually heard very near the sternum. Although they may occur on either or both sides, more are found on the right side. Therefore, if auscultation is limited because of the cat's temperament, auscultation of the right side is more likely to be rewarding. Murmurs are graded on a scale from 1 to 6, with 6 being the loudest. Most detected feline murmurs are grades 2, 3, or 4. There is only a mild correlation with the grade of the murmur and the presence of clinically significant heart disease.

Nursing the Feline Patient, First Edition. Edited by Linda E. Schmeltzer and Gary D. Norsworthy.
© 2012 John Wiley & Sons, Inc. Published 2012 by John Wiley & Sons, Inc.

Figure 20-1 Blood flow through the heart. (1) Oxygen-depleted blood enters the heart through the vena cava (VC). (2) It flows into the right atrium (RA), flows through the tricuspid valve (TCV) (3) into the right ventricle (RV). The right ventricle pumps blood through the pulmonary valve (PulV) into the pulmonary artery (PA) (4) on its way to the lungs. (5) Oxygenated blood returns from the lung via the pulmonary veins (PV) into the left atrium (LA). (6) It is pumped through the mitral valve (MitV) into the left ventricle (LV). (7) The left ventricle contracts forcibly sending oxygenated blood through the aortic valve (AorV) into the aorta (A) (8) on its way to the distant parts of the body. IVS, interventricular septum; LVFW, left ventricular free wall.

Electrocardiogram

An electrocardiogram (ECG) records the electrical activity of the heart on a beat-by-beat basis (Fig. 20-2). The important features to recognize include:

- The P-QRS-T waves are created when the atria contract (P wave), the ventricles contract (QRS complex), and the ventricles repolarize or recharge themselves for the next contraction (T wave).
- The intervals between the P, QRS, and T waves have normal ranges; variation from the established normal is indicative of disease.
- The amplitudes of the five waves are considerably less than that of the dog.

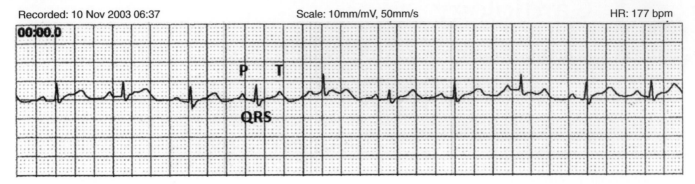

Figure 20-2 Normal electrocardiogram (ECG). The three components of the ECG are the P wave (contraction of the atria), the QRS complex (contraction of the ventricles), and the T wave (repolarization of the ventricles).

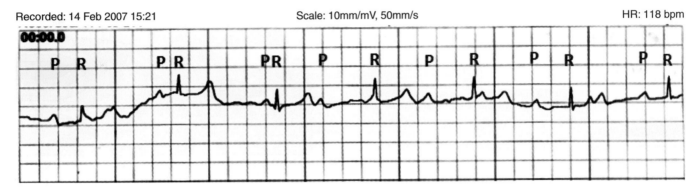

Figure 20-3 P and QRS noncorrelation. The P-R interval should be fixed; however, a heart block will result in variation of this interval.

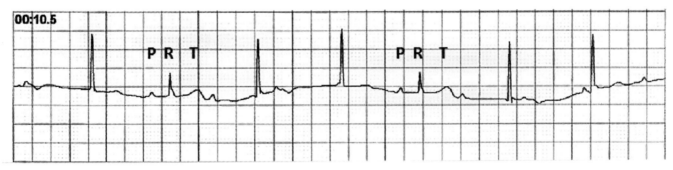

Figure 20-4 Escape beats. This ECG tracing shows only two normal P-QRS-T complexes. The ventricles are not being properly stimulated to contract so they contract spontaneously as a life-saving measure. The ventricular escape beats in this tracing they are tall and irregular in occurrence.

- The cat's heart rate is considerably faster than the dog. A medium-sized dog has a rate of 60–160 beats per minute (bpm); the cat's resting heart rate is 140–220 bpm.
- The QRS complex is often not as distinct as that of other species. Q waves are rare, and the ECGs of many cats have only an R wave or an S wave.
- The dog's heart rate changes during the respiratory cycle (sinus arrhythmia) resulting in an increase in heart rate during inspiration and a decrease during expiration. However, there is no sinus arrhythmia in the cat. The intervals between heart contractions are regular and not influenced by normal breathing.

ECG Abnormalities

ECG abnormalities are commonly found in cats with asymptomatic heart disease. The most common are:

- An abnormal heart rate, either less than 140 bpm or greater than 220 bpm. It should be noted that, by definition, 10% of normal cats fall slightly out of this range. Also note that excitement and stress accelerate the heart rate. However rates greater than 260 bpm should be considered abnormal in all but the most stressed cats.
- Lack of P wave and QRS complex correlation. This situation occurs when the electrical impulse is blocked (heart block) after leaving the atria. Electrical stimulation to the ventricles does not occur so the QRS complex is not formed (Fig. 20-3).
- Ventricular escape beats occur when an undue amount of time occurs after the last ventricular contraction. The ventricles spontaneously contract producing a beat that is life-sustaining but atypical (Fig. 20-4).
- The amplitude of the R and S waves should not exceed two large boxes (1 mV) on the ECG strip. Tall R waves and deep S waves usually represent thickening of the ventricular walls (Fig. 20-5).

(a)

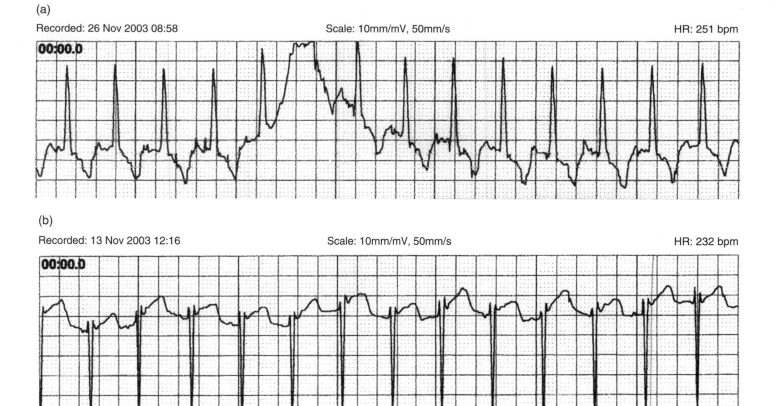

Recorded: 26 Nov 2003 08:58   Scale: 10mm/mV, 50mm/s   HR: 251 bpm

00:00.0

(b)

Recorded: 13 Nov 2003 12:16   Scale: 10mm/mV, 50mm/s   HR: 232 bpm

00:00.0

Figure 20-5   Tall R and S waves. When the R (a) and S (b) waves exceed two boxes, they represent left ventricular hypertrophy. This occurs in hypertrophic cardiomyopathy, hypertension, and hyperthyroidism. When extreme, as shown here, and combined with tachycardia, hyperthyroidism should be the first differential. That was the diagnosis of both of these cases.

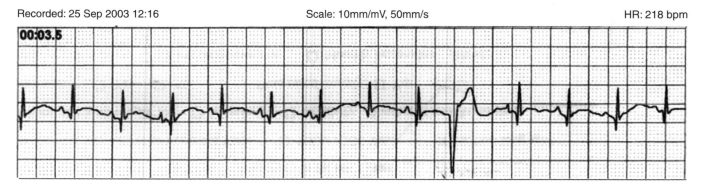

Recorded: 25 Sep 2003 12:16   Scale: 10mm/mV, 50mm/s   HR: 218 bpm

00:03.5

Figure 20-6   Ventricular premature complexes. These are as a result of electrical conduction disturbances or ventricular disease but not a specific disease. They are usually infrequent and clearly different from the P-QRS-T complexes, which are typically normal.

- Ventricular premature contractions (VPCs) are atypical beats that occur as a result of electrical conduction disturbances and ventricular disease. They are not characteristic of any specific heart disease (Fig. 20-6).

It is unlikely that specific heart diseases will be diagnosed with an ECG; however, the ECG is an important screening tool to identify the presence of early cardiac disease. It serves as a basis for recommending further cardiac workup.

Thoracic Radiographs

These radiographs allow one to visualize the outline of the heart (cardiac silhouette). Changes in overall size and in the size of certain chambers

can be appreciated. In addition, it allows one to visualize the major vessels (aorta, caudal vena cava, caudal pulmonary arteries), the trachea (size and position), and the lung fields (Figs. 20-7a,b). It also permits identification of fluid within the lungs (pulmonary edema) (Figs. 20-8a,b) or within the pleural space (pleural effusion) (Figs. 20-9a,b).

However, most cats with early or asymptomatic heart disease will have normal thoracic radiographs.

Ultrasound

Ultrasound of the heart (echocardiogram or "echo") allows measurement the thickness of the heart walls, measurement of the diameter of the

(a)

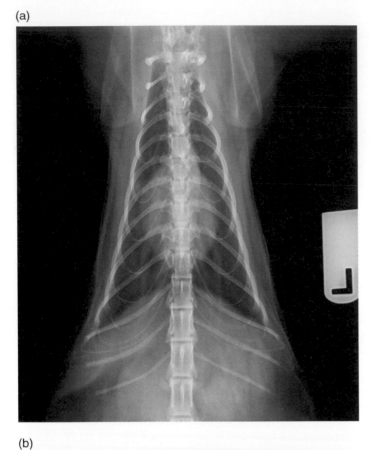

(a)

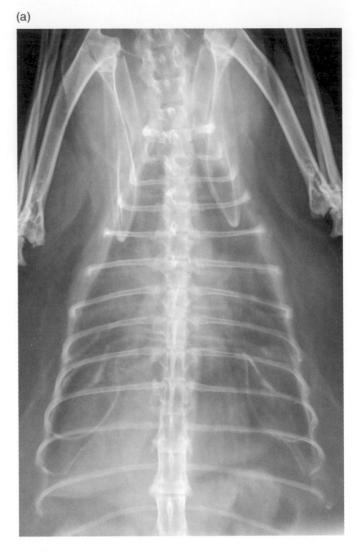

(b)

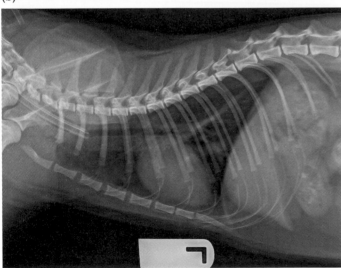

Figure 20-7 Normal thoracic radiographs. Ventrodorsal (a) and lateral (b) radiographs clearly show the cardiac silhouette, lung fields, trachea (containing an endotracheal tube), and major blood vessels.

(b)

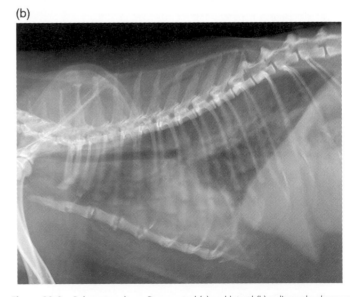

Figure 20-8 Pulmonary edema. Dorsoventral (a) and lateral (b) radiographs show an interstitial lung pattern because fluid is within the lungs. This makes the cardiac silhouette difficult to clearly define.

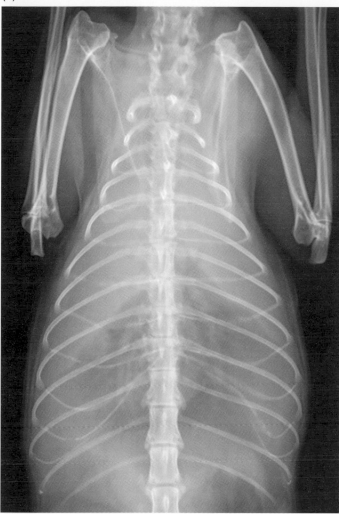

(a)

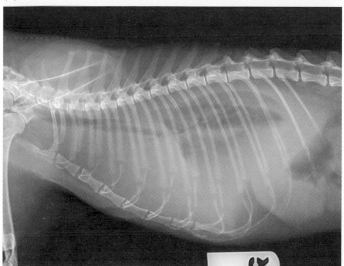

(b)

Figure 20-9 Pleural effusion. Dorsoventral (a) and lateral (b) radiographs show compressed lung lobes (dark) as a result of fluid in the pleural space. The cardiac silhouette has the radiographic same density as the fluid so it is not identifiable. This cat has less than 20% normal lung capacity and is struggling for every breath.

chambers, and observation of the structure and function of valves. None of these are possible with a thoracic radiograph. These criteria are vital in documenting the presence of heart disease in asymptomatic cats and cats in heart failure. An echocardiogram is considered the definitive test for heart disease, and if possible, should be employed when the history, physical examination (auscultation), ECG tracing, or thoracic radiographs is suggestive of heart disease.

Symptomatic Cats

Clinical Signs

Early clinical signs often include gradual weight loss and decreased activity or stamina. However, these signs are subtle and often undetected or unappreciated by owners. The onset of congestive heart failure can take several days or can occur within a 24-hour period. Cats are usually presented with clinical signs of severe respiratory compromise resulting from either pulmonary edema or pleural effusion. Profound lethargy, rapid, shallow breathing, cyanosis of the tongue, and open mouth breathing are typical. Physical examination reveals one or more of the following: hypothermia, dull lung sounds, a murmur, tachycardia, and an arrhythmia. Thus, careful thoracic auscultation is imperative. Ascites (accumulation of fluid in the abdomen), a common finding in dogs with congestive heart failure, is only rarely seen in cats with congestive heart failure.

ECG

An ECG may reveal any of the aforementioned abnormalities. In many cats, several are present; however, in some cats the ECG findings are normal.

Thoracic Radiograph

The most meaningful diagnostic tool is a thoracic radiograph. In addition to various degrees of cardiomegaly, pulmonary edema or pleural effusion is expected; uncommonly, both occur simultaneously. Ascites is not an expected finding. Because these cats are struggling to breathe, radiography may need to be delayed until treatment with an oxygen cage and furosemide improves respiratory efforts. A dorsoventral (DV) view is usually the least stressful and may be the only view that is initially feasible. A combination of DV and lateral views is the most diagnostic.

Ultrasound

An echocardiogram is not needed to establish a diagnosis of congestive heart failure; however, it is needed to diagnose the specific cardiac disease present. It can be helpful in establishing a prognosis, so it is desirable to have this study performed as soon as the cat is clinically stable enough and an ultrasonographer is available. Unlike radiographs, visualization of the heart in the presence of pleural effusion is enhanced with ultrasound.

Therapeutics

Asymptomatic Cats

Therapy for cats with asymptomatic heart disease is controversial. Depending on the specific disease present, some veterinarians elect no treatment. Others preemptively treat with angiotensin-converting enzyme inhibitors (ACEi), calcium channel blockers, or beta-blockers. Diuretics are rarely indicated because asymptomatic cats do not have pulmonary edema or pleural effusion.

Congestive Heart Failure

Congestive heart failure (CHF), or heart failure, is the end point of heart disease. It results in the heart's inability to move blood, oxygen, and nutrients well enough to sustain life. It causes pulmonary edema (Fig. 20-8) or pleural effusion (Fig. 20-9). Severe respiratory distress occurs. Without successful treatment, the cat dies of respiratory failure or cardiac arrest.

Diagnosis

The history and clinical signs of CHF include an often rapid onset of respiratory distress (open mouth breathing, cyanosis of the tongue), profound lethargy, and hypothermia due to poor perfusion. Unlike dogs, coughing does not occur. Auscultation often reveals a murmur and dull lung sounds. ECG findings may include many or all of the abnormalities listed previously. Thoracic radiographs usually find cardiac enlargement and either pulmonary edema or pleural effusion, but usually not both. Ascites is uncommon in feline heart failure. An echocardiogram usually reveals abnormal thickness of the left ventricular walls, an increase or decrease in the left ventricular chamber diameter, enlargement of the left atrium, and pleural effusion. When present, pulmonary edema is not well recognized with ultrasound.

Treatment

In general, CHF is treated the same regardless of the underlying cardiac disease. There are three drugs that should be given immediately. Oxygen is administered either with a face mask, oxygen tent, or oxygen cage. One should be attentive to the degree of resistance the cat offers to the chosen route of oxygen administration. Struggling to fight a face mask is not uncommon; if it occurs, another method should be employed. Nitroglycerin is given for its vasodilation properties. It is administered in the form of a transdermal ointment and applied to the concave surfaces of the pinnae. If the pinnae are cold (because of vasoconstriction) they will not absorb the drug well so they should be warmed with hot packs first. Furosemide is given intravenously (IV) if possible; however, intramuscular (IM) administration may be more feasible because of the stress of giving an intravenous injection to a dyspneic patient. This drug stimulates the kidneys to remove fluid from the lungs or pleural space (diuresis). It may also create or aggravate dehydration so hydration status should be monitored and free choice water should be available.

Other drugs are used to break the renin-angiotensin-aldosterone system (RAAS) or to improve cardiac function. ACEi, notably benazepril or enalapril, and spironolactone are used for RAAS interruption. They should be given to all cats in CHF. Atenolol, a beta blocker, is used for tachycardia or arrhythmias; however, it should not be given in a cat with a respiratory crisis resulting from CHF. If it is not effective, diltiazem, a calcium channel blocker is used in its place. Pimobendan is a drug that helps to stimulate the cardiac muscle to contract (positive inotrope). It is used for some cases of dilated cardiomyopathy. Aspirin and clopidogrel are given to prevent blood clot formation in cats with a dilated left atrium. They are also given following a thromboembolic (blood clot) event.

Major Feline Cardiac Diseases

Hypertrophic Cardiomyopathy

Overview

Hypertrophic cardiomyopathy (HCM) is a disease that causes thickening of the muscle walls of the left ventricle (interventricular septum and left ventricular free wall; Fig. 20-10). As in humans, most cases are genetically driven; therefore, when it is diagnosed littermates and parents should also be examined for the disease.

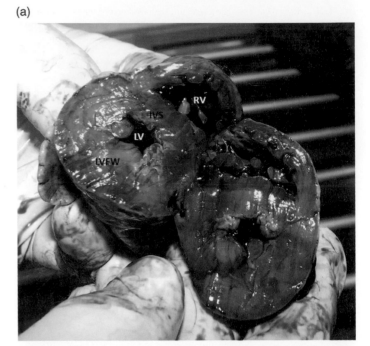

(a)

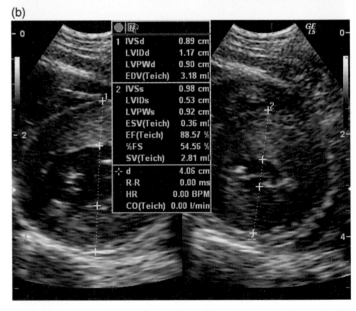

(b)

Figure 20-10 Hypertrophic cardiomyopathy. (a) The diameter of the left ventricle (LV) is very small because the left ventricular walls have thickened and compressed it. The interventricular septum (IVS) is thickened but not as much as the left ventricular free wall (LVFW). Asymmetric thickening is not unusual. Note that the diameter of the left ventricle is much less than that of the right ventricle (RV). (b) The short-axis ultrasound view of the left ventricle shows thickening of the IVS and LVFW. They should measure less than 0.6 cm. Instead they measure 0.89 and 0.90 cm, respectively.

Disease Progression

A progression of events occurs that ultimately terminates in CHF and usually death. The first event is thickening of the left ventricular walls. Usually both are affected, but asymmetric thickening is not uncommon. Because left ventricular thickening is primarily directed inward, the left ventricular chamber's internal diameter gets smaller. As blood is pumped into the left ventricle from the left atrium, some of it is forced backward through the mitral valve because there is not room for all of it in the left ventricle. This damages the mitral valve creating a leak; a leaky valve causes the sound we call a murmur. The left atrium contains regurgitated blood from the left ventricle; more blood arriving from the lungs (pulmonary veins) causes it to overfill and dilate. The left atrium enlarges because of volume overload. Soon afterward, ventricular failure occurs leading to reduced cardiac output and CHF.

Diagnostics

HCM is the most common heart disease of cats. Early changes in the heart often begin during the first 1–2 years of life. Young cats with murmurs are at high risk of developing HCM and should be monitored closely for it. ECG tracings of these cats often show tachycardia, arrhythmias, or VPCs. An echocardiogram should be recommended when a murmur or an ECG abnormality is found.

Treatment

Treatment of cats in CHF proceeds as described; however, pimobendan is not indicated for this disease.

Thromboembolic Disease

A potential sequel to HCM is the formation of blood clots in a dilated left atrium as described. See p. 163.

Dilated Cardiomyopathy

Overview

Dilated cardiomyopathy (DCM) is a disease that causes thinning of the muscle walls of the left ventricle (interventricular septum and left ventricular free wall; Fig. 20-11). It can be caused by a deficiency of taurine, an essential amino acid; however, it also occurs in cats with normal dietary and blood levels of taurine. Because the level of taurine in commercial cat foods was raised to feline-sufficient levels in the late 1980s, the incidence of DCM is much less than it was prior to that.

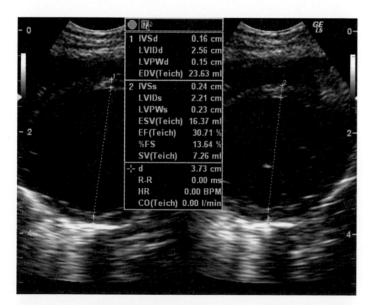

Figure 20-11 Dilated cardiomyopathy. In contrast to Figure 20-10b, these left ventricular walls are very thin, measuring 0.16 and 0.15 cm (N = 0.30–0.55 cm). Note that there is little difference in the left ventricular internal diameter between systole (left) and diastole (right). This is represented in the fractional shortening being 13.64% (N = 35%–55%) and results in reduced cardiac output.

Diagnosis

Because the walls of the left ventricle are thinner than normal, they are also weaker and less able to contract with the force needed to move blood well. This results in reduced cardiac output and CHF. Measurement of the left ventricular walls with an echocardiogram is the confirmatory test.

Treatment

Treatment of cats with DCM is the same as described in CHF. Pimobendan, a drug with proven efficacy for DCM in dogs, is often used in cats. Documentation of efficacy is pending.

Restrictive Cardiomyopathy

Overview

Restrictive cardiomyopathy (RCM) is an uncommon heart disease characterized by fibrosis (scarring) of the myocardium (muscular heart walls). The cause has not been documented; however, inflammation of the cardiac walls (myocarditis) is present in many cases. It can have characteristics of HCM and DCM so it is classified as an intermediate form of cardiomyopathy. RCM ultimately causes CHF; treatment is as described for CHF.

Primary Mitral Insufficiency

Overview

The mitral valve is a one-way valve. When the left atrium contracts, blood is forced through it into the left ventricle. When the left ventricle contracts, blood is refused re-entry into the left atrium because of the mitral valve; instead, blood is forced through the aortic valve into the aorta. If the mitral valve leaflets do not close completely, blood re-enters the left atrium, and a murmur occurs. Incompetence of the mitral valve that occurs without other cardiac disease being present is termed primary mitral insufficiency (PMI).

PMI is a common disease in small breeds of dogs that is most likely controlled by genetics. It occurs infrequently in cats and is most likely unrelated to genetics.

Diagnosis

PMI is virtually always accompanied by a 2+ grade murmur. Clinical signs are often not present. An echocardiogram is used to confirm the diagnosis.

Treatment

Treatment is generally not instituted unless clinical signs of heart failure or ECG (tachycardia, bradycardia, arrhythmia, etc.) abnormalities occur. When CHF occurs, treatment proceeds as described previously.

Ventricular Septal Defect

Overview

The most common congenital heart disease of kittens is ventricular septal defect (VSD). A hole occurs in the interventricular septum. When systole occurs, blood is forced from the left to right ventricle because the contraction velocity is greater in the left ventricle. A loud murmur occurs. Kittens may exhibit this murmur as early as a few weeks of age; it may be detected on the first kitten vaccine examination. They usually have a very loud murmur (Grade 4 or 5). Finding a murmur in a kitten less than 3 months old justifies a diagnostic workup.

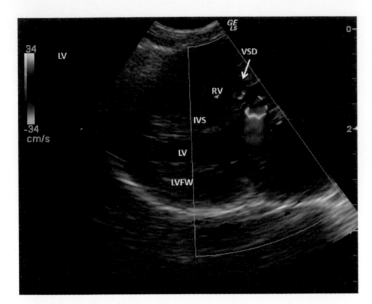

Figure 20-12 Ventricular septal defect (VSD). Blood can be seen flowing from the left ventricle (LV) through the defect into the right ventricle (RV). IVS, interventricular septum; LVFW, left ventricular free wall.

Diagnosis and Treatment

Diagnosis is confirmed with ultrasound using color-flow Doppler. The defect (hole) in the septal wall can usually be seen; blood can be visualized going through it from the left to right ventricle (Fig. 20-12). Most septal defects occur high on the septal wall near the aortic valve. Some small VSDs close as the kitten grows; however, most do not. Surgery to repair the defect is not feasible at the present time so medical management if CHF occurs is the mainstay of treatment.

Pericardial Diaphragmatic Hernia

Overview

The diaphragm is a thin sheet of muscle that separates the chest from the abdomen. It stretches from side to side and from dorsum to ventrum. The pericardium is a thin sac that surrounds the heart. A pericardial diaphragmatic hernia (PDH) is a hole in the diaphragm that communicates with the pericardium. Depending on its size, it may permit much of the liver and loops of intestines into the pericardium.

Clinical Signs and Diagnosis

When stressed, affected kittens have little stamina. They may breathe heavily and rapidly, even with their mouths open. Cyanosis of the tongue is possible. A chest radiograph reveals a very large, usually round cardiac silhouette (Fig. 20-13). The disease is confirmed with an echocardiogram that reveals abnormal structures (liver, small intestine) within the pericardium (Fig. 20-14).

Cats with PDH that live indoors may not show clinical signs; the abnormality may be detected when a thoracic radiograph is made for other reasons.

Treatment

Most PDHs can be surgically corrected. It is technically easier in cats more than 6 months of age, and most cats survive well until this age if they are not physically stressed.

(a)

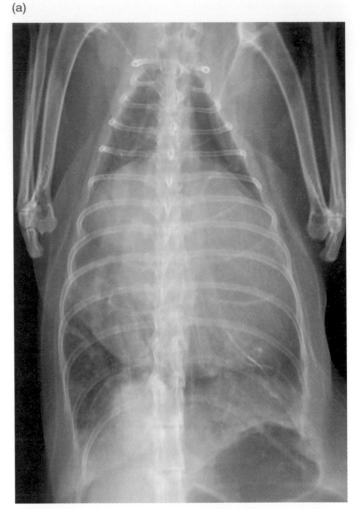

(b)

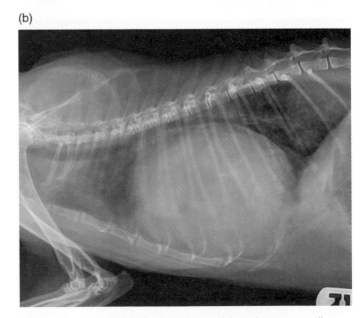

Figure 20-13 Pericardial diaphragmatic hernia. Abdominal contents, usually one or more lobes of the liver, have moved through the rent in the diaphragm and entered the pericardium giving it a global appearance in the dorsoventral (a) and lateral (b) radiographic views.

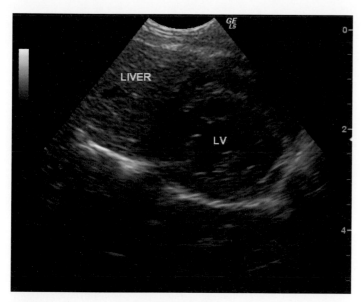

Figure 20-14 Ventricular septal defect. Ultrasound of the pericardium shows liver adjacent to the heart. LV, left ventricle.

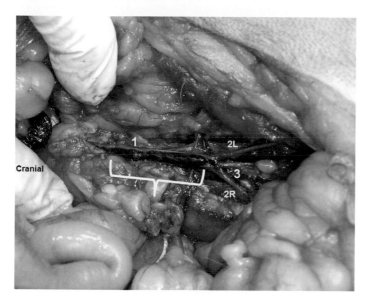

Figure 20-15 Saddle thrombus. A very large thrombus (brackets) is seen in the longitudinally split aorta (1). Blood flow through the internal iliac arteries (2L and 2R) and the median caudal artery (3) is occluded causing acute onset of paralysis and severe pain in the rear legs.

Thromboembolism

Overview

Thromboembolism is a disease that results from a blood clot (thrombus) that accesses circulation and becomes lodged somewhere downstream. The most common scenario is formation of a thrombus in an enlarged

left atrium. Initially it is usually attached to the inner left atrial wall or the mitral valve; however, as it enlarges it breaks free, goes through the mitral valve into the left ventricle, and then exits the heart into the aorta.

The most common route taken is the descending aorta. Because it decreases in diameter as it traverses caudally, the thrombus usually lodges when the aorta splits into three arteries – one to each rear leg and one to the tail. This is called a saddle thrombus (Fig. 20-15). When this occurs, flood flow is terminated to the rear legs and the tail. These parts are paralyzed and become painful. Over a few hours the feet and rear legs get cold. Femoral pulses are no longer palpable.

There are other locations a thrombus can lodged. If it travels cranially it usually obstructs much of the blood flow to the right front leg resulting in sudden-onset lameness. If it enters the renal artery, acute renal failure may occur.

Diagnosis

Diagnosis is based on appropriate clinical signs, which may be dramatic. If the diagnosis is questionable, ultrasound of the abdominal aorta can be confirmatory. Successful ultrasound of other thrombus locations is usually not possible. Nonselect angiography of the abdominal aorta is another test that can be used.

Treatment

The first part of treatment is directed at relieving the resulting pain and restoring leg function. Analgesics are given, and heat is applied to the legs. The legs are massaged several times per day to encourage formation of collateral circulation. The second part of treatment is to address the underlying heart disease. An echocardiogram should be performed so the cardiac disease can be understood; most of these cats have HCM. If the cat is in CHF, treatment for that is instituted. If the cat is not in CHF, there may be no immediate need for cardiac drugs.

About 50% of cats with a saddle thrombus will die within the first 24 hours. If they survive that long and their underlying heart disease can be controlled, function of the rear legs usually returns in 2–3 weeks, and the prognosis is good as long as another clot does not form and pass.

Suggested Readings

Norsworthy GD. 2010. Diaphragmatic Hernia. In GD Norsworthy, ed., *The Feline Patient*, 4th ed., pp. 121–23. Ames: Wiley-Blackwell.

Norsworthy GD. 2010. Plueral Effusion. In GD Norsworthy, ed., *The Feline Patient*, 4th ed., pp. 412–13. Ames: Wiley-Blackwell.

Tilley LP. 2010. Dilated Cardiomyopathy. In GD Norsworthy, ed., *The Feline Patient*, 4th ed. pp. 129–30. Ames: Wiley-Blackwell.

Tilley LP. 2010. Hypertrophic Cardiomyopathy. In GD Norsworthy, ed., *The Feline Patient*, 4th ed., pp. 261–64. Ames: Wiley-Blackwell.

Tilley, LP. 2010. Ventricular Septal Defect. In GD Norsworthy, ed., *The Feline Patient*, 4th ed., pp. 546–47. Ames: Wiley-Blackwell.

Tilley LP. 2010. Thromboembolic Disease. In GD Norsworthy, ed., *The Feline Patient*, 4th ed., pp. 506–8. Ames: Wiley-Blackwell.

Tilley LP, Smith FWK. 2010. Arrhythmias. In GD Norsworthy, ed., *The Feline Patient*, 4th ed., pp. 26–27. Ames: Wiley-Blackwell.

Tilley LP, Smith FWK. 2010. Mumurs. In GD Norsworthy, ed., *The Feline Patient*, 4th ed., pp. 334–35. Ames: Wiley-Blackwell.

Dermatology

Gary D. Norsworthy

Introduction

Skin disease is not as common in cats as in dogs, but it is still a significant part of feline practice.

Skin Anatomy and Function

The skin is comprised of two distinct layers, the epidermis and the dermis. Immediately below the skin is a layer of tissue known as the subcutis.

The epidermis is comprised of four or five microscopic layers depending on location with the nonhaired areas of the pads and nasal planum having the fifth layer.

The dermis is comprised of collagen, elastic and reticular fibers, interstitial ground substance, nervous tissue, blood vessels, lymphatics, arrector pili muscles, and various cellular components.

A hair follicle is the hair and the immediate surrounding structures. Hair follicles extend from the epidermis to the deep layer of the dermis. Feline hair shafts grow to a genetically determined length grouping cats into short-haired, medium-haired, and long-haired breeds. After several weeks to months a hair will be released (shed); soon it will be replaced by a new one. Shedding may be spontaneous, seasonal, or induced by stress or excitement. The latter explains why cats are always shedding when they visit a veterinary hospital.

The skin's thickness varies from one location to another. In general, the skin is thickest on the dorsum of the trunk and on the proximal aspects of the limbs. The latter has clinical significance when venipunctures are made. Because the skin is thinnest in the more distil aspects of the limbs, it is easier to make a venipuncture in these locations.

Allergic Dermatitis

The concept of allergy is based on an exaggerated, abnormal response of the immune system to a substance not normally found in the body. Only rarely are cats born with allergies. Rather, allergies are developed after weeks to months to years of exposure to the foreign material. Thus, it is unusual to find a cat younger than 1 year of age with an allergic condition.

Feline allergies are typically three types: food, flea, and inhalant. Contact allergy is another type that is uncommon in cats. Unlike humans, the primary, and usually only, manifestation of allergy is itching. Respiratory manifestations (sneezing, wheezing) are not typical finding in allergic cats.

Food Allergy

A food allergy is an abnormal response of the immune system to a food component going through the digestive tract. Food intolerance also causes distress but is caused by an adverse response not controlled by the immune system. Because it can be difficult to separate

Nursing the Feline Patient, First Edition. Edited by Linda E. Schmeltzer and Gary D. Norsworthy.

the two in some cases, the term *food reaction* is often used to include both types of adverse response.

In theory, cats may be allergic to any type of food product. However, the allergen most commonly causing a food reaction is the protein source. This is an important concept for testing purposes.

Although there are blood tests available to determine a food allergen, the accuracy of these tests has been questioned repeatedly in humans, dogs, and cats. Therefore, most veterinarians rely on food trials to diagnose food allergy and to determine the specific offending foods. This means feeding a protein source never before eaten by the cat. Because it can take 4–6 weeks for all present food to be eliminated from the body, a food trial lasts for 6 weeks. During this time a special diet is fed with either a protein never before eaten (rabbit, duck, venison) or a food composed of protein molecules that have been broken down (hydrolyzed) to components too small for the immune system to recognize. During these 6 weeks, the diet must be limited exclusively to the test diet; no other cat food, dog food, table food, or treats should be fed. A positive result is the elimination of the clinical signs. A failed food trial means that the clinical signs persist. If that occurs, the trial can be repeated using another food product; however, it is unusual for a second trial to be successful.

The most common clinical sign of food allergy is itching. The cat scratches, licks, or bites the skin resulting in hair loss. Most cases of food allergy have itching limited to the head and neck (Fig. 21-1). Uncommonly, hair loss may be on other parts of the body or vomiting or diarrhea may occur. Chronic rhinitis (sneezing and nasal discharge) has also been induced by food allergy in a few cats. Respiratory signs are unlikely. Cats may also have food allergy and another form of allergy simultaneously, which may result in itching and hair loss on other parts of the body.

Treatment for food allergy is withdrawal of the offending food. This may mean continuing the food trial diet on a long-term basis. Because of the expense of these diets, clients may wish to try other commercial foods. If so, direct them away from protein sources the cat has eaten in the past. Have them read the label on the package to determine ingredients.

Typically, cats with food allergy do not respond well or at all to oral or injectable corticosteroids. Because the skin lesions of food allergy may be similar to inhalant allergy, lack of response to corticosteroids can be an important negative finding that should prompt the veterinarian to consider a food trial.

Inhalant Allergy (Atopy)

Inhalation of offending substances can trigger a strong allergic response. Unlike humans, this response is typically manifested as itching in the skin and not respiratory signs. There is no body region that is typical for inhalant allergy. Because many of the allergens are airborne and plant related (pollens), many cats with inhalant allergy have seasonal disease. However, many of these cats will develop allergies to other substances over time; therefore, what may begin as a seasonal disease may morph into a year-round problem.

Diagnosis of inhalant allergy begins with the recognition of the clinical sign of itching, which may be severe in some cats. Following suspicion of allergy, clinical confirmation can be made in one of two ways. Relief of clinical signs within hours to a few days after corticosteroids are given is a strong indicator of inhalant allergy (Fig. 21-2). Intradermal or blood testing are also ways to identify allergens that may be causing the problem. Intradermal testing is based on injecting small amounts of

(a)

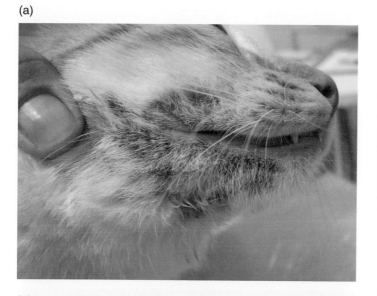

(b)

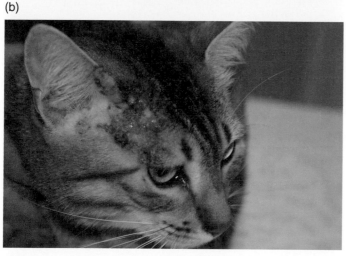

Figure 21-1 Food allergy produces pruritus and results in scratching and hair loss. Most lesions are located on the head and neck. (a) This cat was allergic to fish. (b) The specific allergen for this cat was not found, but the lesions are typical of a food allergy.
(a) courtesy Dr. Vanessa Pimentel.

(a)

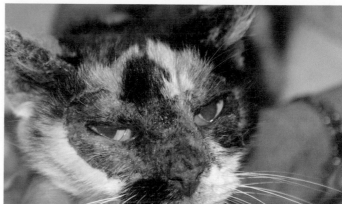

(b)

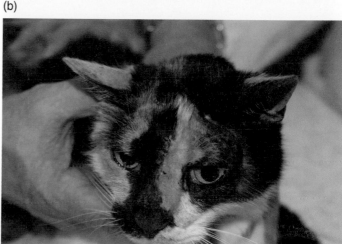

Figure 21-2 (a) This cat had hair loss and signs of self-trauma in many locations including the head and neck. (b) After treatment with corticosteroids for 6 weeks the itching, self-trauma, and hair loss were gone. Inhalant allergies often respond dramatically to corticosteroids.

many potential allergens into the skin and observing for an abnormal response at each injection site. The blood tests are based on detecting immunoglobulin E (IgE) levels specific for various allergens.

Treatment can be performed in three ways: (1) The ideal approach is to remove the cat from its allergens. This requires no further treatment, but it may not be possible in many cats. (2) Because the side effects of corticosteroids are not as severe in cats as in dogs, intermittent treatment with injectable or oral corticosteroids can be effective and safe. The dose and frequency should be the minimum amount and frequency required as determined by the veterinarian. (3) Hyposensitization is an attempt to "reprogram" the immune system so it no longer overreacts to the allergens. Small amounts of the allergens are injected subcutaneously once or twice per week over weeks to months. Unfortunately, this approach is not always successful.

Flea Allergic Dermatitis (FAD)

When fleas bite a normal cat little local reaction occurs. It is likely that the cat is unaware of the bite. However, after the cat has been bitten repeatedly over weeks to months, it may develop an allergic reaction to the saliva in the flea's mouth. At that point, each bite evokes a strong, pruritic response resulting in itching and self-trauma.

Clinical signs of FAD are hair loss and inflamed skin. Because fleas have a propensity to bite just cranial to the base of the tail (tail head), this location is likely to experience the reaction and hair loss first. Scabs and flea dirt are often present followed by hair loss. Scratching this area with one's fingers usually stimulates to cat to turn and lick further or to lick it front feet (Fig. 21-3a).

Diagnosis is based on the presence of fleas or flea dirt, the characteristic skin lesions, especially at the tail head, and response to therapy. Although these may be sufficient for a diagnosis, confirmation may be made with intradermal skin testing or blood tests for allergy.

The most important aspect of treatment is to remove existing fleas and prevent further exposure to fleas. If these are both possible, further treatment is not needed. However, in most cases it is not possible to completely control flea exposure so corticosteroids can be used to stop the reaction and give the cat relief. Even in the presence of further flea bites, corticosteroids will bring the cat relief because it blocks the allergic reaction that causes itching.

(a)

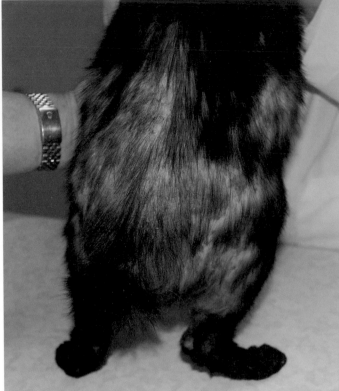

(b)

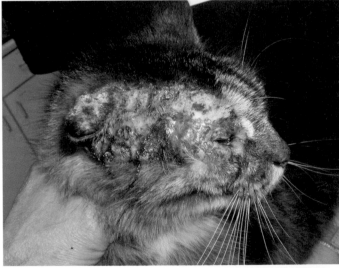

Figure 21-3 Flea allergic dermatitis causes intense pruritus, chewing, scratching, and hair loss. (a) The most common location is the tail head. (b) However, other areas may itch intensely, including the head and face.

(a)

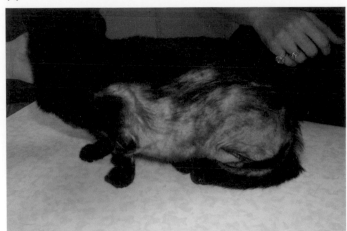

(b)

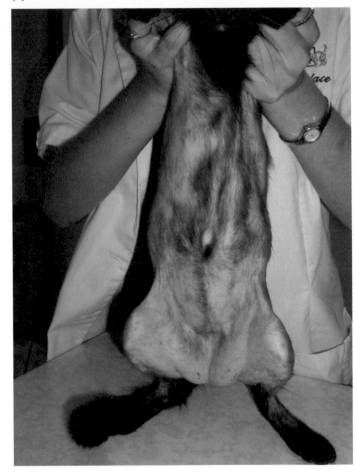

Figure 21-4 Bilateral truncal alopecia is characteristic of obsessive-compulsive alopecia. (a) This cat had symmetrical alopecia on its sides. (b) It also had hair loss on its ventral abdomen and the caudal aspect of the rear legs.

Obsessive-Compulsive Alopecia

Some cats with pruritic skin disease from any cause (food allergy, inhalant allergy, flea-bite dermatitis) will lick and scratch long enough to develop a compulsive desire to continue licking even if the itching is relieved. This is also called psychogenic alopecia. The cat will lick, chew, or scratch compulsively. This results in hair loss that is usually bilaterally asymmetrical. The areas most commonly affected include the caudal aspects of the rear legs, the ventral abdomen, and the flanks (Fig. 21-4).

Treatment is based on treating any skin disease that is causing itching and controlling the obsessive-compulsive aspect of the disorder. Treatment of the former is described previously. Treatment of the latter is based on centrally acting drugs, such as phenobarbital, clomipramine, or others. One of these drugs is usually given for 4–6 weeks while pruritus is controlled appropriately. If the cat is normal at 4–6 weeks, the centrally acting drug is withdrawn. If compulsive licking returns, the drug is reinstated for another 4–6 weeks. In a few cats, therapy may be needed for months to break the compulsion.

Acne

Acne is a proliferation of the glands in the skin of the chin. It is usually found in adult cats; however, it has been reported in a few cats younger than 1 year of age.

Acne causes comedones (black heads) to form in the hair follicles of the chin. Rarely, they may also form on the lower or upper lips. Hair loss begins so the cat's chin has a peppered appearance. Infection can occur resulting in swelling of the chin and purulent drainage from the hair follicles (Fig. 21-5).

Treatment begins with clipping the hair from the chin to assess the degree of the disease and to permit better application of topical medications. Prior to application of a topical antibiotic, the chin should be

(a)

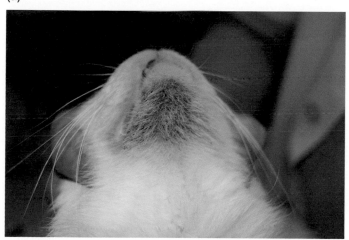

(b)

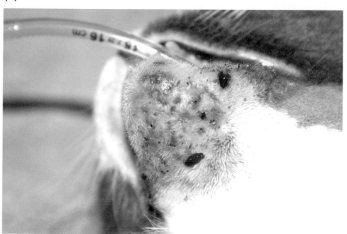

Figure 21-5 Acne causes comedones to form on the chin (a) and can become infected (b).

hot-packed to open the pores for better penetration. A warm, moist cloth should be applied to the chin for 30–60 seconds prior to application of a topical antibiotic such as clindamycin. If infection is present systemic antibiotics that are likely to be effective against *Staphylococcus* are used. In some cases, a 2- to 3-day course of a corticosteroid may be helpful to relieve swelling and pain so the cat will permit topical therapy.

Dermatophytosis

Dermatophytosis is an infection with a cutaneous (affecting the skin) fungus. It is commonly called *ringworm*. The circular shape of the lesions is the basis for the *ring* portion of this term, but the disease is not due to a worm. Although the term is both incorrect and misleading, it is in widespread use.

There are two primary fungal species that infect the hair, skin, and nails of cats. *Microsporum canis* is diagnosed in about 90% of feline cases, and *Trichophyton mentagrophytes* accounts for the majority of the remaining 10%.

The fungus invades growing hairs, causing them to fall out. Then the fungus spreads to the more peripheral hairs, usually resulting in a circular lesion. However, the lesions are not always circular and can be irregular in shape (Fig. 21-6a). Immunosuppression or open skin lesions make active infection more likely.

Transmission of the fungi is by direct contact, fomite contact, or via a contaminated environment. Thus, animal (cat, dog, or other)-to-animal, human-to-cat, or environment-to-cat transmission is possible. The fungi can live in the environment 12–24 months, making environmental decontamination an important aspect of control.

Diagnosis begins with the observation of focal alopecia (hair loss), often with crusts on the skin. The lesions are so nonspecific that they can mimic almost any skin disease. A Wood's light examination of the skin causes affected hairs to fluoresce with a characteristic apple-green color (Fig. 21-6b). Note that many topical medications also fluoresce, so it is important to observe fluorescence of individual hair shafts that have been broken just above the skin surface, leaving stubble. Fungal culture is the only method of confirming dermatophytosis. Dermatophyte test media (DTM™) and Sabouraud's dextrose agar are the most commonly used media. A positive culture results in a change of the media color from yellow to red, followed by a white cottony growth of the fungus (Fig. 21-6c). Saprophytes (fungal skin contaminants) will cause the red color change after colony growth. Direct microscopic examination of the hair shafts revealing arthrospore invasion into the hair shafts can also confirm diagnosis.

Treatment is multipronged. Systemic fungal drugs are almost always required to eliminate the infection and prevent the carrier state. Griseofulvin and itraconazole are the most commonly used drugs. Griseofulvin can be dangerous in a pregnant cat or a cat infected with the feline immunodeficiency virus. It can also cause liver or bone marrow toxicity, although these occur infrequently when the drug is administered at proper doses. Fat in the stomach is required for good absorption. Itraconazole is much more expensive and can cause liver toxicity and birth defects in some cats. The chosen oral drug should be given a minimum of 30 days and longer if active lesions persist. Topical antifungal drugs are also useful, but cats are often not tolerant of topical drugs and will lick them off quickly.

It is important to prevent spread of fungal spores because they become the source of future infections. Lime sulfur dip or enilconazole are used for this purpose. Clipping long-haired cats can be beneficial, but extreme care must be taken to prevent skin abrasions that can result in increased growth and spread of the fungus. Environmental control is also central to stopping this disease. Vigorous vacuuming of exposed areas, especially those with carpet or upholstery, is important. A solution of 1 part bleach and 10–30 parts water should be used on bleachable surfaces.

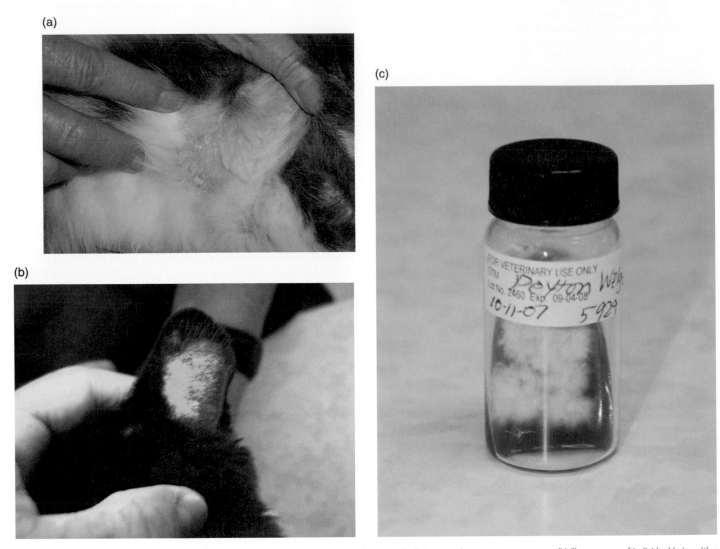

Figure 21-6 (a) Round, focal areas of crusty alopecia are the typical ringworm lesions; however, the lesions can have many appearances. (b) Fluorescence of individual hairs with a Wood's light is typical for *Microsporum canis* but not for *Trichophyton mentagrophytes*. (c) A white cottony growth will occur after the agar turns yellow to red for a diagnosis of dermatophytosis to be confirmed.

(a)

(b)

(c)

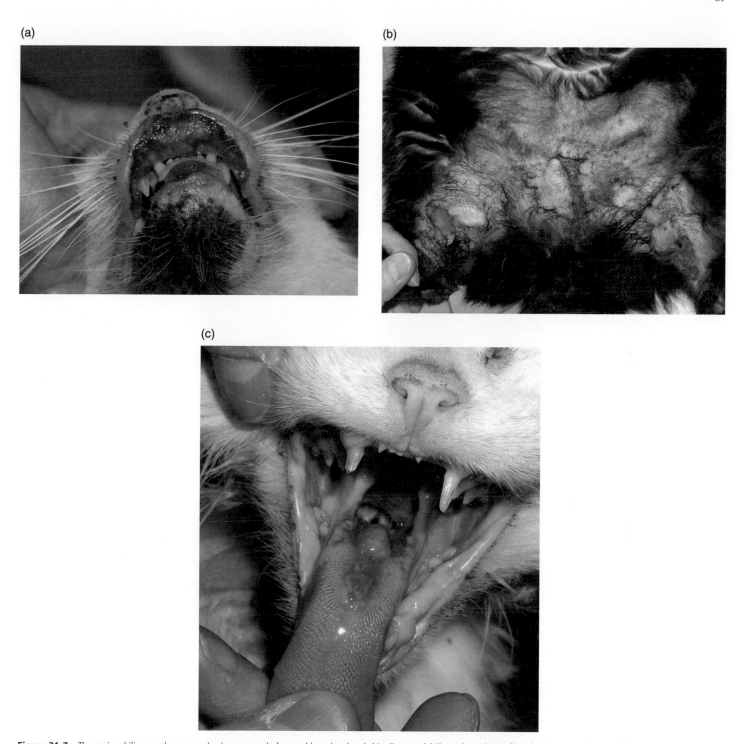

Figure 21-7   The eosinophilic granuloma complex is composed of several loosely related skin diseases. (a) The rodent ulcer is found on the upper lips and, when severe, may extend past the upper canine teeth. (b) Eosinophilic plaques most commonly occur on the ventral abdomen, although they may also occur at the base of the tongue (c).

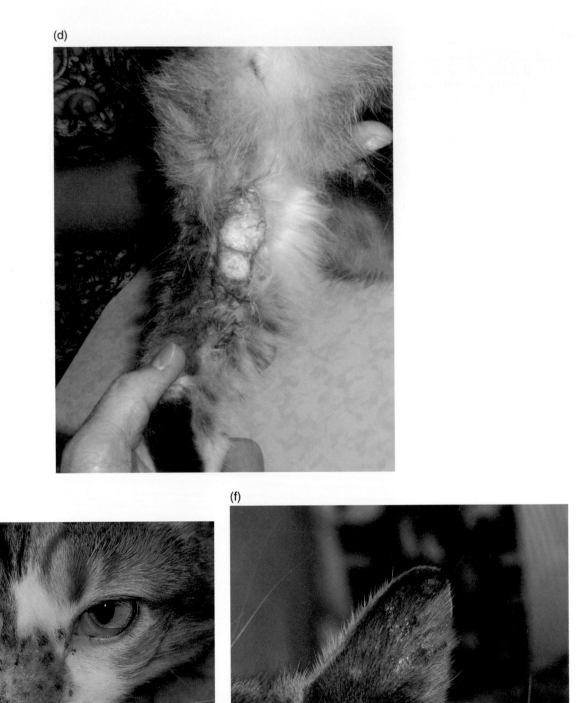

Figure 21-7 (cont'd) (d) An eosinophilic granuloma is a raised, linear mass or collection of masses usually found on the caudal aspect of the rear legs. In this location it is sometimes called a linear granuloma. Mosquito-bite hypersensitivity is a local reaction that occurs on the bridge of the nose (e) and the pinnae (f).

Eosinophilic Granuloma Complex (EGC)

The EGC is a group of somewhat-related diseases that cause characteristic, local skin reactions. Most are infiltrated with eosinophils suggesting an allergic component, and most respond well to corticosteroids. Some of the more common manifestations will be described.

An eosinophilic ulcer ("rodent ulcer") is a unique disease that occurs on the upper lips of the cat and is usually bilateral. A small to very large ulcer occurs resulting in pain and odiferous breath. Some cats are so painful that eating becomes problematic (Fig. 21-7a).

Eosinophilic plaques are masses that form on the ventral abdomen (Fig. 21-7b), between the toes, and on the base of the tongue (Fig. 21-7c).

An eosinophilic granuloma is a linear-shaped row of raised lesions that typically occur on the caudal aspect of the rear legs (Fig. 21-7d).

Mosquito-bite hypersensitivity is the reaction that occurs in some cats to mosquito bites. The primary locations are the areas with thin hair, notably the bridge of the nose (Fig. 21-7e), the pinnae (Fig. 21-7f), or the thin-haired area between the eyes and the ears.

Treatment for the various forms of the EGC is based on corticosteroids. Because there is likely an allergic component to most of these, identification of allergens, including food, is also indicated. Unless an underlying disease can be identified and controlled, intermittent or long-term use of corticosteroids may be needed as these are all recurrent diseases. If corticosteroid use is not feasible (ineffective or side effects) other immunosuppressants, including cyclosporine, should be tried.

Suggested Readings

Horwitz DF. Psychogenic Alopecia. 2010. In GD Norsworthy, ed., *The Feline Patient*, 4th ed., pp. 587–90. Ames: Wiley-Blackwell.

Rees CA. Acne. 2010. In GD Norsworthy, ed. *The Feline Patient*, 4th ed., p. 7. Ames: Wiley-Blackwell.

Rees CA. Atopic Dermatitis. 2010. In GD Norsworthy, ed., *The Feline Patient*, 4th ed., pp. 33–34. Ames: Wiley-Blackwell.

Rees CA. Eosinophilic Granuloma Complex. 2010. In GD Norsworthy, ed., *The Feline Patient*, 4th ed., pp. 154–56. Ames: Wiley-Blackwell.

Rees CA. Flea Allergy Dermatitis. 2010. In GD Norsworthy, ed., *The Feline Patient*, 4th ed., pp. 189–90. Ames: Wiley-Blackwell.

Rees CA. Food Reaction. 2010. In GD Norsworthy, ed., *The Feline Patient*, 4th ed., pp. 195–96. Ames: Wiley-Blackwell.

Diseases of the Digestive System

Linda E. Schmeltzer and Gary D. Norsworthy

Overview

The primary function of the digestive system is to break down food into smaller particles that the body can absorb and use for nutrition and energy at a cellular level. The digestive system consists of a continuous tube – the gastrointestinal (GI) tract – that extends from the mouth to the anus. The process of digestion within the GI tract is aided by secretions from accessory digestive organs: the salivary glands, liver, gall bladder, and pancreas. This overview covers the basic structure of the GI tract and the functions of the liver, bile duct, and gall bladder.

Gastrointestinal Tract: Basic Structure

The organs of the GI tract include the mouth, pharynx, esophagus, stomach, small intestine, cecum, and large intestine. The wall of the GI tract is made up of four layers. From inside to outside they are the mucosa, submucosa, muscularis, and serosa. The mucosa is a moist layer of semi-permeable tissue. In the stomach and intestine the mucosa also contains exocrine cells that secrete mucus and fluid into the GI tract. The submucosa is a layer of dense irregular connective tissue that contains glands, nerves, and blood vessels and joins the mucosa to the muscularis. The muscularis is two thin layers of smooth muscle. The inner circular muscle layer prevents food from traveling backward, and the longitudinal muscle layer shortens the digestive tract. Involuntary contraction of these layers is called peristalsis. Peristaltic contractions help to physically break food down, mix it with digestive secretions, and propel it along the GI tract. The serosa, the outermost layer of the GI tract, secretes a lubricating fluid that reduces friction with the other organs due to muscle movement.

Hepatobiliary Function

Hepatobiliary refers to the liver, gall bladder, and bile duct. These three organs work together to produce, store, and secrete bile into the GI tract.

The liver is the largest gland in the body. It performs numerous vital functions. One function is to break down toxins, including many medications, absorbed from the GI tract. Liver cells are also known as hepatocytes. Hepatocytes synthesize (build) plasma proteins such as albumin, prothrombin, and fibrinogen. Prothrombin and fibrinogen are needed in the process of coagulation (formation of blood clots). The liver stores and breaks down triglycerides. Hepatocytes synthesize lipoproteins to transport triglycerides and other fats to cells in the body. In the cells fat is processed into energy. Vitamins A, B_{12}, D, E, and K, and some minerals, such as iron, are also stored in the liver.

The gall bladder is a small sac that stores bile until it is needed. Bile contains water, electrolytes, bile acids, cholesterol, and conjugated bilirubin. The gall bladder is connected to the duodenum (upper portion of the small intestine) by the bile duct.

Bilirubin is the yellow pigmented breakdown product of heme. Heme is found in hemoglobin, the oxygen-binding component of red blood cells. Red blood cells are produced in the bone marrow. Their average life span in a cat is about 70 days. Red blood cells must be disposed of when they get old or damaged. The body breaks these cells down into iron,

from the heme, and amino acids, from globin molecules. Iron, amino acids, and globin are recycled. The non-iron protein portion of the heme is converted to unconjugated bilirubin. Unconjugated bilirubin is not water soluble. It is carried to the liver by attaching itself to the plasma protein albumin. In the liver unconjugated bilirubin combines with an acid formed by glucose (glucuronic acid) and becomes conjugated bilirubin making it water soluble. Conjugated bilirubin is stored in the gall bladder as part of bile until it is needed.

The liver makes bile continuously, but bile is needed only when food is in the upper intestine. Normal bacteria in the intestines convert conjugated bilirubin into urobilinogen. Some of the urobilinogen will be absorbed and eliminated in the urine as urobilin. The rest will be converted to stercobilinogen and excreted as stercobilin in the feces. These pigments – urobilin and stercobilin – help give urine and feces their normal colors.

Icterus

Icterus, also known as jaundice, is not a disease; it is a sign that disease is present. Icterus occurs when excess bilirubin is deposited in the tissues. Yellowing of the tissue will first be seen in the soft palate, the soft tissue of the roof of the mouth. Icterus may also be easily seen on the gums; skin, especially the pinnae or ear flaps; third eyelids; sclera, white part of the eyes; and irises, colored portion of the eye (Fig. 22-1).

Normal serum bilirubin in cats is less than 17 umol/L (1.0 mg/dL). The serum of a cat with an elevated serum bilirubin will not appear icteric (yellow) until the levels measure 25–35 umol/L (1.5–2.0 mg/dL). Tissues will not be visibly icteric until serum bilirubin levels exceed 35 umol/L (2.0 mg/dL).

Diagnosis of icterus is simple: a visible yellow color is seen in the tissues or serum. The causes of icterus fall into three main categories.

Prehepatic

An excess breakdown or destruction (hemolysis) of red blood cells will result in an excess amount of unconjugated bilirubin. The liver is not able to conjugate all of the unconjugated bilirubin, and the excess is deposited in the tissues. Hemolysis may be caused by toxic plants, chemicals, drugs, parasites on red blood cells, heartworms, autoimmune diseases, or cancer. Immune-mediated causes of hemolysis are less common in cats than in dogs.

Hepatic

This category is the most common cause of icterus in cats. Any disease that causes destruction or decreased function of liver cells will prevent the liver from conjugating even the normal amount of unconjugated bilirubin. The unconjugated bilirubin from normal red blood cell breakdown will be deposited in the tissues. This may be caused by a disease that primarily involves the liver, such as cholangiohepatitis, or be a secondary symptom of a different disease process, such as feline immunodeficiency virus.

Posthepatic

An obstruction preventing conjugated bilirubin from being passed into the intestines will eventually result in a back up of conjugated bilirubin in the blood stream and the tissues. Obstructions can occur within the

(a)

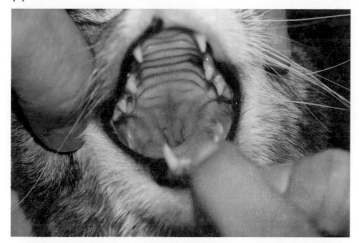

(b)

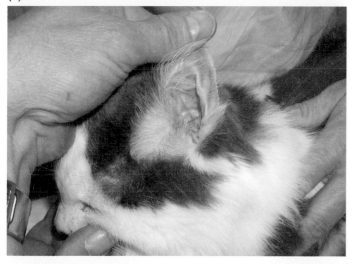

(c)

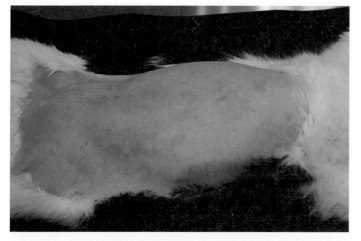

Figure 22-1 (a) Icterus is first seen as two linear streaks in the soft palate. (b) Another common early location for observing icterus is the skin cranial to the pinna or on the pinna itself. (c) Severe icterus results in all of the skin becoming visibly yellow.

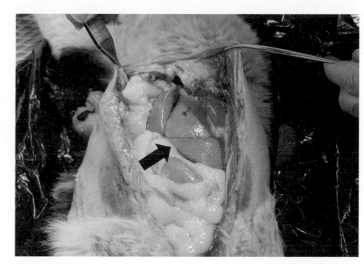

Figure 22-2 This necropsy specimen shows an enlarged and yellow liver (arrow).

gallbladder or anywhere along the bile duct. Such obstructions are less likely to occur in cats than in dogs. Pancreatitis, cholelithiasis (stones in the gall bladder), trauma, cancer, and liver flukes are all possible causes of obstruction.

The Workup

Determining the cause of icterus can be difficult and usually requires several tests. Initial tests may include a complete blood count (CBC), chemistry profile, urinalysis, and screening for feline leukemia virus and feline immunodeficiency virus. Once the probable cause is placed into one of the three categories (prehepatic, hepatic, or posthepatic), additional tests may be needed to determine the specific disease causing the icteric state. Abdominal ultrasound or radiography to evaluate the liver, pancreas, and gall bladder may be ordered. Biopsies of the liver or aspiration of the bile in the gall bladder may also be needed to diagnose specific diseases.

There is no treatment for icterus itself. Treatment for the underlying disease is required for icterus to resolve. The prognosis will depend on the underlying cause.

Hepatic Lipidosis

The most common liver disorder in cats is hepatic lipidosis, also known as fatty liver syndrome. It is caused by an excessive accumulation of triglycerides within the liver. When a cat does not eat for an extended period of time, stored fat (triglycerides) will be broken down in the liver to supply energy to the body's cells. Without an adequate source of dietary protein, the liver is not able to efficiently convert triglycerides into usable energy. The liver will take in fat at a faster rate than it is able to convert and export it causing an excess accumulation of fat in the liver (Fig. 22-2).

The origin of this disease is not well understood. Obesity will make a cat more susceptible to hepatic lipidosis. In many cats a thorough history and diagnostic workup will expose a primary disease or circumstance that caused the anorexia; however, the anorexia-inducing disease will not always be present or diagnosed. Circumstances, such as a new diet, harassment by another pet, or separation from the owner, can cause anorexia. Diseases such as cholangiohepatitis, pancreatitis, and diabetes mellitus have been reported as primary causes leading to hepatic lipidosis.

Clinical signs of hepatic lipidosis can include anorexia, weight loss, icterus, and vomiting. When taking a history, questions about the cat's living environment and habits prior to the onset of anorexia will be helpful in determining a primary cause. Any cat with a history of obesity and a period of anorexia lasting at least 1 week should be suspected of hepatic lipidosis.

A comprehensive blood profile will show a marked alkaline phosphatase increase (two to five times normal). More than 50% of affected cats will have hypoalbuminemia (low blood albumin). A mild nonregenerative anemia may also be present. A urinalysis may reveal bilirubinuria (the presence of bilirubin in the urine). Microscopic evaluation of the hepatocytes will be required to confirm a diagnosis of hepatic lipidosis. Cells or tissue may be collected by a fine-needle aspirate, fine-needle biopsy, core needle biopsy, or wedge biopsy. See Chapter 9. Some patients may require several days of hospitalization and treatment before they are stable enough to undergo anesthesia for any procedures.

Treatment: Phase One

Treatment for hepatic lipidosis occurs in two phases. The first phase, stabilization, lasts approximately 2–7 days and involves hospitalization. Almost all deaths from hepatic lipidosis occur during this phase. Minimizing patient stress as much as possible can increase the survival rate. This phase of therapy may include:

- Control of vomiting: Antivomiting medication may be needed to control vomiting. The stomach of cats with hepatic lipidosis may have a small capacity. Feeding small quantities of food frequently will help prevent vomiting caused from feeding too large of a meal.
- Intravenous or subcutaneous fluids are used to correct dehydration.
- Potassium may be added to the fluids or given orally. Serum potassium levels should be monitored and potassium supplementation adjusted as needed.
- Nutrition is the cornerstone of treatment. A balanced diet containing adequate protein is needed to form the lipoproteins necessary to transport triglycerides out of the liver. Nutritional support begins with the use of syringe feeding or orogastric tube feeding to efficiently deliver a balanced diet. The daily nutritional goal is 60–90 kcal/kg of ideal body weight.
- Antibiotics, usually amoxicillin or metronidazole, are recommended to treat possible underlying infection. Avoid antibiotics that have vomiting as a side effect.
- S-adenosylmethionine (SAMe) and milk thistle are nutraceutical agents that have been shown to have anti-inflammatory and antioxidant properties within the liver. These medications are best absorbed when given on an empty stomach, preferably at least 1 hour before food.
- Vitamin K supplementation is important because absorption is impaired as a result of decreased bile flow and lack of fat ingestion. Bleeding from a liver biopsy site is much less likely if vitamin K is given prior to biopsy.
- Vitamin B$_{12}$ is used as an appetite stimulant and to further support liver function.

Treatment: Phase Two

The second phase of treatment, long-term care, can last for several weeks until the cat's appetite returns.

- Antibiotics and medications to support hepatocyte function will be continued for 2–4 weeks.
- Nutritional support is still of primary importance. An indwelling feeding tube, such as an esophagostomy tube or gastrostomy tube, will be needed to efficiently deliver nutrition. The use of these tubes allows owners to take their cat home and still manage feedings successfully. Feeding small quantities three to six times per day is recommended because the stomach will take time to return to normal capacity. Veterinary technicians should become familiar with the

(a)

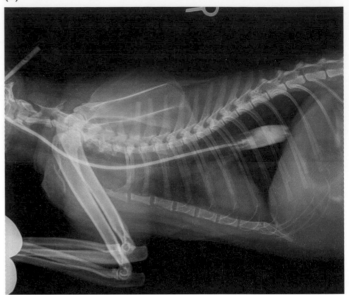

(b)

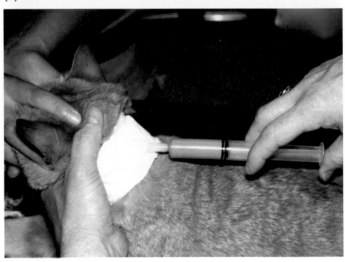

Figure 22-3 (a) An esophagostomy tube is placed through an incision in the neck and extends to the lower esophagus. Injected contrast material shows its placement. (b) Feeding is as simple as injecting food through the tube. Most clients can do this without assistance.

type of indwelling feeding tube used in their practices. Proper care and maintenance of these tubes is important for the patient's well-being. Understanding how the tube is placed and what problems can occur after placement is important so owners' questions may be answered properly and potential problems that need veterinary attention can be quickly identified (Fig. 22-3).

Completion of Therapy and Prognosis

When a cat returns to eating normally, treatment is discontinued. On average it takes about 6 weeks for the appetite to return. Liver function will eventually return to normal; there is no long-term damage.

The prognosis is good with aggressive therapy and treatment of the underlying disease or circumstance that caused the anorexia. The most common reason for failure is the inability to successfully treat an underlying disease that perpetuates anorexia. It is possible for hepatic lipidosis to recur if there is another episode of prolonged anorexia.

Inflammatory Hepatitis

The second most common liver disease in cats is inflammatory disease. The liver produces bile needed for digestion. Bile is stored in the gall bladder and transported to the intestine through the bile duct. In addition to bile the small intestine needs bacteria. The bile duct is a one-way conduit for bile to pass into the duodenum. Inflammatory hepatitis begins when normal bacteria leave the duodenum and ascend the bile duct to the gall bladder and liver.

Inflammatory hepatitis is separated into two types: cholangitis/cholangiohepatitis complex and lymphocytic portal hepatitis. Clinical signs of the diseases may include anorexia, fever, icterus, vomiting, and weight loss. Cholangiohepatitis means inflammation or infection of the liver, gall bladder, and bile duct. CCH is further divided into acute and chronic forms.

Acute Cholangitis/Cholangiohepatitis

Bacteria are the primary cause of acute cholangitis/cholangiohepatitis (CCH). Most access the gall bladder and bile duct by ascension from the duodenum; however, bacteria may also reach the liver via the blood stream from infections elsewhere in the body. Cats with acute CCH typically exhibit anorexia, vomiting, lethargy, fever, icterus, and sometimes abdominal pain. Confirmation is by liver biopsy, with the predominant inflammatory cells seen on histopathology being neutrophils.

Chronic Cholangitis/Cholangiohepatitis

It is unknown whether chronic CCH is a continuation of acute CCH or an immune-mediated condition. Some cases have been linked to infection and parasites. Fever does not usually occur with chronic CCH. Icterus and hepatomegaly (liver enlargement) are common findings. Ultrasound can reveal changes typical of chronic CCH (Fig. 22-4). Confirmation is by liver biopsy, with the lymphocyte being the predominant inflammatory cell seen on histopathology or cytopathology.

Lymphocytic Portal Hepatitis

Lymphocytic portal hepatitis (LPH) is inflammation of the area around the portal triad. The portal triad contains branches of the hepatic artery, hepatic portal vein, and bile duct bound together within the liver by fibrous tissue. Common clinical signs of LPH are anorexia, weight loss, and hepatomegaly. Illness resulting from LPH is usually not as severe as with CCH.

Diagnosis

Diagnostic tests will be ordered to classify the type of inflammatory hepatitis so the proper treatment may be administered. Coagulation profiles to determine the presence of clotting abnormalities may be requested prior to surgery because clotting abnormalities can significantly complicate any surgical procedure. Tissues are collected though fine-needle aspirates or biopsies. Comprehensive blood profiles, urinalysis, abdominal ultrasound, liver biopsy, and gall bladder aspirates may be among the first tests ordered. Aerobic and anaerobic cultures of the bile aspirated from the gall bladder may be requested to isolate the type of bacteria causing the infection.

Treatment

Treatment for inflammatory hepatitis is determined by the type of disease diagnosed. Depending on the severity of the disease some patients will need to be hospitalized initially for supportive care including fluid therapy and nutritional support.

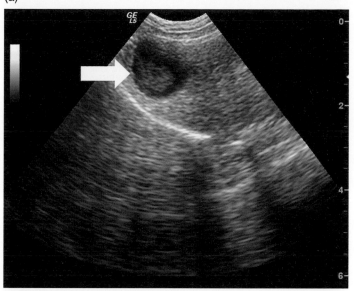

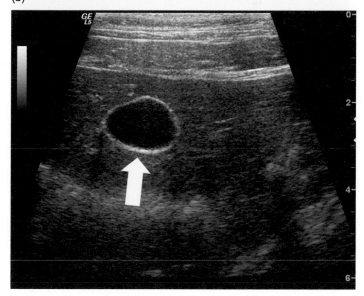

Figure 22-4 Ultrasound findings typical of chronic cholangitis/cholangiohepatitis (CCH) include (a) sludged bile in the gall bladder (arrow) and (b) thickening of the gall bladder walls (arrow).

Acute Cholangitis/Cholangiohepatitis

- Antibiotics for treating the infection are the foundation of the treatment protocol. Up to 12 weeks of antibiotic therapy may be needed to eliminate the infection. A combination of antibiotics may be prescribed at the discretion of the veterinarian.
- Ursodeoxycholic acid is a bile acid that improves the flow of bile, promotes the production of less toxic bile acids, and decreases the immune response to hepatocytes.
- S-adenosylmethionine (SAMe) and silybin (flavonoid extracted from milk thistle) are nutraceutical agents that have been shown to have anti-inflammatory and antioxidant properties within the liver. These medications are best absorbed when given on an empty stomach at least 1 hour before food.

Chronic Cholangiohepatitis

- Antibiotics are usually included in treatment even though most cats do not have active liver or bile infections. Up to 6 weeks of antibiotic therapy may be needed.
- Glucocorticoids, such as prednisolone, are used to decrease inflammation. Prednisolone is created when prednisone is metabolized by the liver. Because the liver is not functioning normally, prednisolone is more likely to be biologically active than prednisone.
- Ursodeoxycholic acid is used for the same effects as in acute CCH.
- S-adenosylmethionine or SAMe plus silybin is used for the same effects as in acute ACH.

Lymphocytic Portal Hepatitis

- Prednisolone is used to decrease inflammation.
- Ursodeoxycholic acid is used as for acute CCH.
- S-adenosylmethionine or SAMe plus silybin is used as for acute CCH.

Prognosis

The prognosis of a cat with inflammatory hepatitis will depend on the severity of the disease, the integrity of the cat's immune system, and the compliance of the owner for medium- to long-term treatment. Many cats with acute CCH recover completely without any long-term effects. Cats with chronic CCH or LPH need long-term or recurrent treatment.

Vomiting

Vomiting may be classified as acute (less than 3 days in duration) or chronic (more than 14 days in duration). Acute vomiting is common in cats to the point that some think (incorrectly) that some vomiting is "normal" for cats, especially when hairballs are involved. Chronic or recurring vomiting is also common and often accepted by cat owners as normal feline behavior.

Irritative Gastritis

There are two things that are commonly swallowed by cats that cause stomach irritation and result in acute vomiting: hair and grass.

Cats shed hair, and cats groom. This results in swallowing of hair. The swallowed hair must either be vomited or pass in the stool. Thus, cats that are compulsive groomers or cats with long hair are predisposed to vomiting hairballs.

Many cats that vomit large hairballs will remain nauseous for 24 hours following hairball expulsion. Symptomatic treatment to prevent further vomiting and correct or prevent dehydration may be need in some cats.

Most cats that eat grass do so because they like the taste of it. Most grasses are hard to digest and irritate the stomach lining. Thus, vomiting of grass and other stomach contents follows. This is contrary to the widely held belief that cats eat grass to cause themselves to vomit.

Foreign Bodies

Cats are not as prone to ingesting foreign objects as dogs. However, this event usually occurs when they are playing with objects and accidently swallow them, resulting in another common cause of acute vomiting. Small objects, such as hair bands and ear plugs, may be swallowed then pass into the small intestine. Obstructions, requiring the need for surgical removal, may result. Swallowing linear objects, such as dental floss, sewing thread, string, and ribbon, is also common. If the linear object is longer than 30 cm (12 inches), it will exceed the length of the peristaltic waves and become trapped in the small intestine. This also requires surgical removal for the cat to survive.

Table 22-1 Characteristics of small dowel diarrhea and large bowel diarrhea. The key to remembering these characteristics is to know that digestion and absorption of nutrients occurs in the small bowel.

Location	Small Bowel	Large Bowel
# BM per day	1–2	5+
Volume of BM	Normal	Small
Mucus in BM	No	Yes
Red blood in BM	No	Yes
Dark blood in BM	Maybe	No
Fat in BM	No	Yes
Urgency	No	Yes
Straining	No	Yes
Weight Loss	Yes	No
Vomiting	Probably	Maybe

BM, bowel movement

Chronic Vomiting

Chronic vomiting is more common than acute vomiting. It is not unusual for cat owners to report vomiting that began infrequently (less than once per 60 days) then slowly (over months to years) increased in frequency to weekly, semi-weekly, or even more than once per day. Some cats have bursts of vomiting that may include several episodes per day for a few days. In general, these cats show little, if any, other clinical signs, which is why owners tolerate it. Because hair is often vomited, owners frequently attribute it to hairballs. These cats need testing to determine the diagnosis because most of them have inflammatory bowel disease or intestinal lymphoma. Both diseases can produce thickening of the small intestinal walls, which can be verified with ultrasound. Both are diagnosed with full-thickness biopsies of the affected areas of the small bowel. Food intolerance is another cause of chronic vomiting, although most of these cats have severe itching in the head and neck area. See Chapter 21. Food trials with novel protein diets (rabbit, duck, or venison) or hydrolyzed diets are used for diagnosis and treatment.

Diarrhea

Diarrhea can also be classified as acute or chronic based on its duration. It is also classified as to the site of origin, being either small bowel diarrhea, large bowel diarrhea, or a combination (Table 22-1).

Acute Diarrhea

Diarrhea of less than 3 days duration is considered to be acute. It is often as a result of dietary indiscretions, but many cases come and go without a confirmed diagnosis. Symptomatic treatment, consisting of antidiarrheal medications and enteric-type diets may be all that is needed for normal stools to return.

Chronic Diarrhea

Diarrhea of 14 days or more duration is considered to be chronic. Intestinal parasites are a common cause, especially in kittens and in cats from multicat situations (shelters, catteries, or homes). Fecal flotation is the first test to be performed. Polymerase chain reaction (PCR) tests for parasites of lesser frequency, such as *Giardia*, *Tritrichomonas*, and *Cryptosporidium*, should be considered if fecal flotation is negative.

Chronic diarrhea may also be diet related or the result of chronic small bowel disease as mentioned previously. Most cases of chronic diarrhea require more than symptomatic treatment. Various tests are indicated based on the characteristics of the diarrhea (*see* Table 22-1), other clinical signs present, and resources available by the client and the veterinarian.

Inflammatory Bowel Disease

Inflammatory bowel disease (IBD) is not a specific disease. The term describes a group of intestinal diseases characterized by chronic abnormal GI signs and infiltration of inflammatory cells into the GI mucosa. These cells can be identified through histopathology. The form of the disease is classified by the predominant inflammatory cells present. For example, the most common form, lymphocytic-plasmacytic IBD, is so named because lymphocytes and plasma cells are the primary types of inflammatory cells present in the mucosa. Eosinophilic IBD is the second most common form. Less common forms include granulomatous, neutrophilic, and histiocytic gastroenteritis.

The most common clinical sign of IBD is chronic intermittent vomiting. Other clinical signs include anorexia, weight loss, and intermittent diarrhea. Vomiting and diarrhea may become more frequent over an extended period of time.

Diagnostic tests to rule out alternative causes of GI disease should be performed. These tests may include a CBC, chemistry profile, total thyroxine, urinalysis, and fecal examination for parasitic and bacterial agents. The most essential diagnostic test for IBD is a microscopic assessment by a pathologist of an intestinal biopsy. Tissue samples may be obtained during exploratory laparotomy, laparoscopy, or endoscopy.

The goals of treatment are to reduce and prevent stimulation and to decrease the overactive immune response of the GI tract. A hydrolyzed diet or a diet containing a unique protein source that is free of milk, wheat, and corn should be fed exclusively. Supplementing additional fiber in the form of psyllium or canned pumpkin has also been beneficial for some cats. Immunosuppressive therapies may be prescribed to suppress the exuberant inflammatory reaction of the GI tract. Secondary therapies that may be prescribed include probiotics, prebiotics, cobalamin, fatty acids, and metronidazole.

IBD is not curable. In most cases diet and medications control the symptoms. Some cats are able to be weaned off medications and remain symptom free with dietary therapy alone.

Suggested Readings

Bassert JM. 2008. Nutrients and Metabolism. In T Colville, JM Bassert, eds., *Clinical Anatomy and Physiology for Veterinary Technicians*, 2nd ed., pp. 283–313. St. Louis: Mosby Inc.

Colville T. 2008. The Digestive System. In T Colville, JM Bassert, eds., *Clinical Anatomy and Physiology for Veterinary Technicians*, 2nd ed., pp. 281–82. St. Louis: Mosby Inc.

Gilbert, SG. 1997. *Pictorial Anatomy of the Cat*, revised ed. Seattle: University of Washington Press.

Grace SF. 2011. Hepatitis, Inflammatory. In GD Norsworthy, ed., *The Feline Patient*, 4th ed., pp. 184–86. Ames: Wiley-Blackwell.

Norsworthy GD. 2010. Hepatic Lipidosis. In GD Norsworthy, ed., *The Feline Patient*, 4th ed., pp. 220–21. Ames: Wiley-Blackwell.

CHAPTER 23

Endocrine Diseases

Linda E. Schmeltzer

Overview

The endocrine system works together with the nervous system to manage the functions of all body systems. The nervous system accomplishes its tasks by sending nerve impulses to muscles or glands. These impulses cause muscles to contract or glands to secrete. The endocrine system releases hormones from glands or organs that are absorbed into the bloodstream and delivered to all of the cells and tissues throughout the body. Hormones have many functions, such as controlling metabolism and regulating growth and development. The endocrine glands include the pituitary gland, thyroid gland, parathyroid glands, and adrenal glands. The organs containing cells that secrete hormones but are not exclusively endocrine glands include the kidneys, stomach, small intestine, and pancreas. For the purposes of this chapter, an overview of the pancreas and thyroid gland will be covered.

The thyroid gland is located in the neck. It consists of a right and left lobe located on either side of the trachea (Fig. 23-1). Iodide is taken from the blood and stored within the thyroid gland. Iodide is then combined with the amino acid tyrosine to produce two of the thyroid hormones: T_3 (triiodothyronine) and T_4 (thyroxine or tetraiodothyronine). The hormone name indicates how many iodine atoms each molecule of hormone contains, three and four, respectively. Most T_4 is converted into T_3 by the removal of one iodine molecule as it circulates in the blood stream and enters cells. T_3 is the active, more potent, hormone. The normal thyroid secretes greater quantities of T_4 than T_3. T_3 and T_4 have several functions, one of which is controlling the conversion of proteins, carbohydrates, and lipids for energy.

The pancreas is located in the abdomen. It is connected to the duodenum by the pancreatic duct. The organ has both endocrine and exocrine functions. The exocrine tissues produce enzymes that aid in food digestion. The endocrine tissues in the pancreas are known as pancreatic islets or islets of Langerhans. The pancreatic islets contain alpha cells that secrete the hormone glucagon, beta cells that produce insulin, and delta cells that produce somatostatin. Insulin moves glucose out of the bloodstream and into the cells, lowering the blood glucose level. Glucagon raises the blood glucose level in two ways: (1) stimulating the liver to convert glycogen to glucose and (2) causing the formation of glucose from lactic acid and amino acids. Somatostatin inhibits the secretion of insulin and glucagon and slows absorption of nutrients from the gastrointestinal tract.

Hyperthyroidism

Hyperthyroidism is caused by an overproduction of the thyroid hormone T_4, resulting in a persistent increase in the metabolic rate. About 98% of affected cats have benign tumors within the thyroid gland; the other 2% have malignant thyroid tumors. The primary cause of hyperthyroidism is unknown. The disease has been reported in cats 4 to 22 years old. The majority of affected cats are older than 10 years old; the average age is 13 years. Males and females are equally affected.

Clinical Signs

The most common clinical sign of hyperthyroidism is increased appetite accompanied by weight loss. Essentially the cat is eating more in an effort to compensate for the weight loss caused by the increase in metabolism. In the early stages of the disease the weight loss may be so gradual that some owners are not aware it has occurred; however, rapid weight loss occurs as the disease progresses. Increased water intake and urine output, vomiting, and diarrhea have also been reported with hyperthyroidism.

Diagnosis

The normal thyroid gland is not palpable; with hyperthyroidism, enlargement of one or both lobes may occur. It is possible to palpate enlarged thyroid lobes (*see* Fig. 1-3). As the thyroid lobes enlarge, they migrate ventrally down the neck. In some cases they may descend through the thoracic inlet, making them nonpalpable. The cat has clusters of ectopic (not in the normal location) thyroid tissue in the neck from the base of the tongue to the base of the heart. About 5% of hyperthyroid cats have a tumor that originates in ectopic tissue instead of one of the thyroid lobes. If an ectopic thyroid tumor is in the chest, it is also not palpable.

Based on clinical signs or thyroid palpation, a veterinarian will order a total T_4 level. This blood test can be run in clinic on some laboratory equipment and is also available at commercial laboratories. In some hospitals, a total T_4 level is part of routine screening in geriatric patients. An elevated T_4 level confirms a hyperthyroidism diagnosis in a cat that has appropriate clinical signs.

In some cats, the T_4 level is within normal range but hyperthyroidism is still suspected because of clinical signs. In these cases, a T_3 suppression test may be ordered. This test requires an initial blood sample collection, followed by the administration of T_3 in tablet form every eight hours for seven doses. A postpill blood sample is collected 2–4 hours after the last dose. Both samples are submitted to a commercial laboratory for total T_4 and total T_3 testing. The timing of medication administration and collection of the postpill sample are extremely important. When the test is performed properly, it is extremely accurate.

The free T_4 (fT_4) is another thyroid test that has been used to diagnose hyperthyroidism. However, free T_4 can be elevated in nonthyroid disease, so its specificity for hyperthyroidism is not ideal.

Secondary Complications

Thyrotoxic Cardiomyopathy

Increased metabolic demand stimulates the heart to pump faster and more forcefully. In response to the increased demand, the heart muscle will enlarge and thicken. Thyrotoxic cardiomyopathy (TCM) is a form of cardiomyopathy resulting in thickening of the left ventricular walls. On an ultrasound study it looks similar to hypertrophic cardiomyopathy (see Chapter 20); however, TCM will resolve when hyperthyroidism is resolved.

Hypertension

Hypertension (high blood pressure) will develop as an effect of increased pumping pressure of the heart. If the blood pressure becomes too high,

Nursing the Feline Patient, First Edition. Edited by Linda E. Schmeltzer and Gary D. Norsworthy.

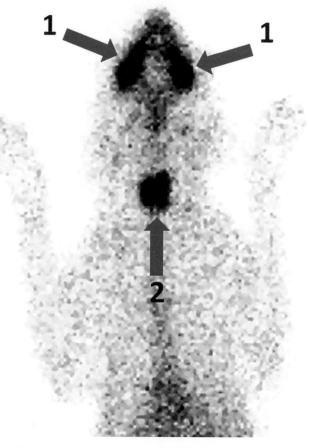

Figure 23-1 The normal thyroid lobes are highlighted in this scintigraphy study. The uptake in the salivary glands (1) and the normal thyroid lobes (2) should be approximately equal. Hyperthyroid cats will have increased uptake in the affected lobe(s).

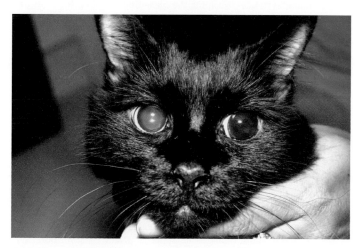

Figure 23-2 Hypertension may be caused by hyperthyroidism and can result in retinal hemorrhage and detachment. Both of this cat's pupils are dilated, and hemorrhage from the left retina has seeped into the anterior chamber.

retinal hemorrhage (abnormal bleeding of the blood vessels in the membrane in the back of the eye) can occur. Retinal hemorrhage will cause blurred or decreased vision. If hypertension becomes too great, retinal detachment can occur, causing the retina to pull away from the outer part of the eyeball. This will result in sudden blindness (Fig. 23-2).

Masked Kidney Disease

Hyperthyroidism can mask kidney disease. High blood pressure increases blood flow through the kidneys, resulting in more efficient function. When hyperthyroidism is treated, the heart rate falls to normal, the blood pressure goes down and the blood flow through the kidneys returns to normal, exposing previously hidden kidney disease.

Treatment

There are two phases to treatment. The initial phase involves administration of methimazole, a drug that directly prevents the production of thyroid hormone by preventing iodine from combining with tyrosine. The purpose of this phase is to stabilize the cat by reducing the elevated heart rate and stopping the weight loss, vomiting, and diarrhea. Methimazole is usually given for 2 to 4 weeks and the dosage may have to be adjusted several times before this is accomplished. The T_4 and kidney function should be rechecked until the T_4 is normal. Some cats experience adverse reactions to methimazole, the most common of which are loss of appetite and vomiting. If kidney insufficiency is revealed, treatment for that disease may need to be started before moving to phase two of the treatment process. See Chapter 30.

There are three treatment choices available in phase two of treatment for hyperthyroidism. Many factors come into consideration when choosing the best therapy for the individual cat, so any one of these may the correct approach to any given cat.

Long-term Medication

Long-term administration of methimazole is an effective treatment for hyperthyroidism. The drug is administered to the cat for the remainder of its life because methimazole only stops the production of thyroid hormone and does not destroy the overactive tissue or the tumor. Side effects to methimazole may begin as long as 6 months after the beginning of the treatment. Because the tumor is not destroyed, it continues to enlarge and produce more T_4. Consequently, the cat will need to have routine examinations and T_4 levels checked so the dose can be adjusted accordingly.

Surgery

Surgical removal of one or both thyroid lobes (throidectomy) is an effective treatment for hyperthyroidism (Fig. 23-3). Anesthesia is necessary,

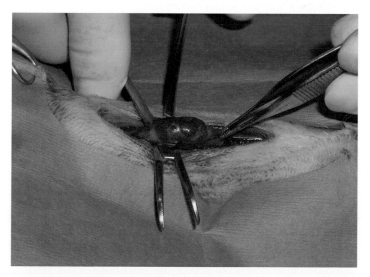

Figure 23-3 Thyroidectomy is the surgical removal of one or both thyroid lobes. It is one of the three treatment options for hyperthyroid cats.

meaning the patient will need to be stable and healthy enough to undergo the procedure. Even if both thyroid lobes are removed, the cat rarely develops hypothyroidism because the ectopic thyroid tissues are stimulated and begin producing thyroid hormone. The most common and severe complication of this surgery is hypocalcemia (low blood calcium levels) as a result of parathyroid damage during thyroid surgery.

Radiation Therapy

Radioactive iodine, radioiodine, or I^{131} (also referred to as ^{131}I) is only available through facilities that have been licensed by the state to administer radiation therapy. When radioactive iodine is injected, the body recognizes it as iodine and directs it to the thyroid gland. Once in the thyroid gland, the radioactive iodine destroys the thyroid tumor and disrupts the function of the overactive cells. Normal thyroid tissue is preserved and continues to function. The treatment is relatively simple, safe, and reported effective in 95% of cats when dosed correctly. The cat must be hospitalized post treatment until the cat's emitted radiation level drops below a certain level, as dictated by the regulations of the state.

Prognosis

Most cats have an excellent prognosis when properly treated for hyperthyroidism. Recurrence is a possibility in some cats but is unlikely.

Diabetes Mellitus

There are two diseases called diabetes: diabetes insipidus and diabetes mellitus (DM). Diabetes insipidus is a rare disorder in cats that originates in the brain or kidneys. DM is fairly common, affecting about 1 in 200 cats. The average onset of diabetes mellitus is 10 to 13 years. Male cats are twice as likely to develop the disease.

DM is failure of the pancreas to regulate blood glucose levels. There are two types of DM in humans: Type I and Type II. Type I DM results from total destruction of the beta cells that produce insulin. Type II DM causes insulin resistance, meaning that insulin, even if produced in sufficient amount, is not able to work properly to control blood glucose levels. Most diabetic cats have features of Type I and Type II diabetes. Insulin production is reduced, and insulin resistance makes that cat's insulin less effective than normal. If the causes of insulin resistance can be determined and reversed, many cats will go into diabetic remission. However, if their insulin production is significantly subnormal, insulin injections will still be needed.

The classic signs of DM are weight loss, polyuria, and polydipsia. Without an adequate amount of insulin, glucose is unable to move from the blood into the cells, leaving them starved for energy. In response to the cells' need for energy, the body begins to break down stored fat and protein as alternative energy sources, resulting in weight loss. The body will try to get rid of the excess glucose in the blood by eliminating it in the urine. Glucose attracts water and will take large quantities of fluids with it, resulting in large amounts of urine production (polyuria). To avoid dehydration, the cat drinks more and more water (polydipsia). Initially the cat may have a ravenous appetite as it tries to make up for the breakdown of energy stores to supply the cells. As the disease progresses without treatment, the cat becomes anorexic and lethargic.

The diagnosis of DM is based upon these three clinical signs and a persistently high blood glucose level accompanied by glucose in the urine. Clinical signs are present once blood glucose concentrations exceed 14–16 mmol/dl (250–290 mg/dL). Stress can also increase the blood glucose level, but it usually returns to normal within a few hours. The kidneys do not filter glucose out of the urine until it has reached excessive levels; therefore, glucose in the urine is used to differentiate DM from stress hyperglycemia. A urine culture may be ordered in addition to a complete blood profile because many cats with DM have a bacterial urinary tract infection. A blood test for pancreatitis (feline pancreatic lipase immunoreactivity [fPLI]) may also be ordered because about 50% of newly diagnosed diabetics have this disease. Bacterial cystitis and pancreatitis are known causes of insulin resistance.

Treatment for newly diagnosed cats may initially require hospitalization if the cat has complicated diabetes, known as diabetic ketoacidosis. Supplemental feeding may be needed until the cat begins to feel better and eat on its own. Short-acting insulin may be administered to stabilize glucose levels during hospitalization.

Once the cat is stabilized, the long-term goal of treatment is to control the clinical signs. This is accomplished by managing the blood glucose level so that it remains within the normal range or as close to normal as possible. This goal is accomplished with insulin, diet, and careful glucose monitoring.

Diet

Research has shown that feeding a low carbohydrate diet can increase chances for remission. There are commercial therapeutic diets available that are specially formulated for diabetic cats. These diets are typically palatable, but not all cats easily accept a new diet. The owner may need assistance in finding an appropriate alternative diet the cat will eat. Diet change alone controls DM in 15% to 30% of cats, and remission is more likely when a canned low carbohydrate diet is fed exclusively.

Insulin

Insulin can be manufactured from the pancreas of pigs (pork insulin), pancreas of cattle (beef insulin), or a combination of the two. It can also be engineered in a laboratory setting (recombinant insulin). Insulins are classified by duration: short-acting, intermediate, or long-acting. Duration refers to how they differ in their onset, peak, and length of time they remain in the cat's body. Insulin is available in concentrations of 40 units/ml (U40) and 100 units/ml (U100). The number identifies the number of active units of insulin in each milliliter of liquid. There are corresponding syringes to use for the measurement of each concentration of insulin. Using the incorrect syringe would result in over- or underdosing the cat.

Long-acting insulin, such as protamine zinc insulin, is prescribed in most cases. Owners may initially be uncomfortable with the thought of giving injections. However, the insulin needle is so small (27- to 29-gauge) that most cats do not react to the injection, helping make the owner feel more comfortable with the procedure. Injections are needed twice a day, preferably 12 hours apart.

Monitoring

Monitoring is a joint project in which owners, veterinarians, and technicians must work together. Home monitoring of the cat's appetite, body weight, water consumption, and urine output are essential. Close monitoring of the cat's daily habits are important for establishing how well the DM is controlled. During each recheck visit in the hospital, the owner should be asked about changes in appetite, water consumption, and urine output. Specifically, whether any of these have increased or decreased since the last check up and how close to normal (pre-illness) they are. The cat's general attitude and activity level are also important indications of how well the DM is controlled. A weight chart should be kept to monitor trends. Adjustment of insulin dosage should be based on clinical signs and blood test results. Rechecks will be scheduled as necessary at the discretion of the veterinarian. Some veterinarians will equip and train diabetic cat owners to collect blood and test glucose values at home. There are pros and cons to this approach that need to be weighed by the veterinarian in charge of the case.

Hypoglycemia

Hypoglycemia, or low blood glucose, can be life-threatening. It is most likely to occur at the peak insulin effect, about 6 hours after an insulin injection. A cat with hypoglycemia may appear tired and be unresponsive when called. It may appear unsteady when it stands and walk with a stagger. If severe hypoglycemia occurs, it may have seizures or lose consciousness. It is extremely important for an owner to understand the clinical signs and to know when veterinary attention should be sought.

Prognosis and Remission

Diabetic remission occurs in some patients. It is likely to occur if the causes of insulin resistance are remedied or if the pancreas spontaneously begins to produce a normal amount of insulin. Remission can occur suddenly, sending the cat into a hypoglycemic crisis after a few doses of insulin. Owners with a cat in remission should monitor closely for the typical signs of DM because it is likely to return within as little as a few days to as long as many months. Prognosis of DM is good if it can be controlled well or if remission can be achieved. Good owner compliance is the greatest determinant of success.

Suggested Readings

Colville T. 2008. The Endocrine System. In T Colville, JM Bassert, eds., *Clinical Anatomy and Physiology for Veterinary Technicians*, 2nd ed., pp. 358–73. St. Louis: Mosby Inc.

Gilbert SG. 1997. *Pictorial Anatomy of the Cat*, revised ed., pp. 40, 48–50, 67. Seattle: University of Washington Press.

Norsworthy GD. 2010. Diabetes Mellitus: Chronic Complications. In GD Norsworthy, ed., *The Feline Patient*, 4th ed., pp. 113–14. Ames: Wiley-Blackwell.

Norsworthy GD, Crystal M. 2010. Hyperthyroidism. In GD Norsworthy, ed., *The Feline Patient*, 4th ed., pp. 256–60. Ames: Wiley-Blackwell.

Rand J. 2011. Diabetes: Uncomplicated. In GD Norsworthy, ed., *The Feline Patient*, 4th ed., pp. 118–19. Ames: Wiley-Blackwell.

Feline Immunodeficiency Virus

Teija Kaarina Viita-aho

Overview

Feline immunodeficiency virus (FIV), formerly known as the T-lymphotropic lentivirus (FTLV), is a retrovirus that belongs to the lentivirus genus. It is closely related to the human immunodeficiency virus (HIV), but because these viruses are species specific, transmission between humans and cats does not occur. FIV was discovered in 1986, but it probably existed for several years, if not decades, prior to that date. The virus is endemic in the cat population worldwide, but the prevalence varies greatly geographically. The prevalence is higher in Oceania and Asia than Europe and North America. FIV is divided in subtypes, also called clades, of which subtypes A and B are most common in Europe and B most common in North America. Only subtype A has been reported in the United Kingdom.

Transmission

The most common route of transmission is via bites because virus is shed in the saliva of infected cats. Cats that show clinical signs, particularly cats with oral lesions, are more infective than clinically asymptomatic cats. Cats that have access to the outdoors where they interact and fight with other cats are at the highest risk for infection. Feral cats, especially intact males and cats with large territories, are the most likely to fight and be bitten. The likelihood of infection increases by age because of prolonged fighting experience. The prevalence of infection is low in cats younger than 1 year of age and highest in cats older than 6 years of age. Nonpedigree cats are more commonly infected as a result of greater exposure to free-roaming cats outdoors.

Transmission from mother to kitten occurs. Infection can be transmitted in utero or later through milk or saliva. If infection occurs in utero arrested fetal development, abortion, stillbirth, and subnormal birth weight may occur, but most kittens are born clinically normal.

Even though virus is shed in saliva, transmission of infection via grooming, food, and water bowls is not likely because the virus does not remain infective long in the environment and is destroyed by common disinfectants such as soap. However, transmission in a closed population of cats without a history of fighting has been reported.

Iatrogenic infection resulting from the use of infected surgical instruments or transmission of infected blood is possible. Penile to vaginal transmission of FIV during mating is unlikely. A greater risk for transmission is as a result of a tom cat's tendency to bite the queen's neck during mating. Transmission by blood-sucking insects is not significant.

Clinical Signs

Infection is lifelong and is divided in three phases: primary phase, prolonged asymptomatic phase, and terminal phase (acquired immunodeficiency syndrome [AIDS]). The primary phase of infection occurs shortly after infection. This phase is followed by a subclinical and asymptomatic phase. Clinical signs during the progressive immunodeficiency syndrome are either the result of an active viral replication or of immune suppression caused by the virus.

Primary Phase

Nonspecific signs, such as lethargy, anorexia, enteritis, or respiratory signs, may occur. In some cats clinical signs of the primary phase are mild and go unnoticed by the owner. A transient period of fever and lymphadenopathy usually begins about 10 days after infection. If the infection occurs during the neonatal period lymphadenopathy may persist for life, whereas it is transient if it occurs in kittens and young cats. In adult cats lymphadenopathy is usually undetectable. In addition to fever and lymphadenopathy neutropenia is a hallmark of this primary phase. Neutropenia occurs 6–8 weeks after infection and increases susceptibility to secondary bacterial infections. A decrease in CD4+ T-lymphocytes begins around 4 weeks after infection. Neurological signs may occur in the primary phase and include anisocoria, delayed pupillary light reflexes, delayed righting reflex, and alterations in the sleeping pattern. Of FIV infected cats, 50% spend more time awake than healthy cats.

Prolonged Asymptomatic Phase of Infection

Following the primary phase of infection there is a prolonged period of asymptomatic infection in most infected cats. Most cats recover from the first phase well and appear normal for months or years before clinical signs related to immunodeficiency appear. The asymptomatic period occurs because the virus can be suppressed at low levels. Nevertheless, total clearance of the virus does not occur, and the cat remains infected for life. The length of the asymptomatic phase varies from several months to several years; the duration is unpredictable because there are many contributing factors. They include the age of the cat at the time of infection, the infective viral dose, the route of infection, and subtype-related pathogenicity. During the asymptomatic phase the cat's immune status progressively deteriorates because the virus destroys CD4+ T-cells eventually leading to development of clinical signs.

Terminal Phase, Progressive Immunodeficiency Syndrome (AIDS)

In the terminal phase clinical signs are the result of immunodeficiency. Clinical signs vary greatly and are nonspecific. They are due to secondary infections and an inappropriate immune response to antigens. Diseases of the oral cavity, respiratory tract, and gastrointestinal tract predominate. Oral cavity diseases such as chronic lymphoplasmacytic gingivitis-stomatitis occur in 56% of the infected cats (Fig. 24-1). Chronic upper respiratory tract disease occurs in 34% of patients (Fig. 24-2), and chronic enteritis causing persistent diarrhea in 19% of patients. Additionally, lethargy, depression, nausea, vomiting, inappetence or anorexia, weight loss, chronic skin disease, recurrent or frequent abscesses, recurrent cystitis, and pyrexia may occur. Chronic conjunctivitis occurs in 11% of infected cats. Other inflammatory ocular diseases may occur including keratitis, uveitis, ocular discharge, glaucoma, chorioretinitis, and retinal hemorrhage. Approximately 5% of cats have neurological abnormalities such as dementia, behavioral changes, ataxia, and anisocoria. Immune-mediated glomerulonephritis leading to renal failure has been reported. FIV is an oncogenic virus; lymphomas, various leukemias, and other tumors may also occur in infected cats.

Nursing the Feline Patient, First Edition. Edited by Linda E. Schmeltzer and Gary D. Norsworthy.

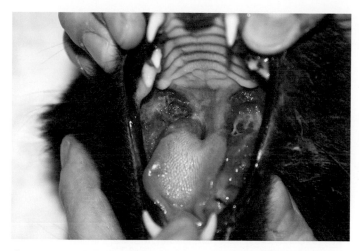

Figure 24-1 Lymphoplasmacytic gingivitis-stomatitis is not directly caused by the feline immunodeficiency virus (FIV), but if the FIV is present the disease is much more difficult to manage.

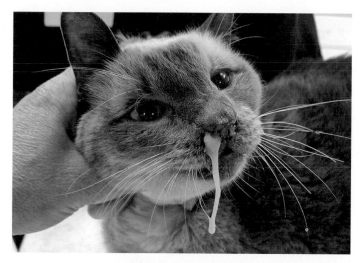

Figure 24-2 Immunosuppression induced by feline immunodeficiency virus (FIV) contributes to various chronic infectious processes, including chronic rhinosinusitis.

Laboratory Changes

Hematologic changes are common but nonspecific and vary depending on the phase of the disease. Multiple abnormalities occur in 54% of infected cats, and 17% of cats have single ones. In the primary phase neutropenia is common. Neutrophilia may follow in the presence of secondary infections. Lymphopenia, progressive anemia, and monocytosis often occur in later stages. Biochemically, elevations in serum proteins, especially globulins, are common. A decreased CD4+ T-cell count is present consistently and is progressive.

Other Concomitant Diseases

Concurrent or opportunistic infections are common because of a suppressed immune system. These include demodicosis, toxoplasmosis, cowpox, notoedric mange, bacterial cystitis, hemotropic mycoplasms, calici virus infection, herpesvirus infection, bacterial pneumonia, systemic candidiasis, coccidiosis, pyothorax, bartonellosis, and otitis externa (Fig. 24-3).

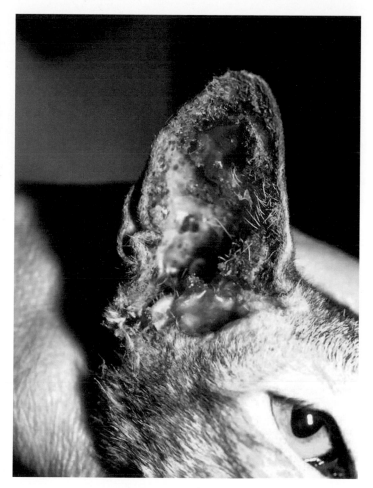

Figure 24-3 Otitis externa is not a common disease in cats as it is in dogs. When present, one should look for an underlying disease or disease agent such as feline immunodeficiency virus.

Diagnosis

Diagnosis of FIV is based on demonstrating FIV-specific antibodies in serum or plasma. There are in-house enzyme-linked immunosorbent assay (ELISA) test kits for FIV that are easy to use and give results within 10–15 minutes. The most commonly used test kit (IDEXX Laboratories) is based on whole blood.

The presence of antibodies is strong evidence of infection. Nevertheless, because false-positives may occur, confirmation should be made with a polymerase chain reaction (PCR) test, which is not as sensitive but is more specific.

In the early stage of infection (during the first 2–4 weeks), antibodies are usually not present in the blood. Most cats have positive test results within 60 days of infection, but rarely, some may require 6 months or more. Therefore, testing should be repeated 60 or more days after the last possible exposure if there is a possibility of infection. Some cats may never produce enough antibodies to be detected by an ELISA test thus creating a diagnostic challenge. Conversely, cats in the terminal phase of infection may have undetectable antibody levels resulting in false-negative test results.

If the cat has been vaccinated with FIV vaccine, the antibody test result will be positive because the test is not able to distinguish vaccine-related antibodies from antibodies of natural infection. Vaccine induced antibodies persist for about 2–3 years. IDEXX Laboratories offers a PCR test for FIV that is not affected by vaccination. It is about 80% sensitive and nearly 100% specific. It should be used in cats with a positive ELISA test and with an unknown vaccination history.

Kittens born to an FIV-infected queen or to a queen that has been vaccinated against FIV usually get FIV-antibodies via colostrum. Therefore, kittens that test positive should be retested immediately with the PCR test or with the ELISA test after 6 months of age. It is highly unlikely for maternal antibodies to persist after 6 months of age.

Other possible means for diagnosis are virus isolation and in situ hybridization. However, these are research tests that are not commercially available to practitioners.

Therapy

FIV is an incurable infection. Currently there are no specific antiviral drugs that are effective against it. Some HIV-drugs may be effective in slowing down the progression of FIV. Nevertheless, none of those drugs can be routinely recommended for cats. Azidothymidine (AZT) is one of the HIV drugs that may be beneficial in cats positive for FIV with chronic gingivostomatitis.

Treatment is mainly symptomatic and supportive including antibiotics when needed for secondary infections, fluid therapy, and possibly blood transfusions in case of severe anemia. Several immune stimulants have been used in cats with FIV, most without significant response. The exception is Oxstrin®, a nutraceutical product that has been shown to improve several immune markers in cats infected with FIV.

Management and Prevention

It is important to understand that FIV infection is not solely a reason for euthanasia. Cats may live normal lives for years despite the infection. Regular check-ups are recommended (at least every 6 months) to detect any changes in clinical status and manage possible secondary infections in their early stage. Appropriate preventative medicine, including dental care and regular vaccinations, is important. It is recommended by some to use inactivated vaccines in cats with FIV because of immunosuppression. Attention should be paid to feeding high quality food, and if weight loss appears, a change to palatable food with high caloric density is recommended. Any unnecessary stress should be avoided because stress is known to suppress the immune system. Keeping the infected cat indoors or only in a restricted area outdoors reduces both the risk for secondary infections and transmitting the infection forward to other cats. If the infected cat still continues go outdoors neutering is essential to reduce the tendency to fight.

Cats that live in the same household with an infected cat have only minimal risk for infection if hostility and fighting do not occur. However, the safest course is to separate the infected cat from noninfected cats. FIV vaccine should be considered for exposed cats, including cats that live with a cat infected with FIV or cats that have unsupervised access outdoors.

There are other preventative measures that should be considered including keeping the cat as an indoor-only pet or having a restricted, enclosed area outdoors to prevent any direct contact with other cats, especially feral and stray. If the cat goes outdoors, keeping it indoors at night helps to reduce fighting behavior. Pure-bred cat breeding colonies should have negative FIV status, and breeding cats should not have access outdoors or have contact with cats that have access outdoors. Additionally, regular testing is important.

Vaccination

There is an inactivated FIV vaccine available in some countries. It contains subtypes A and D, and there is cross-protection against subtype B. The American Association of Feline Practitioners considers it a "noncore" vaccine because many cats are not at risk of FIV infection; therefore, a cat's need for FIV vaccine should be evaluated on an individual basis. FIV vaccination should be started at 8 weeks of age or older. Three injections should be given at 2- to 3-week intervals followed by annual boosters.

Prognosis

FIV is lifelong, progressive infection that often leads to severe illness or death. As the disease progresses the clinical signs become more persistent and more severe. Approximately 20% will die during the first phase of the infection, but up to 50% of cats will remain asymptomatic for 4–6 years after infection. The prognosis depends on when the diagnosis is made related to disease phase. If the diagnosis occurs during the first or asymptomatic phase, there may be many years of normal life ahead. But if the diagnosis is made when the cat already has signs related to immunodeficiency the prognosis is poor. The average life expectancy in the terminal stage of the disease is less than a year.

Suggested Readings

Harbour DA, Caney SMA, Sparkes AH. 2004. Feline Immunodeficiency Virus Infection. In EA Chandler, CJ Gaskell, RM Gaskell, eds., *Feline Medicine and Therapeutics*, 3rd ed., pp. 607–22. Ames: Blackwell.

Sparkes AH, Hopper CD, Millard W, et al. 1993. Feline Immunodeficiency Virus Infection: Clinicopathologic Findings in 90 Naturally Occurring Cases. *J Vet Intern Med*. 7:85–90.

Grace SF. 2010. Feline Immunodeficiency Virus Infection. In GD Norsworthy, ed., *The Feline Patient*, 4th ed., pp. 179–80. Ames: Wiley-Blackwell.

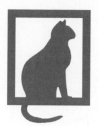

CHAPTER 25

Feline Infectious Peritonitis

Linda E. Schmeltzer

Overview

Feline infectious peritonitis (FIP) is a fatal viral disease of domestic cats. It is caused by the feline infectious peritonitis virus (FIPV), a virus in the coronavirus family. FIPV is a mutation of the feline enteric coronavirus (FECV), another virus in the coronavirus family.

Transmission and Prevalence

FECV is an intestinal virus that usually causes either no symptoms or mild symptoms, such as diarrhea. The virus is shed through feces, urine, and nasal and salivary secretions and is easily passed to other cats on objects such as clothing or countertops. It is especially difficult to control exposure in shelters, catteries, or households with large numbers of cats. Kittens become infected with the virus about 3 to 5 weeks of age if their mothers are shedding it. Once a cat is infected with FECV it will carry the virus for the rest of its life.

At some point during an infected cat's life, the virus within the cells may mutate from FECV to FIPV. This is more likely to occur in kittens, presumably because of their reduced immunity and the rapid replication of the virus. The cause of the mutation is not known and happens to about 20% of cats infected with FECV. However, only a small number of cats that carry the FIPV actually become ill with FIP because most cats have a rapid and strong immune response. Male and female cats are affected equally. The mutation and onset of FIP illness usually occurs in cats younger than 2 years old.

Clinical Signs

There are two forms of FIP. The most common form is the effusive, or wet, form. Fluid may accumulate in the chest, causing dyspnea (difficulty breathing), or in the abdomen, causing a bloated appearance (Fig. 25-1).

(a)

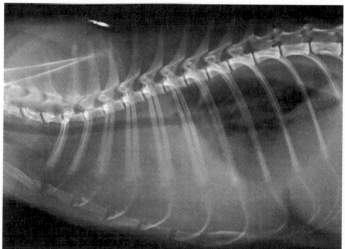

Nursing the Feline Patient, First Edition. Edited by Linda E. Schmeltzer and Gary D. Norsworthy.
© 2012 John Wiley & Sons, Inc. Published 2012 by John Wiley & Sons, Inc.

Fever, lethargy, and appetite suppression are also common. The dry, or noneffusive, form primarily affects abdominal organs, the eyes, and the central nervous system (CNS). There may be symptoms related to failure of multiple organs. Fever, lethargy, appetite suppression, and weight loss are also associated with this form of FIP (Fig. 25-2). CNS signs may include personality change, weakness in the hind legs, lack of coordination, head tilt, circling, or seizures.

Diagnosis

Diagnosis can be difficult because there are no specific tests reliable for diagnosis other than histopathology with immunohistochemical staining of an affected organ. Unfortunately, relevant organ biopsy is not always

(b)

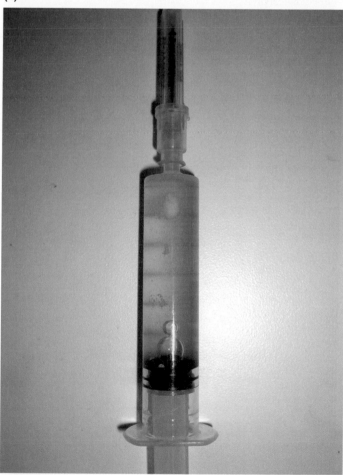

Figure 25-1 The effusive ("wet") form of feline infectious peritonitis (FIP) causes fluid to collect in the thoracic or abdominal cavities. (a) This lateral thoracic radiograph shows pleural effusion causing compression of the lung lobes; however, pleural effusions can be caused by many diseases. (b) Thoracentesis of a few milliliters of fluids provides a sample for analysis. Removal of 100–300 ml improves breathing.

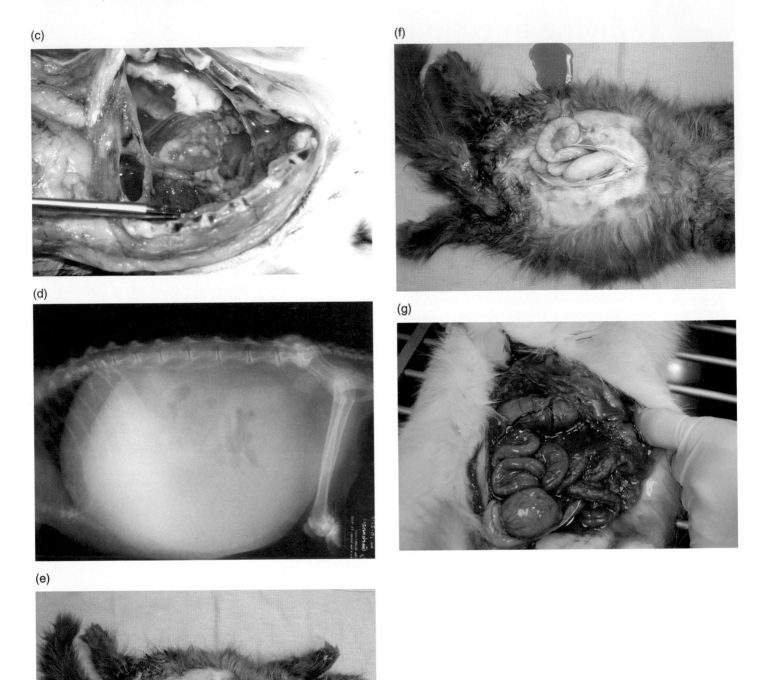

Figure 25-1 (cont'd) (c) The thorax has been opened showing white granulomas on the pericardium (center of the picture) and free fluid within the pleural space. (d) This lateral abdominal radiograph shows ascites (fluid) in the abdomen. It has the same radiographic density as the abdominal organs so there is a uniform white appearance present. The dark lines are gas pockets in the intestinal tract. (e) Abdominal distension is obvious in this kitten as a result of fluid buildup in the abdomen. (f) When the abdomen is opened at necropsy, fluid runs out. (g) This abdomen has free fluid present. Note the white granulomas on several loops of small intestine.

Images courtesy Dr. Gary D. Norsworthy.

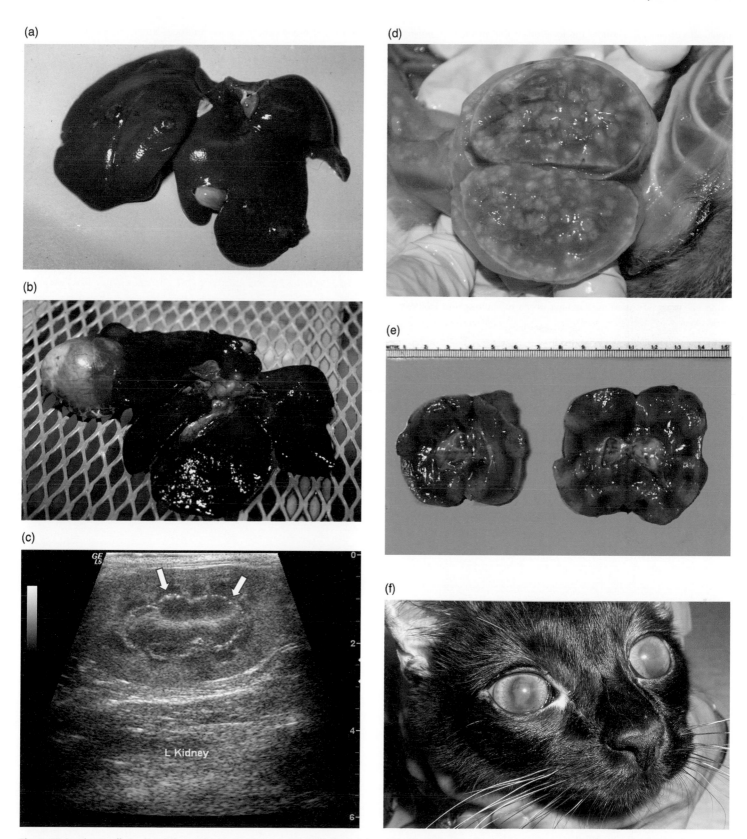

Figure 25-2 The noneffusive ("dry") form of feline infectious peritonitis (FIP) affects various organs causing masses (granulomas) to form. (a) This liver has several small granulomas. (b) This liver has several very large granulomas. (c) The medullary rim sign can be caused by several diseases including FIP. The arrows point to the hyperechoic line that occurs in the outer zone of the medulla parallel to the corticomedullary junction. (d) Small FIP granulomas are seen throughout the cortex and medulla of this young cat. (e) Several large granulomas are seen in these kidneys. When this size the kidneys have a "lumpy, bumpy" feel when palpated. (f) Dry FIP may also be a cause of uveitis. The irises change colors and white precipitates form in the anterior chamber.

practical either as a result of the location of the affected organ (brain, retina) or the cat's declining health condition making it too high a risk for anesthesia and surgery. There is a blood test, the coronavirus titer, that detects the presence of coronavirus antibodies, but this test does not discriminate between FIPV and FECV. Antibodies may be present in the blood even when the virus is no longer present. A positive test indicates that the cat was exposed to or is infected with one or both viruses. A veterinarian will interpret the results in conjunction with results of other tests to make a definitive or reasonable diagnosis. A decrease in the white blood cells in combination with a low lymphocyte count is fairly consistent with FIP. However, not all cats will have abnormal white blood cell counts, and other nonfatal diseases may also cause these changes. The accumulated fluid in cats with the wet form of FIP will be a characteristic yellow-tinged, stringy or mucous-like fluid, and is of great benefit in diagnosis.

Prevention

A preventive vaccine is available for FIP, but there is much debate regarding its safety and effectiveness. The most effective way to prevent FIP is to minimize or avoid situations that have been proven to spread FECV:

- Do not breed cats that have produced kittens that have developed FIP. Some evidence points to a genetic factor.
- Eliminate overcrowding. This can be difficult in a cattery.
- Reduce fecal-oral transmission by cleaning litter boxes several times per day.
- Regularly disinfect surfaces.
- Strictly isolate queens and their kittens. Wean kittens at 3–5 weeks of age and isolate them from other cats, including their mother. Continue isolation of the kittens until they are 16 weeks old.

Treatment and Prognosis

There is no effective treatment for FIP. When a veterinarian is reasonably sure of the diagnosis euthanasia is generally recommended.

Suggested Reading

Norsworthy GD. 2011. Feline Infectious Peritonitis. In GD Norsworthy, ed., *The Feline Patient*, 4th ed., pp. 181–83. Ames: Wiley-Blackwell.

Feline Leukemia Virus Diseases

Linda E. Schmeltzer

Overview

In the 1970s and 1980s the feline leukemia virus (FeLV) was the most common fatal infectious disease of cats. Because infected cats can now be identified by testing and healthy cats can be protected with leukemia virus vaccine, fewer cases of this disease are being seen. However, it is still one of the common infectious diseases of cats.

The FeLV is classified as a retrovirus. Retroviruses are species specific. These viruses produce an enzyme (reverse transcriptase) that permits them to insert copies of their own ribonucleic acid (RNA) genetic material into the deoxyribonucleic acid (DNA) of the cells they have infected. Once FeLV produces DNA from its RNA, it incorporates its DNA into the host cat's DNA. There it can remain dormant, giving no sign of its presence, or it can take over the host cell's genetic machinery to produce more of the virus.

Transmission

Large amounts of the FeLV virus are shed in saliva. The most common source of transmission is through social interaction such as mutual grooming or sharing food and water dishes. It may also be transmitted by biting. Transmission may also occur through blood, nasal secretions, feces, and milk. Sharing a common litter box, nose-to-nose contact, bite wounds, and nursing are also possible routes for infection. The virus may also be passed from mother to kitten across the placenta during pregnancy and from donor to patient in a blood transfusion.

The FeLV does not survive for more than a few hours on dry surfaces outside the body, and it is easily killed using standard disinfectants. It is possible for FeLV to survive outside the body for up to several weeks when it remains moist and at room temperature. Transmission can occur through contaminated needles, endotracheal tubes, and surgical instruments.

Testing

There are three tests that can be used to detect FeLV. Positive test results will vary depending on the stage of the disease, the organs involved, and the outcome of the infection. Vaccination for FeLV will not interfere with any of the test results.

Enzyme-linked Immunosorbent Assay

The enzyme-linked immunosorbent assay (ELISA) test is the most commonly used screening test; it detects free FeLV antigen in plasma. This test is easily performed in a clinic setting, with results available in about 10 minutes. In-clinic test kits can be run on plasma or anticoagulated whole blood. It is possible for a cat to test positive and then later test negative. *See* Outcomes of FeLV Infections.

Immunofluorescent Assay

An immunofluorescent assay (IFA) test is performed by a commercial laboratory on a blood or bone marrow smear. It will detect the presence of FeLV antigen within the blood cells. FeLV antigen is mixed with a fluorescent compound and then with a sample of the patient's blood. If FeLV antibody is present in the white blood cells (WBC) of the patient sample, the WBCs will fluoresce when examined with an ultraviolet microscope. A positive test result occurs in the later stages of infection, approximately 3 weeks after the virus enters the blood stream. False-negatives may occur if the number of leukocytes in the sample is low (leukopenia).

Polymerase Chain Reaction Test

Polymerase chain reaction (PCR) test is another laboratory performed test that is highly sensitive for FeLV antigen. It can be performed on blood or other body fluids. Unfortunately, its relatively high cost prohibits it from being a routinely performed test.

Outcomes of FeLV Infections

There are several possible outcomes for cats infected with FeLV. Understanding these will explain the wide variation in clinical signs.

Regressor

Following infection by the FeLV through the oronasal route (mouth or nose), the virus will replicate in the lymphoid tissues in the mouth and throat (oropharynx). An immune response is initiated within the cells, virus replication is stopped, and the virus is completely eliminated from the cat's body. Regressor cats will test negative on ELISA and IFA tests because they have high levels of antibodies and no presence of the FeLV antigen in their blood.

Transient Viremia

Viremia is defined as the presence of the virus in the blood stream. If the initial immune response is not successful the cat will become infected with FeLV. The virus will spread within the lymphatic tissue to other organs including the lymph nodes and spleen. The cat can develop fever, poor appetite, lethargy, and swollen lymph nodes. During the next 3–16 weeks, the immune system may still be able to produce antibodies and eliminate the virus resulting in transient viremia. For this reason, ELISA tests can turn positive within 1–3 days of infection but will later turn out negative. The IFA test will be negative during this phase. Until the virus is completely eliminated, the cat will shed the virus and be able to infect other cats.

Latent Infection

Some cats are able to mount an immune response and eliminate the virus after it has entered the blood stream but not before it invades the bone marrow. These cats do not actively produce or shed the virus. Cats with a latent FeLV infection may appear healthy. They will test negative on ELISA and IFA tests. A stressful event can cause the virus to be reactivated, at which time the tests will turn positive. These cats may develop neoplasia (abnormal growth of cells, such as malignant tumors). The longer the virus remains latent, the less likely it is to reactivate.

Nursing the Feline Patient, First Edition. Edited by Linda E. Schmeltzer and Gary D. Norsworthy.

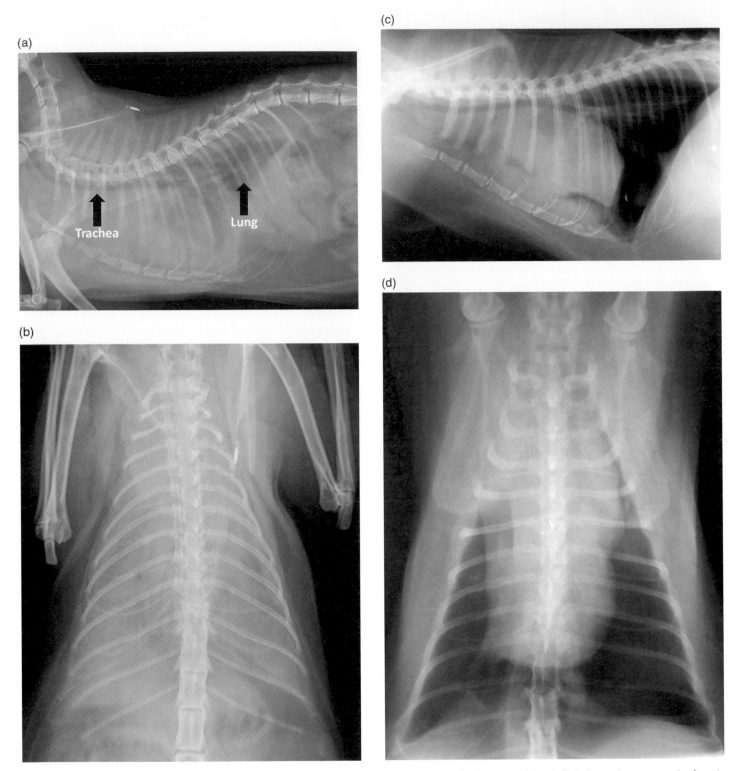

(a)

Trachea   Lung

(b)

(c)

(d)

Figure 26-1 Thoracic lymphoma. (a) (b) The most common form of thoracic lymphoma causes fluid to form in the pleural space (pleural effusion) secondary to a mass that forms in the anterior mediastinum. Masses in this area elevate the trachea (left arrow) so it is nearly against the thoracic spine. The lungs become compressed by the surrounding fluid. The only functional lung tissue is seen a black (right arrow) because it is filled with air. (c) (d) This cat also has a mediastinal mass but only a minimal amount of fluid. Note the elevated trachea.

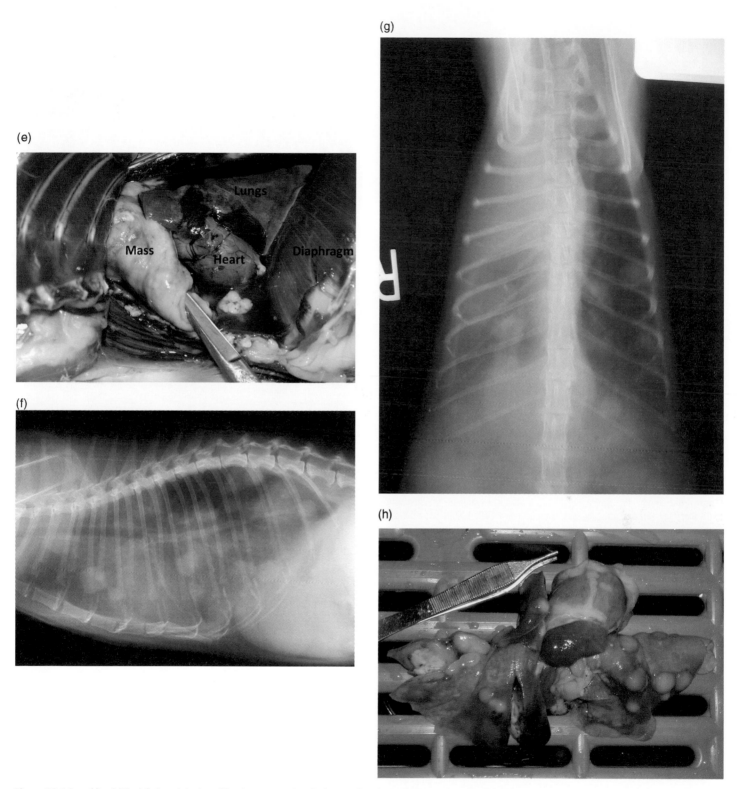

Figure 26-1 (cont'd) (e) The left thoracic body wall has been removed so the heart and mediastinal mass can be seen. (f) (g) Discrete masses can be seen in the thoracic radiographs of this cat. (h) At necropsy, the white masses are seen in the lung lobes. This is an unusual form of lymphoma.

Images courtesy Drs. Gary D. Norsworthy and Vanessa Pimentel.

(a)

(b)

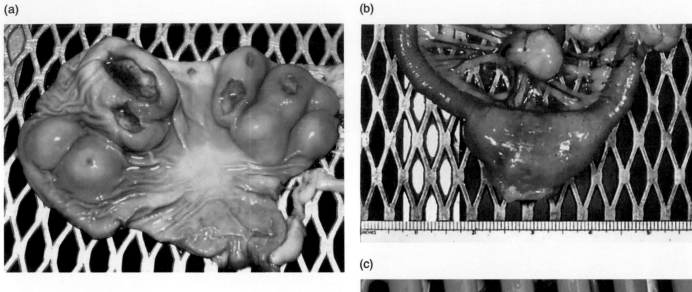

(c)

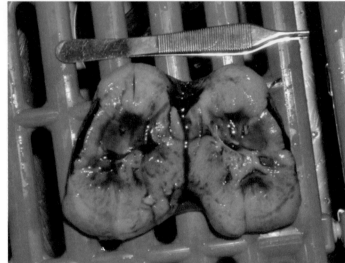

Figure 26-2 Abdominal lymphoma. (a) This is an opened stomach showing several large, ulcerated lymphomatous masses in the stomach wall. (b) This large mass is a lymphoma in the small intestine. (c) Lymphoma in the kidneys causes discrete masses, making the kidneys "lumpy and bumpy."

Images courtesy Dr. Gary D. Norsworthy.

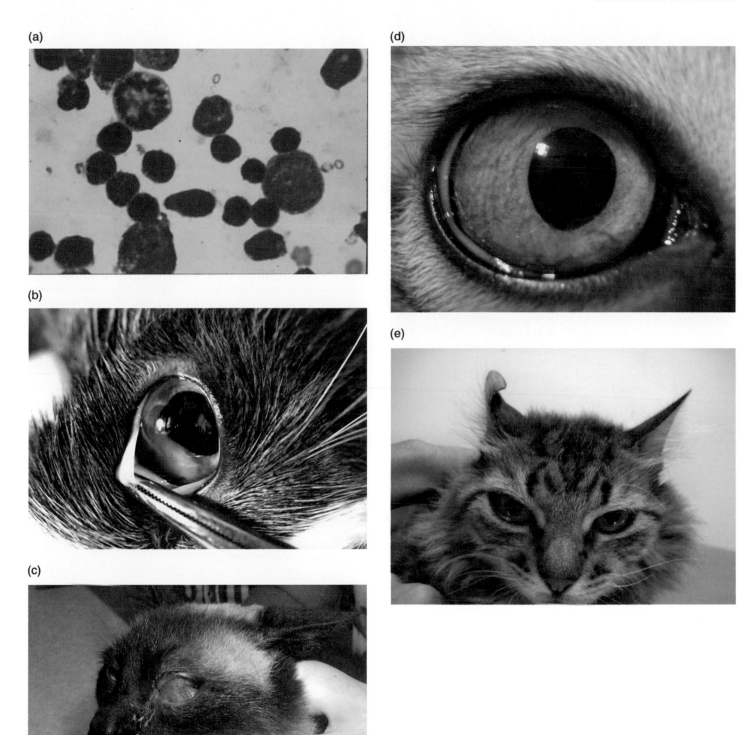

Figure 26-3 Unusual manifestations of lymphoma and the feline leukemia virus (FeLV). (a) True lymphoblastic lymphoma (cancer of the blood cells) occasionally occurs as a result of FeLV. (b) This cat has a lymphomatous mass in the anterior chamber. (c) This cat has a lymphoma on the lymphoid tissue (gland of the third eyelid) of the third eyelid. (d) FeLV uveitis causes the iris to change color and for the blood vessels in it to become enlarged. (e) A curled pinna is one of the unusual manifestations of FeLV.

Images courtesy Drs. Gary D. Norsworthy and Vanessa Pimentel.

Persistent Viremia

When the virus reaches the bone marrow it is then released into the blood. This results in a permanent infection, and affected cats will test positive on ELISA and IFA tests. Most of these cats die from a FeLV-associated disease within 3 years of infection.

Diseases

The FeLV causes a wide variety of diseases. Lymphoma (cancer), anemia, abortion, and immunosuppression are a few examples (Figs. 26-1, 26-2, and 26-3). Immune suppression will cause the cat to be more susceptible to many diseases that would ordinarily be successfully eliminated by the immune system. Commonly mild diseases, such as upper respiratory infections, can become fatal because of the immune system's inability to mount a proper response and eliminate the disease.

Lymphoma is commonly caused by FeLV, but not all cats that develop lymphoma have FeLV infections. Lymphoma is a cancer that can occur in many different organs, including the blood, bone marrow, brain, intestines, kidneys, liver, lymph nodes and spinal cord.

Maintenance of a Cat Infected with FeLV

Cats infected with FeLV should be kept indoors and separated from noninfected cats. The client should be educated on a proper nutrition program for the cat infected with FeLV. Raw meat, raw eggs, and unpasteurized milk should be avoided because they can contain bacteria that an immune-suppressed cat may be unable to successfully eliminate. Water and food bowls should be changed and washed regularly to prevent bacterial or fungal growth. Litter boxes should be scooped at least daily and thoroughly cleaned at least weekly. Preventive health programs, including regular vaccinations, should be followed. Heartworm and parasite prevention is extremely important. Biannual wellness visits can be recommended to detect weight loss or early stages of secondary diseases. Regular dental prophylaxis should be performed to prevent dental related diseases. Routine screening of the blood, urine, and feces can be recommended as a means to detect problems early. Medications to aid immune system support are available and can be recommended by the veterinarian. It is important for a client to understand that these medications are not a substitute for proper nutrition and care.

Prognosis and Prevention

There is no cure for a FeLV infection. Cats with persistent viremia and latent infection will always be infected. Some of the diseases caused by FeLV can be successfully treated with aggressive therapy; however, the virus will remain in the cat.

FeLV vaccination is considered a noncore vaccine by the American Association of Feline Practitioners (AAFP). Outdoor cats and cats that live with cats infected with FeLV are at risk for exposure. Owners who foster cats with unknown history of exposure to FeLV may unintentionally expose their own cats to FeLV and should consider vaccinating the resident cats as well. If an owner chooses not to vaccinate, he or she should be counseled to isolate fostered cats to prevent passing infection to unvaccinated cats. Vaccination for FeLV is not 100% effective; a small percentage of vaccinated cats do become infected. This is most likely to happen when daily exposure to the virus occurs.

Suggested Readings

Amorim de Costa FV, Norsworthy GD. 2011. Feline Leukemia Virus Diseases. In GD Norsworthy, ed., *The Feline Patient*, 4th ed., pp. 184–86. Ames: Wiley-Blackwell.

Colville T. 2008. Blood, Lymph and Immunity. In T Colville, JM Bassert, eds., *Clinical Anatomy and Physiology for Veterinary Technicians*, 2nd ed., pp. 221–46. St. Louis: Mosby Inc.

Levy J, Hartmann K, Hofmann-Lehmann R, et al. 2008. 2008 American Association of Feline Practitioners' feline retrovirus management guidelines. *J Fel Med Surg.* 10(3):300–316.

CHAPTER 27

Parasitology

Teija Kaarina Viita-aho

Overview

Feline parasitology is a broad topic with significant variation in parasite prevalence in different parts of the world, largely depending on the climate and other environmental factors. Cats are definitive hosts to many parasites, but some parasites occasionally infect cats even though cats are not their primary host.

Parasites always have a definitive host or primary host, which is required for maturation and completion of the parasite's life cycle. Many parasites additionally require an intermediate host or secondary host, which the parasite infects for some time period during which some stage of the life cycle is completed. Paratenic or transport hosts are similar to intermediate hosts, but they are not required for the parasite's life cycle to progress. Paratenic hosts may transport the infection to intermediate or definitive hosts or act as a reservoir of the parasite.

Parasites are divided into ectoparasites and endoparasites. Ectoparasites live on the host animal's external surfaces: on or within the skin, within the ear canal, and on the hair coat. Endoparasites live inside the host: in the gastrointestinal tract, the respiratory tract, and within various organs, including those of the cardiovascular system.

Ectoparasites

Ctenocephalides Felis (Cat Flea)

Fleas are blood-sucking parasites. They are easily recognized by their laterally flattened shape and their ability to jump. Only adult fleas are found on the cat; the remainder of the life cycle is completed in the environment. Adult fleas live on the cat's skin where they suck blood. Female fleas lay eggs on the cat. Eggs drop off and hatch into larvae within a few days. Larvae develop to pupae before maturation to adult fleas. The duration of the pupae stage varies; it can take more than 100 days. However, in a warm and humid environment the life cycle can be completed in 2–4 weeks.

The flea population is enormous; however, adult fleas compromise only 5% of the entire flea population. The largest segment of the population consists of eggs (50%), larvae (35%), and pupae (10%). Therefore, the most important aspect of flea control is controlling the eggs and juvenile fleas.

Diagnosis of a flea infection is usually straightforward. Fleas or flea feces ("flea dirt") is usually seen on cat's hair coat. To determine if the dark dirt on the cat's hair coat is flea dirt, comb it off, and drop a small amount of water on it. If it is flea feces, the water will change to red as the blood is resuspended.

Some cats become hypersensitive to flea bites resulting in flea allergic dermatitis (FAD). FAD causes pruritus, alopecia, and dermatitis and may be severe. The pruritus results in scratching and licking and may lead to secondary infections (Fig. 27-1).

In areas where fleas are common it is recommended to use regular flea control. There are several spot-on products available.

Ctenocephalides Canis (Dog Flea)

This dog flea may also infect cats. The life cycle is similar to cat flea.

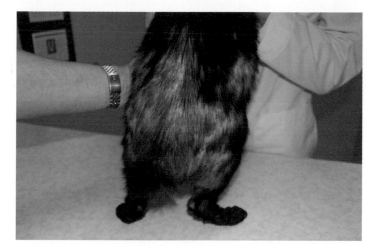

Figure 27-1 Flea allergic dermatitis (FAD) creates intense itching on many parts of the skin. The most intense reaction for most cats is at the tail head, just cranial to the base of the tail. Image courtesy Dr. Gary D. Norsworthy.

Otodextes Cynotis (Ear Mite)

These small (~0.5 mm) mites live in the external ear canal. They are distributed worldwide and infect cats, dogs, foxes, and ferrets. Humans may also get rashes and pruritus when bitten. Ear mites are the most common cause of otitis externa in young cats. Infection is transmitted through direct cat contact. Female mites lay eggs in the ear canal. The life cycle, consisting of eggs, larvae, two nymph stages, and adult mites, takes 3–4 weeks. The primary clinical sign, pruritus, is usually bilateral and results in head shaking and intense scratching of the ears. This self-trauma contributes to secondary infections and aural hematomas (Fig. 27-2). Infection may even spread into the middle ear (otitis media) resulting in a head tilt, circling, and ataxia. Chronic infections may result in hyperkeratosis of the pinna. Occasionally mites can be found elsewhere on the skin leading to regional pruritus or dermatitis.

Diagnosis is suspected based on the presence of black ear discharge. Close examination of the ear canal with an otoscope or microscopic examination of the discharge may reveal motile mites and confirms the diagnosis. The mites are tiny, white, organisms. The heat of the otoscope light may encourage their movement, making diagnosis easier. When treating ear mite infection it is recommended that all in-contact dogs and cats be treated; however, transmission does not occur readily.

Cheyletiella Blakei

These grey, white, small (0.3–0.5 mm) mites are also known as "walking dandruff" because of their appearance on the hair coat. Mites live on the skin-surface keratin and get nutrition from tissue fluids and skin debris. The life cycle is completed on the host in approximately 35 days. Eggs are attached to the cat's hair, which serves as the means for contaminating the environment. Infection is highly contagious and spreads easily by direct contact. Indirect contact may also be a source of infection because adult female mites may survive up to 14 days in the environment. Males and juveniles die within 48 hours outside the host. Eggs shed in the environment can also be a source of infection. Infection can also spread

Nursing the Feline Patient, First Edition. Edited by Linda E. Schmeltzer and Gary D. Norsworthy.
© 2012 John Wiley & Sons, Inc. Published 2012 by John Wiley & Sons, Inc.

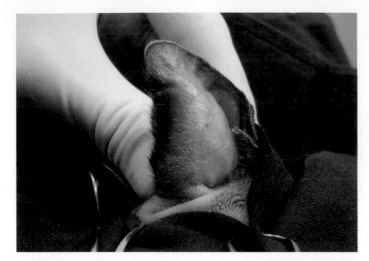

Figure 27-2 Ear mites cause severe itching in the ear canals. Cats respond to that with scratching and head shaking. The latter can result in broken blood vessels in the pinna; and aural hematoma results.

Image courtesy of Dr. Vanessa Pimentel.

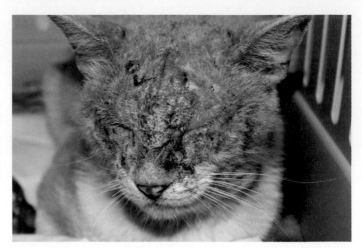

Figure 27-3 The *Notoedres cati* mites live on the head and cause intense itching. Crusty lesions are common. Scratch marks as the result of self-trauma are seen on this cat's head.

Image courtesy Dr. Gary D. Norsworthy.

to other animals and humans. Additionally, the canine (*Cheyletiella yasguri*) and rabbit (*Cheyletiella parasitovorax*) species can infect cats.

Infection is more common in long-haired cats. Clinical disease is typically mild, and asymptomatic carriers are possible. The clinical signs include scaling of the tail from where it spreads cranially resulting in crusting of the dorsum. Pruritus is variable. If it occurs, secondary infections as a result of scratching usually develop. In human infections there usually appear small, erythematous, pruritic papules in groups of two or three on the skin of the arms and abdomen. Diagnosis is made by sticky tape preparations or superficial skin scrapings in which the mites can be seen on microscopic examination. In heavier infestations white moving keratin scales (walking dandruff) can be easily seen when the coat is brushed over a black sheet of paper. A flea comb can be used to collect mites and eggs from the coat. When a cat is diagnosed with cheyletiellosis all in-contact animals should be treated.

Notoedres Cati (Feline Scabies)

Notoedres mites are 0.2 mm long and live under and on the skin. Female mites burrow under the skin and lay eggs. In these subcutaneous tunnels eggs hatch into larvae that then mature to nymphs. Nymphs reach the skin surface and mate. Mites survive less than 48 hours in the environment; therefore, the entire life cycle is completed on the host animal. Cats are natural hosts of these mites, but host specificity is poor. Infection is highly contagious; transmission is by direct contact. Young and debilitated cats are most susceptible to disease, and humans can also be infected. In the cat skin lesions usually start at the margins of the pinna with crusting and papules and then spread to the face, head, and neck. There is hair loss, erythema, and scaling initially, but as the disease progresses thick crusts, very heavy scaling, and lichenification develop (Fig. 27-3). In severe cases the lesions spread from the head and neck to other parts of the body, and local lymphadenopathy may occur. Infection causes severe pruritus and self-trauma frequently leading to secondary bacterial infections. Diagnosis is made based on clinical signs and microscopic examination of skin scrapings. All in-contact animals should be treated.

Sarcoptes Scabiei (Canine Scabies)

Cats are not natural hosts of these mites, but they may become infected from dogs or foxes. The life cycle is similar to feline scabies. Compared to *N. cati*, in *S. scabiei* infections pruritus is usually absent or is mild. Skin

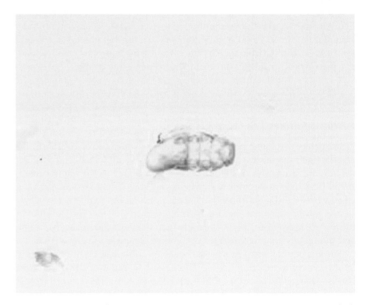

Figure 27-4 *Demodex gatoi* is shorter and thicker than D. *cati* and lives in the skin's keratin layer (stratum corneum), not in the hair follicles.

Image courtesy Dr. Gary D. Norsworthy.

lesions, which are similar to *Notoedres* infection, occur usually around the head and neck but can also be found on the paws and elsewhere in the body, possibly through grooming. Diagnosis is made with skin scrapings, and all in-contact animals should be treated simultaneously.

Demodex Cati and Demodex Gatoi (Cigarette Mites)

D. cati can be regarded as normal fauna. These cigarette-shaped mites are 0.2–0.4 mm in length and live in the hair follicles and sebaceous glands, usually a few millimeters under the skin surface (Fig. 27-4). Kittens get infected from their mother by direct contact. Infection lasts for life, but transmission between cats does not occur again in later life. In healthy cats there are no clinical signs of infection. Clinical disease appears only if the cat's immune system is compromised, most commonly by a

(a)

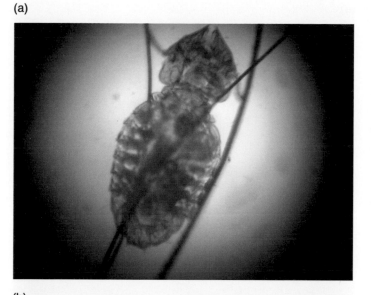

(b)

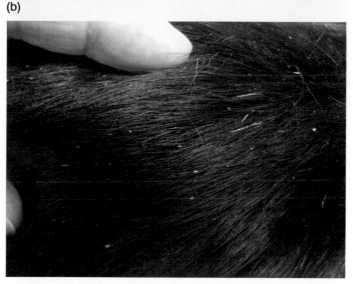

(c)

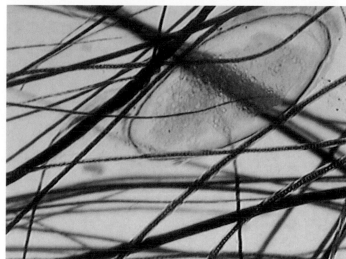

Figure 27-5 *Felicola subrostratum* is the louse of the cat. It can be found on the skin or hair. (a) This is a louse attached to a hair and seen under 40× magnification. (b) The eggs (nits) of the louse can be seen as tiny white objects attached to the hair. (c) The attached eggs are seen under 40× magnification.

Images courtesy Dr. Gary D. Norsworthy.

retroviral infection, immunosuppressive medication, stress, or severe systemic disease. Clinical disease can also be idiopathic.

D. gatoi is not a normal inhabitant of the cat. It is shorter and thicker than *D. cati* and lives in the skin's keratin layer (stratum corneum), not in the hair follicles. It is an infective disease that is highly contagious between cats. It can cause clinical disease without concomitant immuno-suppressive disease. Most cases of clinical demodicosis are caused by *D. gatoi.*

Clinical demodicosis is divided into focal and generalized forms. In focal disease there is alopecia or thinning of the hair coat or reddish, scaling dermatitis on the head and front limbs. It usually affects the eyelids, face, or ears. Demodicosis can also cause ceruminous otitis. Generalized disease starts as focal disease but extends wider and deeper becoming generalized folliculitis or pododermatitis. It causes usually symmetrical alopecia or barbered hair. Of affected cats, 50% have significant pruritus that leads to self-trauma and secondary infections.

Diagnosis is made by finding the organism with skin scrapings. However, because all cats potentially have a few mites present the clinical signs described previously and several mites must also be present. Focal and idiopathic demodicosis are usually self-limiting diseases, and

they are not treated if pruritus is not present. Nevertheless, it is crucial to treat the underlying disease that caused the clinical signs to erupt. Generalized demodicosis requires treatment.

An unnamed "long" *Demodex spp.* has also been discovered that may be found in conjunction with *D. cati.*

Felicola Subrostratum (Louse)

Lice are host-specific insects that spend their whole life cycle on the skin and hair coat. They are about 1 mm long, wingless, and dorsoventrally flattened, and their life cycle is completed within 3 weeks. Transmission between cats occurs by direct contact or by grooming with contaminated brushes and combs. Eggs are attached to the hair. Eggs hatch into nymphs which undergo several moults prior to becoming adults. Clinical disease varies from asymptomatic carriers to pruritus, alopecia, papules, and severe inflammation. Diagnosis is made by finding lice (Fig. 27-5a) or eggs on the skin or hair (Fig. 27-5b,c). Infection should be always treated because lice are intermediate host to the tapeworm *Dipylidium caninum.* Cats can also be infected by dog louse *Tricodectes canis.*

Ixodes Ricinus

These blood-sucking ticks are oval and dorsoventrally flattened. Prefeeding, the female is 2.5–5.0 mm in length, but after sucking blood it can grow up to 15 mm long. Male ticks are 2–4 mm and do not suck blood. Adult ticks live in a moist environment that includes long grass. They attach to animals and humans and mate. Female ticks suck blood up to 14 days, then drop off the cat, lay eggs, and die. Eggs become larvae that become nymphs and then mature to adults. A new blood meal is needed for completion of each stage in the life cycle. The duration of the entire life cycle depends on environmental conditions. In cooler climates and locations where the summer is short it takes up to 3 years to complete the life cycle.

Ticks do not cause any symptoms to the host besides local irritation. However, their significance is in disease transmission including bordetellosis and tick-borne encephalitis, some of which can affect humans. Cats may carry ticks inside the house resulting in human infections. Fortunately, there are products available for effective tick control.

Trombicula Autumnalis (Harvest Mite, Chiggers)

Adult *T. autumnalis* are not parasites, but their larvae infect cats with outdoor access causing small pruritic erythematous papules on the ventrum or on the feet. Some papules may have small orange-red spots at the place where the larva is embedded into the skin, or there may be clusters of larvae seen on the affected area. Pruritus can be intensive, but some cats remain asymptomatic. Diagnosis is made according to appropriate clinical signs that occur seasonally and direct visualisation of red-orange larvae or by visualization of the larvae on skin scrapings. Sometimes the larvae have already abandoned the cat prior to presentation so the diagnosis will be presumptive.

Endoparasites

Gastrointestinal Tract

Roundworms or Ascarids

Toxocara Cati

This roundworm is the most prevalent of all endoparasites in cats. It is a white and large arrow-headed worm. Males are usually 5–6 cm in length but may be up to 10 cm. Females are longer, 4–10 cm, but may be up to 15 cm (Fig. 27-6a). Adult worms live in the small intestine where females lay eggs, which are passed to the environment via feces (Fig. 27-6b). Eggs need to embryonate before becoming infective; this takes at least 4 weeks and longer in colder temperatures. During embryonation infective second-stage larvae (L2) develop within the egg, and after a cat ingests these infective L2 eggs the larvae migrate from the intestine to the liver and lungs. In the lungs the L2s mature to third-stage larvae (L3), which eventually are coughed up and swallowed returning to the small intestine. There the L3 mature, and female worms start laying eggs about 6–11 weeks after infection.

If infective L2 eggs are ingested by a paratenic host (earthworm, beetle, rodent, bird) L2s migrate into tissues and remain there until a cat eats this paratenic host. When a cat eats an L2-containing paratenic host there is no liver-to-lung migration; maturation occurs entirely in the intestine.

In adult cats most of the roundworm larvae migrate from the intestine to other parts of the body and encapsulate, most commonly in mammary tissue. Larvae are passed in the milk during lactation, infecting the kittens. When infestation occurs from the milk there is no liver-to-lung migration. Intrauterine infection does not occur in cats even though it may occur in dogs infected with *T. canis*.

Toxocara spp. can also infect people causing visceral larva migrans. This disease occurs mainly in small children who have ingested large quantities of eggs. It may cause fever, pneumonitis, hepatomegaly, and even encephalitis. Rarely, larvae may migrate to the eyes (ocular larva migrans) and cause blindness.

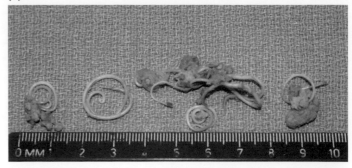

(a)

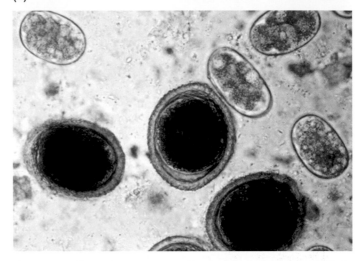

(b)

Figure 27-6 (a), Roundworms are so named because of their propensity to curl. (b), The three large eggs are those of *Toxocara cati* seen under 100 × magnification. The four smaller eggs are hookworm eggs.

Images courtesy Dr. Gary D. Norsworthy.

Toxascaris Leonina

This ascarid is smaller than *T. cati*. Male worms may grow up to 7 cm and females up to 10 cm. The life cycle is similar to *T. cati*, but it occurs only in the small intestine; there is no liver-to-lung migration or transmammary infection. Infection occurs by ingestion of embryonated L2 eggs or by ingestion of a paratenic host that harbors infective L2 in its tissues. The L2s become L3s in the cat's intestine and undergo maturation. The prepatent time, which is the time from ingestion to shedding of eggs, is at least 8 weeks. Because infection does not occur via milk and the prepatent period is long, *T. leonina* infection is only rarely seen in kittens younger than 6 months of age.

T. cati and *T. lenonina* are common roundworms in cats. In adult healthy cats infection is usually either asymptomatic or mild. There may be vomiting with or without the worms being expelled and some degree of diarrhea. The hair coat may be poor, and weight loss may occur in chronic infestations. Clinical signs of roundworms occur often in kittens that have acquired heavy infestations via milk. In addition to diarrhea and vomiting kittens usually have abdominal distension (pot-bellied abdomen) and failure to gain weight. Intestinal obstructions occur rarely. Because of lung migration *T. cati* infection may also cause coughing because of larva-induced pneumonitis or pneumonia; this is the most common cause of coughing in young kittens.

Diagnosis is made easily if worms are found in feces or vomitus. Eggs can also be found in the feces by fecal flotation but not until 6–8 weeks after infestation. There are good deworming medications available.

Because of infection acquired via milk, all kittens should be dewormed starting at 4–6 weeks of age and followed by retreatment every 3 weeks until 4 months of age. During adulthood the need for deworming depends on the cat's lifestyle. For outdoor, hunting cats regular dewormings are recommended.

As previously mentioned *T. cati* has public health significance because it may cause visceral and ocular larva migrans in humans. However, the opportunity for humans to obtain a roundworm infection from cats is less than from dogs (*T. canis*) because cats bury their feces. Therefore, *T. canis* is the most important roundworm regarding human larva infections.

Ollulanus Tricuspis

These small roundworms live in the cat's stomach wall. Males are only 0.7–0.8 mm and females 0.8–1.0 mm in length. Usually this is a nonpathogenic parasite, but it may cause vomiting, anorexia, weight loss, and chronic fibrosing gastritis. Infective L3 forms may be passed either in the vomit or with feces, but usually the entire life cycle occurs in the stomach, and intermediate hosts are not needed. Therefore, diagnosis is challenging because worms, larvae, or eggs may never leave the stomach. Direct microscopic examination of vomits or stomach washings or direct endoscopic visualization can be performed for diagnosis.

Physaloptera spp.

This is another roundworm of the feline stomach that is acquired by ingestion of an infected intermediate or paratenic host (reptile, insect, or small mammal). Typical clinical signs include chronic or intermittent vomiting. Melena and anemia may occur in heavy infestations. Diagnosis is difficult to confirm from a fecal sample because eggs do not float in routine fecal flotation solutions. Worms may be found in the vomitus. Direct visualization via gastroscopy is the preferred diagnostic method.

Strongyloides spp.

These small threadworms live in the crypts of the small intestine. There are four species that can infect cats: *Strongyloides felis*, *Strongyloides planiceps*, *Strongyloides tumefaciens*, and *Strongyloides stercoralis*. Females lay eggs containing first-stage larva (L1). Depending on the species, eggs are hatched either in the gut or passed in the feces and hatch in the environment. In the environment, larvae can take two routes in their development. they can become infective larvae or develop into free-living adults and lay eggs that hatch and become infective larvae. When the larvae become directly infective the life cycle is called homogonic, and the life cycle involving development of free-living adults is called heterogonic.

Infective larvae penetrate the skin of cats in skin locations that contact the soil. The larvae travel to the lungs from where they are coughed up and swallowed. After skin penetration, infective larvae may also travel randomly until they reach the small intestine. The prepatent period is approximately 2 weeks. *S. stercoralis* and *S. felis* have also the capability for autoinfection. Autoinfection happens when L1s become infective inside the cat's gut. These infective larvae penetrate the gut wall or perianal skin and re-enter the blood stream. They travel to the lungs then are coughed up and swallowed returning them back to the small intestine. In healthy adult cats clinical strongyloidosis usually causes mild clinical signs consisting of local skin irritation and respiratory and gastrointestinal signs.

Spirocerca Lupi

S. lupi is a bright red worm that lives in the esophagus and stomach and is much more common in dogs than in cats. Eggs are passed in the feces, and beetles act as an intermediate host. When a beetle eats the eggs, infective L3s develop and become capsulated in beetle's body. Chickens,

reptiles, and rodents may act as paratenic hosts if they eat an infected beetle. Cats become infected by eating either an intermediate or paratenic host. Larvae are released in the stomach, penetrate the stomach wall arteries and migrate to the aorta from where they migrate to esophagus and stomach after 2–3 months. Eggs are passed in the feces 5–6 months after infection. Clinical signs are usually absent or mild, but vomiting and dysphasia may occur. Infection provokes the development of fibrous nodules, which may be related to esophageal sarcoma. Diagnosis is made by finding eggs in the feces or by esophagoscopy or gastroscopy.

Tapeworms

Usually tapeworm infections are asymptomatic; therefore, infection remains undetected in cats that bury their feces outdoors. Abdominal discomfort may be occasionally seen. The most dramatic occurrence is the reaction of the client to seeing the segments.

Taenia Taenieformis

Tapeworms live in the small intestine. Small numbers are usually present in each host; there is rarely more than three to four worms in a cat. Adult tapeworms consist of segments that break off and pass in the stool (Figs. 27-7a,b). They may be seen on the surface of the stool or attached to the hair near the anus (Figs. 27-7c,d). Each segment contains many eggs. These gravid proglottid segments are passed with the feces. When a proglottid segment comes in contact with water it disintegrates and releases infective eggs (Fig. 27-7e). In water, eggs become larvae. When an intermediate host (rat, mouse, vole, squirrel, or rabbit) ingests this larva, a metacestoid cyst develops in the intermediate host's liver. This cystic stage is infective for cats after 60 days. Cats get infected by eating an intermediate host. After ingestion, the adult tapeworm is mature in 4–8 weeks. Usually a tapeworm infection in cats is asymptomatic, but proglottid segments may cause local perianal irritation.

Dipylidium Caninum

Adult worms live in the small intestine and are usually less than 25 cm in length. In most cases, the more worms a cat has the shorter the worms are. Like *T. taenieformis*, proglottid segments are passed in the feces, and they can also pass directly from the rectum and are seen crawling out the anus. The intermediate hosts for this tapeworm are fleas (*Ctenocephalides* spp.) and lice (*Felicola subrostratum*) in which cysticercoids are developed after ingestion of eggs. Cats get infected via ingestion of an infected flea or louse.

Spirometra spp.

These are tapeworms found in southeast United States. Their life cycle resembles that of *Diphyllobothrium latum*. Copepods act as primary and small mammals and reptiles as secondary intermediate hosts. Adult worms are about 25 cm in length and live in the small intestine. Infections are rare and remain usually asymptomatic. In more severe cases, cats may have weight loss and changes in appetite. Diagnosis is based on finding eggs in the feces.

Diphyllobothrium Latum (Broad Fish Tapeworm)

The broad tapeworm lives in the intestine of cats and may grow up to the whole length of cat's intestine. Proglottid segments are 1–1.5 cm long and are usually shed in chains. When eggs access water, larvae are hatched. Larvae are eaten by shellfish, which are then eaten by fish. Infective forms for cats (and dogs and humans) are plerocercoid cysts that are found in the muscles, intestine, and roe of fish. Cats get infected when they eat raw or undercooked fish. Salt water prevents the maturation of

(a)

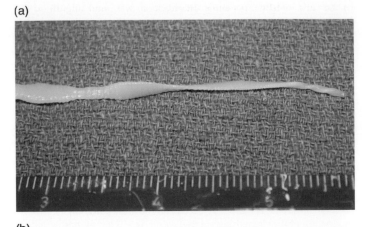

(b)

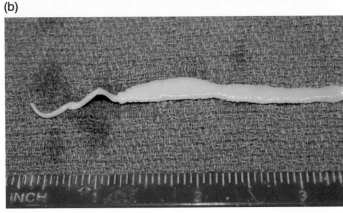

(e)

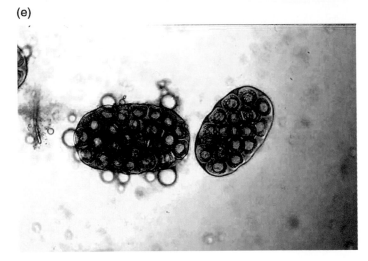

(c)

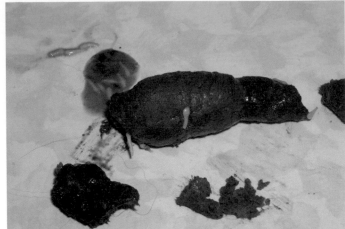

(d)

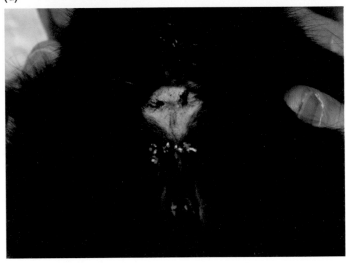

Figure 27-7 *Taenia taeniaeformis* is a segmented worm. (a) The head attaches to the intestinal wall. (b) The tail end terminates in segments that break off and pass in the stool. (c) They are often seen on the surface of the stool or attached to the hair near the anus (d). (e) When segments are ruptured, eggs are released.

Images courtesy Dr. Gary D. Norsworthy.

this worm; therefore, fish from sea water are not a source of infection. Infection is usually asymptomatic, but it may cause mild diarrhea and in chronic infections, anemia and deficiency of vitamin B_{12} may occur.

Echinococcus spp.

Echinococcosis is an infection caused by the tapeworms *Echinococcus granulosus* and *Echinococcus multilocularis*. Cats, dogs, and foxes are hosts for these tapeworms, and other mammals, including humans, are intermediate hosts. Hundreds of infective eggs are produced by these worms in the cat's intestine, and eggs are passed with the feces. Infective eggs are resistant in the environment and may remain infective for up to 1–2 years, but heating and drying will destroy them. Eggs are easily spread via

insects, wind, and rain. An intermediate host becomes infected by ingesting infective eggs; following and after ingestion hydatid cysts forms in tissues. Cats get infected by eating this tissue cyst contained within the intermediate host. Usually infection is asymptomatic for the host animal, but because it causes life-threatening disease to humans, this is a disease that should be prevented by regular dewormings in the endemic areas of echinococcosis.

Joyeuxiella Pasqualei

This tapeworm resembles *Dipylidium caninum* and is especially common in Africa and the Middle East. Beetles and lizards act as intermediate hosts.

Hookworms

Ancylostoma Tubaeforme

This feline hookworm lives in the small intestine where they suck blood. Adult worms are 7–12 mm long. Female worms lay eggs, which are passed in the feces into the environment from where the eggs are ingested by cats. Rodents and other transport hosts may also be a source of infection. Sometimes the infection may be acquired via skin penetration. In the cat's small intestine, larvae hatch, the worms mature, and new eggs are produced. The life cycle takes 2–3 weeks and does not include an extra-intestinal migration. A hookworm infection is significant only in kittens and young cats because age immunity develops. Clinical signs include diarrhea, vomiting, dark stools (*see* Fig. 27-6b), and weight loss or failure to gain weight. Diagnosis is made with a fecal flotation, but clinical signs may develop before eggs are detected in the feces. *Ancylostoma braziliense* is the canine hookworm; it has been reported in cats. *Uncinaria stenocephala*, which is a canine hookworm of colder climates, may also infect cats even though it is rarer.

Whipworms

Trichuris Serrate

Whipworms live in the colon. They are quite rare among cats. Infection occurs when a cat eats an infective egg from which a larva is hatched. The larva enters the small intestine and moves to the large intestine where maturation occurs. Worms suck blood from the intestinal epithelium, which causes local inflammation. Clinical signs are result of colitis including frequent, bloody, and mucoid diarrhea. Cats may also be inappetent and depressed. Diagnosis is made from a fecal sample, but because eggs are not shed continuously, it may be necessary to examine fecal samples for several consecutive days.

Lungs

Aleurostrongylus Abstrusus (Lungworm)

Adult lungworms are small (male 5 mm, female 9 mm) and live in the terminal bronchioles, alveolar ducts, and smaller branches of the pulmonary arteries. Eggs are laid in the alveoli. After the first-stage larvae have hatched they are coughed up into the pharynx, swallowed, and passed in the feces. Further development only occurs in the intermediate hosts, which are slugs and snails. The L1s survive for months in the environment. L3s develop in the intermediate host. Cats acquire infection by eating either an intermediate host or a paratenic host (rodent, amphibian, reptile, bird) that has ingested a slug or a snail containing L3. The L3s are not infective to paratenic hosts; they remain unchanged within the paratenic hosts. In the cat L3s penetrate the intestinal wall and migrate to the lungs via lymph and blood vessels. Egg production is started four weeks after infestation.

Most infections are mild and self-limiting in 3–4 months because of an effective immune response. Nevertheless, in heavy infestations respiratory signs may be severe consisting of dyspnea, coughing, harsh respiratory sounds, sneezing, and oculonasal discharge. Diagnosis is made based on clinical signs and demonstrating L1s in fecal samples. After the first infection occurs cats tend to be resistant to reinfection.

Eucoleus Aerophila (Formerly *Capillaria Aerophila*)

These larger (25–30 mm) lungworms live on the mucous membrane of the trachea and bronchi of the dog, cat, and fox. Disease is quite rare among cats and is most likely found in cats sharing the same environment with foxes. Eggs are laid in the trachea and bronchi. They are coughed up, swallowed, and passed in the feces where they become infective and can survive in the environment for more than a year. When a cat eats eggs or a paratenic host (earthworms and rodents), larva hatch in the cat's intestine, penetrate the intestinal wall, and migrate to the lungs where maturation occurs. Egg production starts 40 days after infestation. This parasite has direct life cycle, which means that it does not need an intermediate host to complete its life cycle. Clinical signs include coughing, sneezing, and nasal discharge. The eggs can be identified from a tracheal wash, bronchoalveolar lavage, and fecal flotation.

Paragonimus Kellicotti (North-American Lung Fluke)

This is lung fluke of cats (and dogs) found in the southern, Midwestern, and Great Lakes regions of the United States and in a few other parts of the world. Adult worms are about 1 cm long and live in the lung parenchyma where they form bullae or cysts. Eggs are laid, coughed up, and swallowed. Freshwater snails and crayfish act as intermediate hosts, which ingest eggs shed in the cat's feces. Cats get infected by ingesting an intermediate host. The typical clinical sign is coughing, which is caused by an inflammatory reaction in the lungs. If a cyst in lung parenchyma ruptures, rapid and usually fatal pneumothorax may develop.

Bladder

Capillaria Feliscati

These small hair-like nematodes live in the surface of the bladder mucosa of cats. Adult females measure 30–60 mm and males 13–30 mm long. The life cycle of bladder worms is not totally understood. Eggs are released in the urine but are not immediately infectious. Eggs are ingested by an earthworm in which infective L1s are hatched. Cats get infected when ingesting this intermediate host. Larvae migrate from the intestine to the bladder. Eggs usually appear in the urine 2 months after infestation. There are usually no clinical signs of infestation, which is usually self-limiting. Treatment is indicated if the cat has clinical signs.

Protozoas

Toxoplasma Gondii

T. gondii is a coccidian protozoan that can infect any warm-blooded animal, but only cats can shed infective oocysts into the environment. *T. gondii* has three infective forms: tachyzoite, bradyzoite, and sporulated oocyst. Tachyzoites are rapidly dividing forms that migrate from the intestine to extraintestinal tissues via blood and lymph during active infection. Damage to these tissues is responsible for the clinical signs of toxoplasmosis and relates to the organ affected. In immunocompromised cats the tachyzoite period can be fatal. In healthy adult animals the tachyzoite phase is eventually changed to slowly dividing bradyzoites, which encapsulate into cysts in tissues. This cyst stage is the chronic phase of toxoplasmosis. If a cat's immune status worsens bradyzoites may reactivate and cause clinical disease. Oocysts are the result of a reproductive cycle, which only takes place in domestic and wild cats. Oocysts are shed in the feces, but they are not readily infective. They need sporulation to become infective. Sporulation occurs when oocysts are exposed to oxygen and takes 1–5 days. Cats shed large numbers of oocysts within 3 weeks after infection. The shedding continues usually a week. Oocyst shedding is heaviest in kittens 6–14 weeks of age.

Cats and other warm-blooded animals can become infected by eating sporulated oocysts, tachyzoites, or meat containing tissue cysts (bradyzoites). Additionally, infection is possible through the conjunctiva, the respiratory tract, and percutaneously. Milk and eggs may be infective, too. If the life cycle begins with the ingestion of tachyzoites or oocysts, it requires 3 weeks for completion. However, if tissue cysts are ingested, the entire life cycle can be completed within 3 days. The most common infection route for cats is eating a tissue cyst usually found in a rodent. In pregnant animals and humans *T. gondii* may infect the fetus transplacentally. For humans the most common route of infection is undercooked meat (tissue cysts) or from vegetables contaminated with oocysts. Direct transmission from cat to humans is rare.

Clinical signs of toxoplasmosis refer to the individual organs affected. The most commonly affected organs are the lungs, liver, intestine, and eye. Anorexia, fever, lethargy, diarrhea, dyspnea (due to pneumonia), ocular signs, and icterus are the most common clinical signs. Toxoplasmosis can also cause neurological signs. Most cats show no clinical signs and spontaneously recover from infection developing good immunity. Susceptible cats may become severely ill and even die.

Diagnosis is made based on clinical signs and serum antibody tests. Immunoglobulin G (IgG) and immunoglobulin M (IgM) antibodies should be measured. IgG antibodies are present for life, and therefore, indicate that the cat has been exposed to *T. gondii* at some point in its life. IgM antibodies are present only for about 3 months after infection and indicate recent or active infection. A fourfold rise in an IgG titer from blood samples taken 2 weeks apart also suggests recent infection.

Toxoplasmosis has human health significance because it may cause abortion if a pregnant woman becomes infected. To prevent infection proper meat handling is critical. Meat should be cooked at temperatures above 70°C (160°F) or frozen at −20°C (−4°F) for at least 24 hours before cooking. Surfaces and utensils that have been in contact with raw meat should be washed adequately. Pregnant women should avoid contact with soil, raw meat, and cat feces. Because oocysts need at least 24 hours to sporulate, litter boxes that are emptied daily should not be means of transmission.

Isospora Felis, Isospora Rivolta

These coccidian protozoans are common and widespread but only rarely cause clinical disease in adult cats. Clinical disease occurs mainly in kittens and usually in poor hygienic conditions. Cats shed infective oocysts in their feces (Fig. 27-8). Oocysts contain two sporocysts each of which contains four sporozoites. Rodents act as paratenic hosts, and when they eat oocysts, sporozoite cysts remain in their tissues. Cats get infected by eating either oocysts or rodents that have eaten oocysts. Because cats develop strong age-related immunity, only kittens usually show significant clinical signs. Mild infections may occur in cats that hunt rodents. Clinical signs include large bowel diarrhea with tenesmus. Infection is usually self-limiting, and reinfections are unlikely. Diagnosis is made by detecting oocysts in fecal smears or by fecal flotation.

Sarcocystis spp.

Sarcocystis is another coccidian protozoa. Cats and human are definitive hosts for some *Sarcocystis* species. In cats they infect the mucosal cells of the intestine. Oocysts are produced in the intestine and passed in the feces. Oocysts release infective sporocysts in the environment. When an intermediate host (cow, pig, rodent, or small mammal) eats these sporocysts, sarcocysts are formed in its tissues, usually muscles or lymph nodes. Inside these resting sarcocysts bradyzoites mature and become infective to the definitive host. This cystic disease of the intermediate host is called sarcosporidiosis, and cysts can be so large that they are visible to the naked eye. When a definitive host eats an intermediate host, oocyst production begins about a week later. Sarcocysts are also formed in cats' tissues (heart, skeletal muscles, or diaphragm muscles), but the infection is usually asymptomatic. Sarcocystis encephalitis has been reported in young cats.

Cryptosporidium Felis and *Cryptosporidium Parvum*

These coccidia usually infect young cats with poorly developed immune system or individuals with compromised immunity. The life cycle is similar to other coccidians, but there are two types of oocysts produced. Some infective oocysts pass in the feces, and others release infective sporozoites within the intestine causing autoinfection. Oocysts are stable

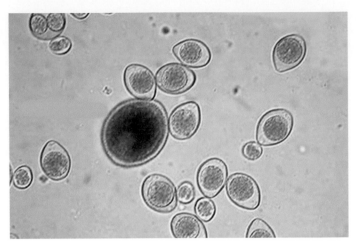

Figure 27-8 *Ancylostoma tubaeforme*, the cat hookworm, lives in the small intestine where it sucks blood. The eggs are passed in the feces. Several hookworm eggs are seen with one roundworm egg.

Image courtesy Dr. Gary D. Norsworthy.

in the environment but can be destroyed by freezing or heating to 60°C (140°F) for 30 minutes. Cats become infected by ingesting oocysts within feces or contaminated food or water. Diarrhea, weight loss, and anorexia are the main clinical signs, but most infections are mild and self-limiting. These asymptomatic carriers spread the infection by shedding oocysts in feces. This is a zoonotic disease. Diagnosis is made by demonstration of oocysts in fecal smears with special staining or by the fecal flotation test. A polymerase chain reaction (PCR) test that detects *Cryptosporidium* DNA in feces is available. Direct fecal ELISA or immunofluorescent antibody tests are also available.

Cytauxzoon Felis

This is a hemoparasite transmitted by tick as vectors with bobcats serving as asymptomatic reservoir hosts. Infection is more common in the spring and summer when ticks are most active. The disease has two phases. In the tissue phase, replication occurs within tissue macrophages leading to vascular obstruction and severe clinical disease or death. In the erythrocytic phase, hemolytic anemia occurs causing severe clinical signs, which are also often fatal. Clinical signs usually occur approximately 10 days after infection and include fever, anorexia, pallor, icterus, dehydration, lethargy, tachypnea, or dyspnea. Diagnosis is made based on clinical signs and identification of the parasites within the red blood cells. Without therapy cats usually die within 1 week. Therapy includes aggressive supportive therapy and antiprotozoal drugs. Clinical signs may worsen during therapy prior to recovery, and many cats still die despite therapy. Therefore, prevention based on tick control is paramount.

Giardia spp.

Giardia is protozoan that infects many mammals and birds and is common in cats. Trophozoites live on the mucosa of the small intestine and occasionally in the large intestine. They encyst in the small or large intestine and are passed in the feces. Oocysts are resistant in the environment. Cysts are infective, and transmission occurs by ingestion of these cysts. Cyst shedding may be continuous or intermittent. After ingestion trophozoites are released from oocysts in the intestine and are responsible for clinical signs. The prepatent period is 5–14 days. Clinical signs include intermittent or continuous diarrhea, steatorrhea, vomiting, fever, and weight loss. Feces are light brown in color, a have strong odor, and are usually mucoid; blood in the stool is common. There are many asymptomatic infections, and clinical signs may appear under stress. Diagnosis is made based on a combination of appropriate clinical signs and a fecal antigen test, fecal flotation, or a direct saline smear. Because *Giardia* cysts are excreted intermittently, several fecal examinations should be performed if giardiasis is suspected.

Tritrichomonas Foetus

T. foetus colonizes the colon of cats resulting in chronic large bowel diarrhea. It is most commonly seen in kittens and young cats and in cat colonies because increased housing density increases the risk for infection. Trophozoites live in the bowel, and cysts are shed in the environment where they can be transmitted by flies and other vectors. Transmission occurs by the fecal-oral route. Incubation time is 4–14 days. The typical clinical sign is malodorous, mucoid, and bloody diarrhea. Flatulence and tenesmus are also common. Infection usually resolves spontaneously, but it may take up to 2 years. Most infected cats continue to shed low levels of the organism in their faeces for many months after the resolution of the diarrhea. Ronidazole can be used to accelerate clearing the infection. Tritrichomoniasis is usually misdiagnosed as giardiasis. Diagnosis can be made by detecting motile trophozoites under the microscope from fresh feces or rectal swab, by culture, or by a PCR test, which is the most reliable test. *T. foetus* may also infect people.

Suggested Readings

Bowman DD, Hendrix CM, Lindsay DS, et al. 2002. *Feline Clinical Parasitology*. Ames: Iowa State University Press.

Crystal MA, Walker MC. 2010. Hookworms. In GD Norsworthy, ed., *The Feline Patient*, 4th ed., p. 234. Ames: Wiley-Blackwell.

Crystal MA, Walker MC. 2010. Roundworms. In GD Norsworthy, ed., *The Feline Patient*, 4th ed., pp. 468–69. Ames: Wiley-Blackwell.

Crystal MA, Walker MC. 2010. Stomach Worms. In GD Norsworthy, ed., *The Feline Patient*, 4th ed., p. 492. Ames: Wiley-Blackwell.

Crystal MA, Walker MC. 2010. Tapeworms. In GD Norsworthy, ed., *The Feline Patient*, 4th ed., pp. 496–97. Ames: Wiley-Blackwell.

Foreyt WJ. 2001. *Veterinary Parasitology Reference Manual*, 5th ed. Ames: Iowa State University Press.

Grace SF. 2010. Fleas. In GD Norsworthy, ed., *The Feline Patient*, 4th ed., pp. 191–92. Ames: Wiley-Blackwell.

Norsworthy GD. 2010. Lung Parasites. In GD Norsworthy, ed., *The Feline Patient*, 4th ed., pp. 306–7. Ames: Wiley-Blackwell.

Norsworthy GD, Grace SF. 2010. Toxoplasmosis. In GD Norsworthy, ed., *The Feline Patient*, 4th ed., pp. 512–14. Ames: Wiley-Blackwell.

Rees CA. 2010. Skin Parasites. In GD Norsworthy, ed., *The Feline Patient*, 4th ed., pp. 483–86. Ames: Wiley-Blackwell.

Robson M, Crystal MA. 2010. Cryptosporidiosis. In GD Norsworthy, ed., *The Feline Patient*, 4th ed., pp. 100–101. Ames: Wiley-Blackwell.

Robson M, Crystal MA. 2010 Cytauxzoonosis. In GD Norsworthy, ed., *The Feline Patient*, 4th ed., pp. 106–7. Ames: Wiley-Blackwell.

Robson M, Crystal MA. 2010. Giardiasis. In GD Norsworthy, ed., *The Feline Patient*, 4th ed., pp. 197–98. Ames: Wiley-Blackwell.

Robson M, Crystal MA. 2010. Tritrichomoniasis. In GD Norsworthy, ed., *The Feline Patient*, 4th ed., pp. 523–25. Ames: Wiley-Blackwell.

Trees AJ. 2004. Endoparasites. In EA Chandler, CJ Gaskell, RM Gaskell, eds., *Feline Medicine and Therapeutics*, 3rd ed., pp. 697–707. Ames: Blackwell Publishing.

CHAPTER 28

Respiratory Diseases

Linda E. Schmeltzer

Overview

The most important functions of the respiratory system are: (1) to supply oxygen to all body cells and (2) to eliminate carbon dioxide produced by cells. Blood is the vehicle used for oxygen and carbon dioxide transport. The respiratory system also filters inhaled air, helps eliminate waste, and contains receptors for the sense of smell.

When a cat inhales air molecules are carried into the upper respiratory tract through the nostrils and into the nasal passages. Within the nasal passages are thin, scroll-shaped bones (turbinates). The turbinates are covered in nasal epithelium, thin moist tissue that contains the receptors for the sense of smell. Microscopic hairs called cilia help trap foreign material on the moist surface of the nasal epithelium. Air is warmed and humidified as it is forced through the twists and turns of the turbinates and nasopharynx into the pharynx. The pharynx, or throat, passes food down to the esophagus and air to the larynx. When the cat swallows, a leaf-shaped piece of cartilage, the epiglottis, is pulled over the opening of the larynx to prevent food from passing into the airway. The larynx is lined with mucous and cilia that trap foreign material before it reaches the trachea. The last structure in the upper respiratory tract is the trachea, a tubular structure that extends from the larynx into the chest and connects to the lower respiratory tract. In the chest, the trachea divides, or bifurcates, into the right and left main stem bronchi. Each main stem bronchus leads directly into the lungs, where it repeatedly divides into many smaller tubes that connect to tiny sacs called alveoli. Deoxygenated blood enters the lungs through the pulmonary artery. The pulmonary artery divides to the right and left lung lobes, continues subdividing into smaller vessels along the bronchi, and eventually enters a network of capillaries around the alveoli. The exchange of carbon dioxide and oxygen occurs through two thin layers of tissue that separate the air in the alveoli and blood in the capillaries. Oxygen-rich blood then travels through venules that join together to become veins. Veins join together and eventually join the large pulmonary vein that leaves the lungs and enters the left side of the heart. When a cat exhales, carbon dioxide and other waste gases leave the body in the reverse pathway.

Asthma

Asthma, also known as allergic bronchitis, is a disorder of the lower respiratory tract caused by a combination of inflammation of the airway and muscle contraction of the bronchi resulting in a restriction of airflow. The inflammation may be the result of exposure to allergens, like pollen or mold, or noxious stimuli, such as ammonia or smoke. The symptoms can subside spontaneously or may need medical treatment to control. The irritation results in a buildup of mucous and cellular material within the bronchi. Severely affected cats may have sudden severe muscle spasms of the bronchi that are life threatening.

The most common clinical sign is coughing (Fig. 28-1). Some cats will only cough occasionally; others will have multiple coughing episodes per day. Wheezing or rapid breathing are commonly reported. More severe cases will have respiratory distress needing immediate treatment.

Several diagnostic tests can be ordered to confirm a diagnosis and rule out other causes of the clinical signs. Radiographs will show characteristic changes in the lungs (Fig. 28-2). The changes will vary with the severity of the asthma. Blood tests to rule out heartworm disease may also be ordered. Bronchoalveolar lavage or tracheal wash for cytology and culture may be performed to rule out bacterial or fungal causes.

Treatment for asthma will vary depending on the severity of the case. Cats with severe, life-threatening disease will be hospitalized and require oxygen administration until they can be stabilized with medications. Corticosteroids can reduce the inflammation. Bronchodilators are given as an inhaler or injectable drug to open the airway and allow air to move more freely in and out of the bronchi. Antibiotics are often needed because the lungs of cats with asthma are susceptible to infection. Once a cat is stabilized, oral medications are used to help reduce symptoms and prevent future episodes of respiratory distress. Oral corticosteroids, such as prednisolone, and bronchodilators, such as terbutaline, will often need to be administered long term. Inhaled corticosteroids and bronchodilators are also available by prescription and may be chosen at the discretion of the veterinarian.

Administration of inhaled medications requires special equipment and technique for cats. The equipment consists of a standard metered dose inhaler attached to a tube called a spacer. On the other end of the spacer is a small face mask. When the inhaler is depressed, the medication is released into the spacer, allowing the cat to breath in the entire dose in 7–10 breaths (Fig. 28-3). The procedure takes very little time, and most cats will be cooperative. Owners should be taught to watch their cat's breathing during treatment because many cats will hold their breath when first introduced to inhalation therapy. Drug dosages and frequency of medications and inhalers will be adjusted as needed at the discretion of the veterinarian.

Asthma is usually a manageable disease. With aggressive treatment and owner compliance the prognosis is good.

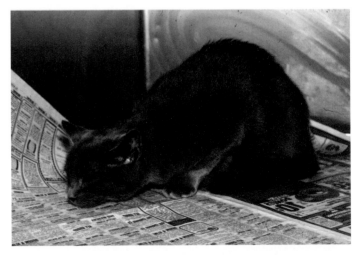

Figure 28-1 The two major differentials for coughing in adult cats are feline asthma and feline heartworm disease. The cat assumes the position shown here, and the cough is generally nonproductive.

Image courtesy Dr. Gary D. Norsworthy.

Nursing the Feline Patient, First Edition. Edited by Linda E. Schmeltzer and Gary D. Norsworthy.

(a)

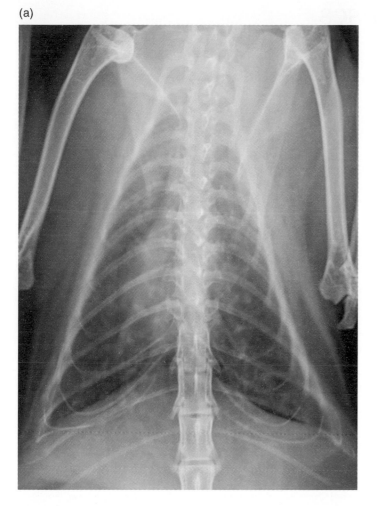

(b)

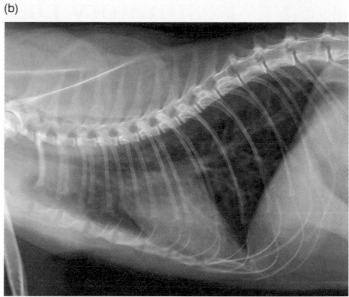

Figure 28-2 The radiographic findings in feline asthma include a bronchial pattern. The major blood vessels are normal in size. (a) Ventrodorsal view. (b) Lateral view.

Image courtesy Dr. Gary D. Norsworthy.

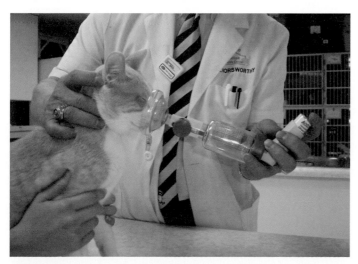

Figure 28-3 Some cats can be treated with inhalant bronchodilators or corticosteroids using a device with a small face mask and a spacer.

Image courtesy Dr. Gary D. Norsworthy.

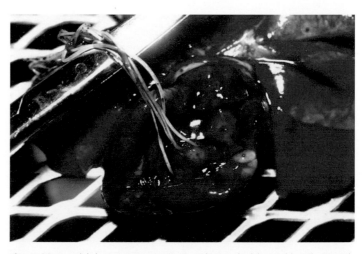

Figure 28-4 Adult heartworms are 10–15 cm (4–6 inches) long. Although primarily found in the pulmonary arteries, they may be in the right side of the heart when there is no room for them in the pulmonary arteries. It is unusual to find this many adult worms in a cat.

Image courtesy Dr. Gary D. Norsworthy.

(a)

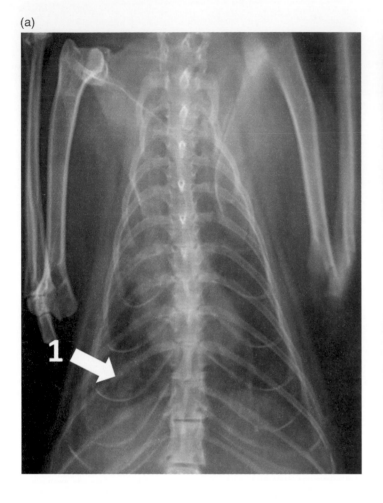

(b)

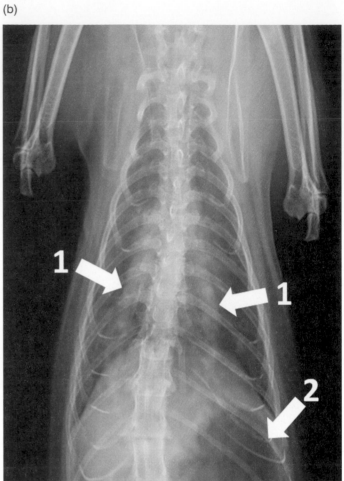

(c)

(d)

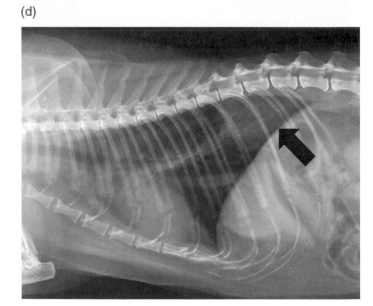

Figure 28-5 Most of the classic heartworm findings are seen in the dorsoventral or ventrodorsal view. (a) A focal interstitial pattern is seen at the end of the arrow. (b) Very large caudal pulmonary arteries (1) and air in the stomach (2), known as aerophagia, are seen in this cat with heartworms. (c) An enlarged and blunted right caudal pulmonary artery (1) and a focal interstitial pattern (2) are seen in this infected cat. (d) The enlarged caudal pulmonary arteries are not appreciated in a lateral view, but areas of focal interstitial disease as the result dead worms are often seen (arrow).

Image courtesy Dr. Gary D. Norsworthy.

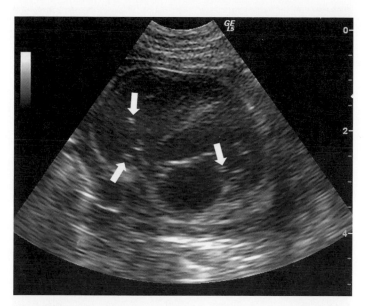

Figure 28-6 When heartworms are in the right side of the heart ultrasound of the right ventricle and pulmonary outflow tract demonstrate adult heartworms as short parallel lines (arrows).

Image courtesy Dr. Gary D. Norsworthy.

Heartworm Disease

Heartworm disease is a potentially fatal infestation by the parasite *Dirofilaria immitis*. The disease occurs in regions where a favorable environment supports the parasite's life cycle and affects cats, dogs, and other mammals in the dog family such as coyotes. The life cycle of the heartworm in cats is similar to that in dogs, but with some notable differences.

The life of a heartworm begins when male and female heartworms living within an infected animal reproduce and release larva (microfilariae) into the bloodstream. A heartworm goes through five stages of development, termed L1 through L4 and juvenile adult, before reaching mature adulthood. When a mosquito bites an infected animal and takes a blood meal it also ingests the microfilariae. Over the next 10–14 days the parasites live inside the mosquito and develop from L1 to L3 larva. When the mosquito bites a cat the L3 larvae enter the skin through the bite. Over the next 75–90 days the parasites develop to L4 and then 2-inch long juvenile adults and migrate to the pulmonary arteries and lungs. Most of the juvenile adults that enter the bloodstream die in the pulmonary arteries before reaching the adult stage. On average, one to three juvenile adults develop into adult worms. Adult heartworms grow to be 4–6 inches long (Fig. 28-4). These worms are usually the same sex, so they are unable to reproduce. It has been reported that adult heartworms can live up to 4 years. As the juvenile and adult heartworms die, they cause an intense inflammatory reaction in the pulmonary arteries. The pumping action of the arteries carries the dead parasites into the lungs where the same intense reaction occurs.

Clinical signs of heartworm infection in cats include coughing (*see* Fig. 28-1), rapid breathing, or respiratory distress. Vomiting may also

occur, although the mechanism is poorly understood. Sudden death as a result of a thromboembolism has been reported.

Diagnosis may occur during the workup for respiratory distress or coughing. It can be an incidental finding in an asymptomatic cat. Radiographs of the chest can be suggestive of a heartworm infection (Fig. 28-5). Enlargement of one or both of the caudal pulmonary arteries can be a sign of heartworm disease. Heartworms in cats are not usually detected during an echocardiogram because the worms are primarily found in the pulmonary arteries. However, sometimes the adult worms become too crowded in the pulmonary arteries, causing one or two to migrate into the right ventricle (Fig. 28-6).

There are two types of blood tests for the diagnosis of heartworm disease: an antigen test and an antibody test. These tests can be helpful in confirming a diagnosis of heartworm disease, but interpretation of the results must be fully understood. A positive antigen test result occurs when the cat is carrying at least three mature adult female heartworms. Unfortunately, most cats with one or more adult heartworms do not have three or more female worms present. The juvenile adult worms will not cause a positive antigen test result. The antibody test identifies proteins released from L3, L4, and juvenile adult stages of development. A positive test indicates that the cat has been infected with heartworms. However, it does not differentiate between a current infection with live worms and an infection in which the larvae or juvenile adult worms have died within 4 months.

It is important to understand that a positive result on either test is confirmation of heartworms, but a negative test result does not rule out heartworms.

Treatment has two parts. The first is geared toward stabilizing the cat and relieving inflammation caused by the worms. Oxygen therapy will be required if the cat is in respiratory distress. Once breathing is normalized, corticosteroids can be prescribed to reduce and relieve inflammation. They may be prescribed long term at the discretion of the veterinarian. The second step is to avoid further infection by using an approved heartworm prevention product. These products will eliminate the immature larva before they reach the circulatory system, thereby preventing further damage to the lungs.

There is not a safe or effective drug for killing heartworms in cats and if there was such a drug, killing many juvenile adults or adults at once would result in acute, severe lung disease. Controlling symptoms and preventing further infestation while the cat's immune system kills the larvae and adults are the recommended approach to the cat becoming heartworm free.

Suggested Readings

Brunt JE. 2011. Heartworm Disease. In GD Norsworthy, ed., *The Feline Patient*, 4th ed., pp. 208–10. Ames: Wiley-Blackwell.

Colville T. 2008. The Respiratory System. In T Colville, JM Bassert, eds., *Clinical Anatomy and Physiology for Veterinary Technicians*, 2nd ed., pp. 247–63. St. Louis: Mosby Inc.

Eddlestone SM. 2006. Small Animal Medical Nursing. In DM McCurnin, JM Bassert, eds., *Clinical Textbook for Veterinary Technicians*, 6th ed., pp. 810–11. St. Louis: Elsevier Saunders.

Padrid P. 2011. Bronchial Disease, Chronic. In GD Norsworthy, ed., *The Feline Patient*, 4th ed., pp. 58–61. Ames: Wiley-Blackwell.

CHAPTER 29

Toxicoses

Sharon Fooshee Grace

Introduction

The cat has unique susceptibility to a variety of toxins. Both metabolic idiosyncrasies and species-specific behavioral characteristics put the cat at risk for toxicosis. Cats have a deficiency of some hepatic glucuronyl transferase enzymes needed for conjugation of compounds to glucuronic acid. Conjugation increases water solubility and promotes elimination of substances in bile or urine. In cats, lack of sufficient enzyme can result in slowed or altered metabolism of some compounds. Also, feline erythrocytes are predisposed to oxidative damage because they have a large number of hemoglobin sulfhydryl groups. Oxidation of these groups leads to development of methemoglobin (hemoglobin which cannot carry oxygen) and formation of erythrocyte Heinz bodies (denatured hemoglobin).

Cats may absorb some toxins through the skin or as a consequence of their grooming habits. Although cats are less likely to have oral exposure to toxins than are dogs, the dermal route may be relatively more important for this species.

Household Toxins

Phenolic Disinfectants

The cat is dependent upon glucuronide conjugation for elimination of phenolic substances. Proximity to household phenols (Lysol®, Pinesol®) puts the cat at risk of poisoning by these agents. Dermal exposure may occur after the cat walks over wet surfaces and then licks the paws or fur. The caustic nature of these agents may cause necrosis of tissue, including in the oral cavity. Also depending upon which phenol is ingested, the liver, kidneys, or nervous system may be affected, leading to ataxia, tremors, seizures, respiratory alkalosis, or methemoglobinemia.

Treatment is nonspecific. Because of the caustic nature of phenols, treatment should *not* include induction of vomition or gastric lavage. Fluid therapy is indicated for support of vascular volume. If methemoglobinemia occurs, N-acetylcysteine (NAC) should be administered. Acid-base status should be monitored, along with biochemical profiles and urinalysis.

Plants

Acute tubular necrosis leading to renal failure can develop in cats following ingestion of certain types of lilies (Figs. 29-1a,b). Although not every lily is associated with renal failure, it is advisable to consider all lily species as potentially toxic. Ingestion of any part of the plant, including pollen, may result in severe toxicosis; death may result from ingestion of part of a leaf. The presence of the yellow pollen on the cat's hair can be an important diagnostic finding. To date, only the cat has been shown to develop renal failure following lily ingestion. The mechanism of toxicity is unknown.

Clinical signs may be apparent within 2 hours and include depression, vomiting, and anorexia. Dehydration, uremic breath, and renal pain are

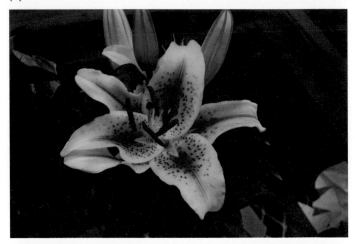

(a)

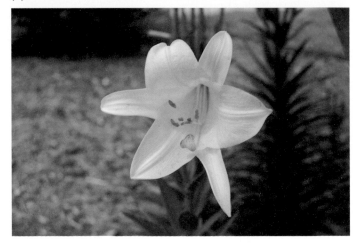

(b)

Figure 29-1 (a) The Easter Lily (*Lilium longiflorum*) and (b) the Stargazer Lily (*Lilium orientalis*) are highly toxic to cats.

noted within 24–96 hours. Azotemia, hyperkalemia, and hyperphosphatemia are detected within 24–72 hours. Epithelial casts may appear in the urine within 2 days of ingestion. Isosthenuria, glucosuria, and proteinuria are other supportive findings.

Treatment is nonspecific because there is no antidote. If exposure is known, vomiting should be induced and gastric lavage considered. Intravenous fluid therapy is critical and must be closely monitored with strict attention to the balance between fluid input and urine output because of the potential for oliguria or anuria. A crystalloid fluid is a reasonable first choice. Electrolytes and acid-base status should be monitored.

The prognosis is good if the cat is presented immediately and the gastrointestinal (GI) tract is successfully decontaminated; prognosis is poor after onset of renal failure.

Nursing the Feline Patient, First Edition. Edited by Linda E. Schmeltzer and Gary D. Norsworthy.

Ethylene Glycol

Cats are commonly poisoned by ethylene glycol (EG) following ingestion of antifreeze and are more easily poisoned than dogs, requiring only one-third to one-half the amount that is fatal for dogs. Ethylene glycol is rapidly absorbed from the GI tract with blood levels peaking in a few hours. Metabolites of EG cause the toxicosis; these form rapidly and persist for several days. Metabolic acidosis and acute renal failure often lead to death.

Clinical signs typically progress through three stages. Stage 1 may begin within 30 minutes and reflects central nervous system (CNS) changes. The cat may have a drunken appearance, as indicated by ataxia, incoordination, vomiting, and depression. Stage 2 develops 12–24 hours after ingestion and is characterized by the onset and progression of acute renal failure. Stage 3 begins approximately 24 hours after ingestion and is marked by oliguria which progresses to anuric renal failure. Cats in Stage 3 will exhibit vomiting and depression, renal pain and palpably enlarged kidneys, coma, worsening azotemia, crystals in the urine and, eventually, death.

Diagnosis may be established by history of possible exposure to EG, consistent laboratory findings, and measurement of blood EG with in-house test kits. Wood's lamp screening of the oral cavity, vomitus, or urine may show fluorescence, a finding which is consistent with EG poisoning.

Nonspecific therapies directed toward GI decontamination are rarely helpful because of the rapid EG absorption and minimal efficacy of activated charcoal in binding EG. Fluids should be initiated and the patient monitored for urine output relative to fluid input. Therapy aimed at interrupting production of toxic EG metabolites may be achieved with intravenous administration of ethanol or fomepizole (4-methylpyrazole). Ethanol may be given as a constant rate infusion or intermittent therapy; it is not without risk because it may lead to further CNS and respiratory depression. Cats require a higher dose of fomepizole than dogs. Therapy is rarely successful if begun more than six hours after ingestion.

Rodenticides

Anticoagulant Rodenticides

Rodenticide poisoning occurs when cats inadvertently ingest rodent bait. Dogs are more commonly poisoned than cats. Relay poisoning (by ingestion of poisoned rodents) is unlikely with the first-generation hydroxycoumarins (warfarin, dicoumarin) and indandiones (diphacinone) but can feasibly occur with the newer, more potent second generation hydroxycoumarins (brodifacoum, bromadiolone).

Several coagulation factors depend upon vitamin K for conversion to functional forms. The anticoagulant rodenticides (ACR) impair clotting by interfering with normal recycling of vitamin K. After ingestion of ACR, vitamin K becomes depleted, and there is an eventual failure of normal coagulation.

Diagnosis may be achieved with a thorough history, potential exposure to bait, appropriate clinical signs, and laboratory abnormalities. Clinical signs are variable but may include cutaneous bruising (Fig. 29-2), prolonged bleeding after venipuncture, dyspnea (bleeding into lungs, pleural space, or mediastinum), hematuria, oral bleeding, seizures (meningeal bleeding), lameness (bleeding in joint), epistaxis, and ocular hemorrhage. Radiographs may provide evidence of blood accumulation in the lung or pleural space.

Clotting tests may be come abnormal within 24 hours while the onset of clinical bleeding may lag for several days, though there is great variation dependent upon the type and amount of bait ingested. It is expected that coagulation tests become abnormal before evidence of bleeding occurs.

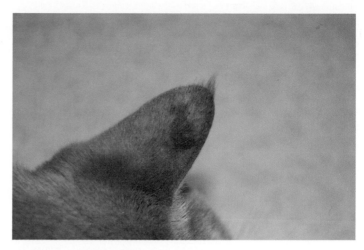

Figure 29-2 This photo shows an ecchymotic hemorrhage on the pinna of a cat that ingested an anticoagulant rodenticide.
Photo courtesy Dr. Gary D. Norsworthy.

Many practices utilize the activated clotting time (ACT) test because it is simple and relatively inexpensive. It evaluates the ability of blood to clot upon exposure to a contact activator (diatomaceous earth). After an atraumatic blood draw, 2 ml is placed into a specialized ACT tube (Becton-Dickinson, Franklin Lakes, NJ). The tube is gently rocked several times and is then immersed in a water bath or placed into a warming block at 37°C. After 60 seconds, the tube is tilted to look for the presence of a gel or clot. If none is observed, the tube is returned to the bath or warming block for another 5–10 seconds and then gently tipped to look for the clot. This continues until a clot is observed. Normal cats have an ACT of less than 75 seconds.

The prothrombin time (PT) detects abnormalities in the factor with the shortest half-life (factor VII) and will identify early or mild cases of toxicity. The activated partial thromboplastin time (APTT) will not prolong until the coagulopathy is more severe. Blood for PT and partial thromboplastin time (PTT) testing should be drawn into a syringe with the original needle replaced by a new one, followed by evacuation into a citrated tube. Tests may be sent out or performed in house with an in-house analyzer.

Vitamin K is the antidote and the mainstay of therapy. It should be initiated whenever ACR poisoning is suspected (especially if lab tests must be sent outside). Initially, it is given subcutaneously, and then the cat can be transitioned to oral therapy. It should *never* be given intravenously because of the risk of anaphylaxis. Length of therapy is dependent upon the bait ingested. In all cases, the ACT should be checked every 3–4 days after vitamin K is discontinued to be sure that the length of therapy has been adequate.

Cholecalciferol Rodenticides

Cholecalciferol, or vitamin D, is contained in a variety of rodenticides. Following ingestion and absorption of the bait, the cat develops hypercalcemia and hyperphosphatemia. Reported signs in cats have included polydipsia, weakness, vomiting, halitosis, and depression. Mineralization of soft tissues is a common necropsy finding. Diagnosis is based upon clinical and laboratory findings and potential exposure to causative baits. Some labs are able to measure vitamin D levels. Treatment is aimed at lowering serum calcium levels. Fluid therapy (0.9% saline recommended), furosemide, and prednisolone are therapies that encourage calcium diuresis. Salmon calcitonin may be helpful in cases that do not respond to other therapies.

Over-the-Counter Medications

Aspirin

Aspirin has a much longer half-life in cats (45 hours) than dogs (7.5 hours) because of the cat's impaired ability to conjugate the drug. Most cases in cats result from unintentional overdosing by owners. This drug can be safely given to cats when dose and dosing interval are carefully monitored. The primary signs of toxicosis are nonspecific and include depression and vomiting.

Treatment of aspirin toxicosis follows the general principles of poison management.

Acetaminophen

Acetaminophen is a human pain reliever that is highly toxic to cats. One regular strength (325 mg) tablet is capable of inducing life-threatening toxicosis in a few hours. Toxic metabolites quickly overwhelm the cat's limited drug conjugation pathways and lead to development of methemoglobinemia and Heinz body hemolytic anemia. Early signs may be nonspecific, but over a period of a few hours, respiratory distress and cyanosis herald the onset of methemoglobinemia. Swelling of the face and paws are sometimes seen and are considered highly correlated with acetaminophen toxicosis. Heinz body hemolytic anemia develops within 24–48 hours (Fig.29-3). Diagnosis can sometimes be confirmed with a thorough history.

Treatment of recent exposure is aimed at gastric emptying through induction of emesis or gastric lavage. Activated charcoal may be helpful if given soon after ingestion. Methemoglobinemia should be treated with NAC to facilitate production of nontoxic metabolites. This drug is available in 10% and 20% solutions and should be diluted to 5% concentration with 5% dextrose. It may be administered orally or intravenously, with a total of five to seven treatments usually given over 48–72 hours. Cimetidine may have additive effects with NAC by inhibiting hepatic drug metabolism and limiting formation of toxic intermediates. S-adenosylmethionine (SAMe, Denosyl® or Denamarin®, Nutramax Laboratories) may help because of its hepatoprotective and antioxidant properties, although it should not be used as sole therapy. Fluid therapy and blood transfusion (or Oxyglobin®) may be indicated if hypoxia persists. Handling of affected cats should be limited because methemoglobinemia alters the ability to handle stress.

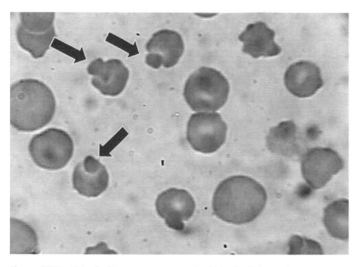

Figure 29-3 Heinz bodies are seen on several red blood cells (arrows).
Photo courtesy Dr. Gary D. Norsworthy.

Phosphorous-Containing Enemas

Phosphate-containing enemas should never be used in cats because they can cause severe hyperphosphatemia and hypocalcemia, sometimes leading to death. Treatment is aimed at restoring normal calcium levels with slow intravenous administration of 10% calcium gluconate. Once the cat is stabilized, continued monitoring of calcium and phosphorous should occur and additional calcium administered as needed. A continuous rate infusion may be prepared with 5% dextrose.

Pharmaceuticals

Methemoglobinemia/Heinz Body-Inducing Drugs

Methemoglobinemia and Heinz body hemolytic anemia may be caused by several pharmaceuticals, which are found in small animal clinics. Topical laryngeal anesthetic sprays that contain benzocaine were once commonly used to facilitate endotracheal intubation of cats. Benzocaine has largely been replaced by lidocaine gel or 2%–4% lidocaine solution. These may be applied to the larynx with a cotton-tipped applicator. The urinary antiseptic methylene blue is another agent that is associated with Heinz body hemolytic anemia in cats.

Insecticides

Permethrin

Permethrin is a synthetic pyrethroid insecticide commonly used in spot-on preparations marketed for flea control in dogs. It has low toxicity in dogs but is highly toxic to cats. Cats are usually exposed when owners fail to read label warnings about its toxicity for cats and inadvertently treat all pets with the same flea product. Veterinary poison control centers report permethrin toxicosis as a common feline poisoning.

Its effects are mediated by continuous stimulation of excitable membranes in muscle and nervous tissue. Consequently, hyperexcitability, muscle tremors, and signs of neurotoxicosis predominate. Other common signs are seizures, twitching, ataxia, and hyperthermia. Signs usually appear within a few hours of application. Diagnosis is based on a history of permethrin application and the presence of typical clinical signs.

Treatment is supportive with a focus on decontamination and control of clinical signs. Dermal decontamination involves bathing the cat with a mild dishwashing detergent and *lukewarm* water, followed by blow drying. The cat should be closely monitored so as to avoid hypothermia after bathing because this can exacerbate the toxicity. Intravenous fluid therapy, muscle relaxants (methocarbamol), anticonvulsants (diazepam or propofol), and hospitalization in a quiet, dark room are the mainstays of therapy because there is no specific antidote. Cats who recover generally have resolution of signs within a few days.

Organophosphates and Carbamates

Organophosphate (OP) and carbamate poisonings have decreased dramatically since safer topical spot-ons have become popular for flea control. These agents bind acetylcholinesterase (AChE), the enzyme that degrades acetylcholine at some receptor sites. Toxic effects are a result of accumulated acetylcholine at nerve endings. Common clinical signs are salivation, lacrimation, urination, and defecation (SLUD). Other findings include vomiting, increased bronchial secretions, bronchospasm, muscle twitching, and weakness. Diagnosis may be confirmed by history of application or determination of blood AChE levels.

Treatment is aimed at decontamination. Bathing with mild dishwashing detergent is indicated. If the cat has been orally exposed, GI decontamination should be considered. In most cases, signs are evident at the time of presentation. Atropine is used to control SLUD signs and is important for relief of respiratory distress but is ineffective against neuromuscular signs (weakness, tremors). Pralidoxime chloride (Protopam chloride [2-PAM]) can relieve the neuromuscular signs not affected by atropine. After a period of time, 2-PAM may be ineffective, but it should be given when OP toxicosis is suspected. It is not effective in carbamate toxicosis. Over-atropinization can be avoided by repeating doses when indicated and not on a prescribed schedule.

General Principles of Poison Management

Initial stabilization and Assessment

Cats with known or suspected toxin exposure should undergo a review of all body systems, with special attention to airway patency, breathing, and circulatory status. Rectal temperature and body weight should be recorded prior to institution of therapy, when possible. Blood and urine should be obtained at this time and, at a minimum, the blood glucose, calcium, packed cell volume (PCV), and total protein determined. In most cases, it is reasonable to place an intravenous catheter to maintain venous access. As soon as possible, a complete blood count, biochemistry profile, and urinalysis should be performed.

Circulation and Cardiovascular Assessment

At presentation, the hydration status, mucous membrane color, capillary refill time, pulse quality, heart rate and rhythm, and mental status should be evaluated. As soon as possible, electrocardiographic monitoring should be initiated.

Breathing and Respiratory Assessment

The respiratory rate and depth should be noted and the patient observed for exaggerated respiratory effort. Lung sounds should be auscultated. Patency of the airway should be determined, and the larynx inspected for edema. During the oral examination, the oral cavity should be examined for debris, ulcers, and oropharyngeal swelling. If indicated, excessive respiratory secretions should be suctioned and oxygen administered via face mask, nasal tube, or intubation.

Neurologic Assessment

The cat's level of alertness should be noted. Seizures should be treated immediately with intravenous diazepam; it may be given rectally if venous access cannot be established.

Nonspecific Therapy

When toxicosis is suspected, nonspecific therapy should be immediately initiated. Good supportive care is essential because the causative toxin may never be identified and, even when known, specific antidotes are rarely available.

Decontamination

Dermal and Ocular Decontamination

Cats in which dermal exposure is suspected should be bathed with a mild dishwashing detergent and clipped, if necessary. Hand soap and shampoos are not recommended as they do not break down greasy substances well. All types of citrus-based products should be avoided. Body temperature should be monitored before and after bathing, and the cat monitored for hypothermia after rinsing. Eyes should be gently rinsed with a saline solution. Gloves should be worn when handling cats with dermal toxins.

Induction of Emesis

Attempts to limit toxin absorption through induction of vomiting are helpful for only the first 1–2 hours after ingestion. Xylazine is the emetic of choice for most clinicians. Some clinicians are beginning to question use of hydrogen peroxide as an emetic because it has been associated with esophagitis in some cats. Apomorphine is a less predictable emetic in cats than dogs and may cause adverse effects in this species. Vomiting should not be induced once signs of poisoning are evident. Contraindications for induction of emesis include weak, depressed, or seizuring patients, those that have ingested petroleum distillates (risk of aspiration), and those that may have ingested a caustic or acidic substance (which may burn the esophagus). Induction of vomiting may add an intolerable level of stress to some patients, especially those with respiratory compromise.

Gastric Lavage

Gastric lavage helps remove ingested toxin from the stomach if induced emesis fails. The cat should be placed under general anesthesia and intubated, with the cuff fully inflated to protect the airway. The head should be lower than the stomach and thorax. A stomach tube with fenestrations on the end should be premeasured; the approximate distance from the oral cavity to the last rib should be determined and the distance should be marked on the tube. The tube is carefully advanced up to the mark, with proper placement confirmed by listening for "bubbling" sounds in the stomach as air is blown into the tube. Small aliquots (5–10 ml/kg) of lukewarm water should be instilled and allowed to drain by gravity. The goal is to retrieve fluid that is clear and free of stomach contents; the majority of lavage fluid should be recovered during the procedure. Activated charcoal may be administered after lavage is complete and while the endotracheal tube is still inflated. Prior to removing the tube, it should be kinked or the end occluded or the syringe left attached to avoid leakage of contents. Complications include water intoxication, esophageal or gastric perforation, and accidental tracheal intubation by the stomach tube. Contraindications to gastric lavage are the same as for induction of emesis.

Activated Charcoal

Charcoal is administered to bind toxic substances in the GI tract, although it does not reliably bind all substances (including EG and plant hydrocarbons). Premixed activated charcoal is convenient and less messy than powdered formulations. Premixed products often contain a cathartic, such as sorbitol, to hasten transit of material through the GI tract. Administering charcoal by syringe is less than ideal because this increases the risk of aspiration. If gastric lavage has been performed, charcoal may be administered before the tube is removed. Charcoal is contraindicated in the vomiting patient. Although charcoal may limit absorption of toxins, it may also interfere with treatment by binding oral therapeutic agents in the GI tract.

Fluid Therapy

Fluid therapy is useful for hastening the elimination of toxins from the body. A crystalloid solution, such as lactated Ringer's solution, is usually a good first choice. Because cats are easily volume overloaded, a conservative rate of fluid administration (10–15 ml/kg/hr) should be adopted until the patient is completely assessed and monitoring parameters are established. Urine output should be recorded. If an indwelling urinary catheter cannot be placed, absorbent underpads should be placed in the cage to subjectively monitor for adequate urination.

Suggested Readings

Crystal MA. 2010. Rodenticide Toxicosis. In GD Norsworthy, ed., *The Feline Patient*, 4th ed., pp. 466–67. Ames: Wiley-Blackwell.

Grace SF. 2010. Acetaminophen Toxicosis. In GD Norsworthy, ed., *The Feline Patient*, 4th ed., pp. 5–6. Ames: Wiley-Blackwell.

Grace SF. 2010. Aspirin Toxicosis. In GD Norsworthy, ed., *The Feline Patient*, 4th ed., p. 32. Ames: Wiley-Blackwell.

Grace SF. 2010. Heinz Body Hemolytic Anemia and Methemoglobinemia. In GD Norsworthy, ed., *The Feline Patient*, 4th ed., pp. 211—12. Ames: Wiley-Blackwell.

Grave T, Boag A. 2010. Feline Toxicological Emergencies. *J Fel Med Surg.* 12(11):849–60.

Lovelace KM. 2010. Hypocalcemia. In GD Norsworthy, ed., *The Feline Patient*, 4th ed., pp. 270–71. Ames: Wiley-Blackwell.

Lovelace KM. 2010. Plant Toxicities. In GD Norsworthy, ed., *The Feline Patient*, 4th ed., pp. 402–11. Ames: Wiley-Blackwell.

Norsworthy GD. 2010. Organophosphate and Carbamate Toxicosis. In GD Norsworthy, ed., *The Feline Patient*, 4th ed., p. 364. Ames: Wiley-Blackwell.

Norsworthy GD. 2010. Pyrethrin and Pyrethroid Toxicosis. In GD Norsworthy, ed., *The Feline Patient*, 4th ed., p. 439. Ames: Wiley-Blackwell.

Norsworthy GD. 2010. Vitamin D Toxicosis. In GD Norsworthy, ed., *The Feline Patient*, 4th ed., pp. 553–54. Ames: Wiley-Blackwell.

Rosendale ME. 2002. Decontamination Strategies. In RH Poppenga, PA Volmer, eds., *Vet Clin North Am Small Anim Pract.* 32(2):311–21. St. Louis: Elsevier.

Weissova T, Norsworthy GD. 2010. Ethylene Glycol Toxicosis. In GD Norsworthy, ed., *The Feline Patient*, 4th ed., pp. 167–68. Ames: Wiley-Blackwell.

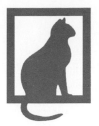

CHAPTER 30

Urinary Tract Diseases

Linda E. Schmeltzer and Gary D. Norsworthy

Overview

The urinary tract consists of the kidneys, ureters, urinary bladder, and urethra. The kidneys and ureters comprise the upper urinary tract; the urinary bladder and urethra comprise the lower urinary tract. Thus, urinary tract diseases are often referred to as upper urinary tract disease or lower urinary tract disease, based on the organ(s) involved.

Kidney disease is a common disorder in cats. It is one of the leading causes of death in geriatric cats. The kidneys serve as a waste filtration and elimination plant for metabolic waste in the blood. The renal artery carries blood into the kidneys. Inside the kidney it divides and subdivides into smaller arteries and capillaries. Blood pressure forces some of the plasma (water and dissolved blood components) to filter out of the blood through fenestrations in the capillaries, a process called glomerular filtration. As the filtrate continues through the kidney, the water and usable blood components are reabsorbed into the blood. The purified blood leaves the kidney through the renal vein. The unusable components filter into the renal pelvis, out through the ureter, and into the urinary bladder as urine. These processes are called tubular reabsorption and tubular secretion. If any of these processes are compromised due to aging, disease, or trauma, filtration becomes less effective and waste products will build up in the blood.

Each kidney has an outflow duct called a ureter. Urine is constantly being produced by the kidneys and channeled through the ureters to the bladder. The ureters are tube-shaped structures consisting of three layers. The outer fibrous layer is made up of connective tissue containing blood vessels and nerves and functions as an anchor to keep the ureters in place. The middle muscular layer contains smooth muscle fibers that move urine through the ureter with peristaltic (wave-like) contractions. The inner mucosal layer is lined with transitional epithelial cells that allow the ureter to inflate and deflate as urine passes through it on the way to and into the urinary bladder. As the bladder fills the opening of the ureter collapses (closes) to prevent urine from flowing back into the ureters. The peristaltic contractions are strong enough to force urine through the collapsed opening.

The urinary bladder is an elastic organ that changes shape according to the amount of urine it contains. It resembles a deflated balloon when empty but becomes somewhat pear-shaped and ascends into the abdominal cavity as the volume of urine increases. The urinary bladder is lined with transitional epithelial cells that allow it to stretch as it becomes filled with urine. The wall of the bladder becomes thinner as the volume of urine within the bladder increases. When the bladder reaches a certain volume muscles in its wall will stretch and stimulate the nerve endings in the bladder wall. Impulses are sent up the nerves to the brain telling the cat that it needs to urinate. When the sensation occurs normal cats are able to voluntarily tighten the muscle around the neck of the bladder. When a suitable place to urinate has been located, the cat will posture and voluntarily relax this muscle to pass urine out of the bladder and through the urethra to the outside.

Kidney function is measured with various blood and urine values. The most commonly used blood values are creatinine and blood urea nitrogen (BUN). The creatinine value is considered more specific for kidney function because it is less influenced by nonrenal factors (diet, dehydration, or liver disease) that often affect the BUN. However, emaciation will result in a lower creatinine value than would be expected; therefore, it is important to consider the body condition score when interpreting creatinine values. The most commonly used urine test for kidney function is a urinalysis, and the most important value in that test group is urine specific gravity. In theory, urine specific gravity less than 1.035 indicates kidney disease; however, the cat is able to concentrate urine better than most species, so that value is not as reliable as in other species.

Kidney insufficiency

Kidney insufficiency occurs when the kidneys are no longer able to efficiently perform their normal function of removing waste products from the blood. Kidney deterioration occurs slowly as the kidneys undergo various disease processes or microscopic, irreversible aging changes. Depending on the cause, this process can take months or years. An elevation in blood values (BUN and creatinine) will not occur until about 75% of kidney function is lost. A cat with a blood creatinine value above normal and up to about 440–530 umol/L (5.0–6.0 mg/dl) has kidney insufficiency. Clinical signs will become more severe as the creatinine value increases. Because the waste product is building up in the blood the body increases blood flow through the kidneys producing more urine. Kidney insufficiency eventually progresses to kidney failure, a state of renal decompensation that usually leads to death.

For most cats, clinical signs will begin to appear between the ages of 9 and 14 years. A gradual decrease in weight and appetite and a gradual increase in water consumption and urine output per day will occur. These signs often go undetected by owners for months. Owners will usually note slight increases in the number or size of urinations, based on the amount of wet litter in the litter box, before noticing slight changes in thirst. Therefore, when taking a history questions about the quantity of wet litter in the litter box are important. Because the change is slight an owner might not realize it is important to mention this to a technician or veterinarian. Multicat households make detection in water consumption and urine output more difficult to detect.

Kidney insufficiency is often identified during routine blood screening. Laboratory findings include a creatinine value between 220 and 520 umol/L (2.5–6.0 mg/dl) and low urine specific gravity on a urinalysis. As the filtering ability of the kidneys declines and creatinine levels increase, anemia, elevation of blood phosphorus, decrease of blood potassium, and metabolic acidosis (imbalance of acid levels) may occur. Because of the flow of blood through smaller kidneys, hypertension (high blood pressure) may be present in many of these cats.

The purpose of treatment is to increase kidney function and slow further deterioration. Treatments are chosen based on clinical signs, test results, capabilities and motivation of the owner, and the cooperation level of the cat.

Kidney Diet

A restricted protein diet helps minimize the waste products filtered through the kidneys. These diets have decreased phosphorus, increased potassium, and are nonacidifying. For a picky eater this can be a difficult transition, so it is important to offer a choice of more than one renal diet and to educate the owner on the proper way to transition to a new food.

Nursing the Feline Patient, First Edition. Edited by Linda E. Schmeltzer and Gary D. Norsworthy.
© 2012 John Wiley & Sons, Inc. Published 2012 by John Wiley & Sons, Inc.

Benazepril

Recent studies have shown benazepril may slow the progression of kidney disease by reducing glomerular blood pressure (renal hypertension). Renal hypertension is likely one of the major causes of progression of kidney disease.

Rehydration and Diuresis

Depending on the creatinine levels, some cats will need to be hospitalized for fluid therapy. Intravenous (IV) or subcutaneous (SC) fluids will correct dehydration and assist the kidneys in flushing out the waste products in the blood. This flushing process, known as diuresis, is designed to maximize the function of all remaining kidney tissue.

Client Administered Fluids

Fluids can be administered subcutaneously two to seven times per week to keep hydration levels up and aid in diuresis. Most owners easily master the technique, and most cats tolerate it well. Technicians and assistants play a vital role in teaching and reassuring owners. It is important to have patience and understanding with them, especially during the initial learning phase. Occasionally an owner will prefer to bring the cat into the office for fluid administration. Performing this treatment with the owner present may serve as a coaching opportunity for him or her to become more comfortable with the technique and can also be used as a time to assess how the cat is doing at home with other prescribed treatments.

Phosphate Binder

If a kidney diet alone does not reduce elevated phosphorus levels in the blood, a phosphate binder can be prescribed. Phosphate binders attach to phosphorus in the intestinal tract, preventing the phosphorus from being absorbed. Blood levels are usually monitored so the dosage can be adjusted properly. Some of the available phosphate binders contain calcium. If a rise in blood calcium levels occurs, a veterinarian can prescribe a product that does not contain calcium, most commonly aluminum hydroxide. The desired serum phosphorus level is less than 1.9 mmol/L (6 mg/dL).

Calcitriol

This drug regulates the parathyroid gland and calcium levels. An increase in blood phosphorus level stimulates the parathyroid gland to increase the blood calcium level by removing calcium from the bones. This helps to normalize the needed 2:1 ratio of calcium to phosphorus. Calcitriol can be used to reduce the function of the parathyroid gland and to increase calcium absorption from the intestinal tract. Data for its efficacy in cats is pending.

Erythropoietin Replacement

Feline red blood cells live an average of 68 days, after which they are broken down and must be replaced by new cells. The kidneys produce erythropoietin, the hormone that stimulates the production of red blood cells by the bone marrow. The presence of a nonregenerative anemia could indicate the production of erythropoietin has been impaired or stopped. Administration of synthetic forms of erythropoietin can help correct this anemia in most cats.

Hypotensive Agent

If testing determines the cat has high blood pressure medication may be prescribed to control the blood pressure, helping to prevent blindness and strokes.

Appetite Stimulant

Imbalance of acid levels caused by decreased filtration in the kidneys may cause an increase of stomach acid resulting in nausea or loss of appetite. An acid reducer (H2 antagonist), such as famotidine, may be helpful in improving appetite. Mirtazapine and cyproheptadine can be effective appetite stimulants for some cats.

Client Education

During the first 3 months of treatment some cats have decreases in creatinine values, even into the normal range. It is important for the owner to understand that this event is an indication that the treatment is working; therefore, treatment should be continued rather than stopped. Regularly scheduled rechecks are important to assess creatinine and other blood values, as well as to monitor weight and clinical signs. Patient history should include questions about diet, appetite, and overall attitude.

Prognosis

The prognosis depends to a large extent on how much kidney tissue is functional, how well the patient adjusts to the prescribed treatment, and how closely the owner follows the treatment plan. In most situations many cats respond well to treatment and have good quality of life. They may often live 1–3 years before the onset of kidney failure.

Kidney Failure, Chronic

Chronic kidney failure is often the result of several diseases or insults to the kidney over many years. These include pyelonephritis, exposure to toxins, normal aging, or trauma. The exact cause usually can not be determined. Chronic kidney failure is typically preceded by kidney insufficiency.

A cat in kidney failure will have a creatinine level higher than 485 umol/L (5.5 mg/dl). The most common clinical signs are weight loss, anorexia, lethargy, increased urination, and increased thirst. Poor hair coat, diarrhea, and bad breath may also be present. Vomiting may occur but is less common than in dogs. Blindness can occur if severe high blood pressure occurs. Many patients will be dehydrated and emaciated and have pale mucous membranes. On palpation, the kidneys are usually smaller than normal. Abnormal kidney size can also be documented with radiographs or ultrasound.

Laboratory findings can include azotemia (increased BUN and creatinine), low urine specific gravity, nonregenerative anemia, hyperphosphatemia (elevation of blood phosphorus), hypokalemia (low blood potassium), and metabolic acidosis (imbalance of acid levels). Because pyelonephritis is a recognized cause of kidney failure, a urine culture can detect bacterial infection. As with kidney insufficiency, these cats may also have systemic hypertension.

Treatment for chronic kidney failure usually requires hospitalization for rehydration and diuresis. If enough functional kidney cells remain they may be able to adequately meet the body's need for waste removal with the help of IV fluids. The purpose is to substantially increase kidney function resulting in a decrease of BUN and creatinine levels. Potassium supplementation may be added to the fluids, if needed.

Nutritional support via orogastric or nasogastric feeding may be needed for anorexic patients. Some patients may have a red blood cell count low enough to require a blood transfusion. Treatments prescribed in the kidney insufficiency section may also be used at the discretion of a veterinarian. Blood profiles should be repeated during treatment to determine progress.

If there is no improvement in blood values after 3–5 days of fluid therapy, the prognosis is poor. If there is improvement in the blood tests and the cat begins eating, treatment can continue at home (see kidney insufficiency section for treatment list), and the prognosis is favorable.

A successfully treated cat will typically have kidney values of kidney insufficiency but not normal kidney values. Thus, it will need long-term treatment.

Kidney Failure, Acute

Acute kidney failure (AKF) is a disease of rapid onset, usually occurring within a few days. It is less common than chronic kidney failure. AKF is the result of an acute disease process that adversely affects kidney function. Some of the possible causes of AKF include toxins (from drugs, chemicals [antifreeze] or plants [lilies]), trauma (resulting in loss or decrease in blood supply), pyelonephritis, hypotension during anesthesia, and urethral obstruction. When taking a history, asking questions about onset, duration, and progression of the illness are important. Also include questions about environment and possible exposure or access to toxic plants, medications, or chemicals. A list of medications the cat has recently taken may also be helpful. Clinical signs can vary but may include anorexia, lethargy, kidney pain, or vomiting.

Laboratory findings will include an elevated BUN and creatinine as with chronic kidney failure. The most reliable way to determine the difference between acute and chronic kidney failure is the red blood cell count. With AKF the red blood cell count will typically be normal; do not fail to account for dehydration when interpreting packed cell volume values. Additional tests, such as urine culture or an ethylene glycol test, may also be required to help determine the cause. Radiographs and ultrasound can be ordered to determine if there are stones causing a blockage in the kidney or ureters.

Treatment will be determined largely by the disease process that caused the acute kidney failure. IV fluid therapy for rehydration and diuresis will probably be prescribed. Antibiotics or medications to reduce vomiting may also be needed. If fluid therapy at a high rate of infusion is prescribed or if cardiac compromise is present, overhydration is a risk. A veterinarian may request weighing the cat frequently, as an increase in weight can be an indication of overhydration. The cat should also be monitored for other signs of overhydration such as elevations in breathing or heart rate, serous nasal discharge, and swelling of the tissue that lines the eyelids and surface of the eye.

Prognosis will vary depending on the cause and how quickly the cat received treatment. A successfully treated cat will usually have kidney insufficiency and will need long-term treatment.

Pyelonephritis

Pyelonephritis is an infection in the kidney. More specifically it is inflammation of the renal pelvis and parenchyma, which is part of the kidney where filtration occurs (Fig. 30-1). Bacteria typically access the kidneys either by ascending up the ureters from the bladder or via the bloodstream from infections elsewhere in the body. Periodontal disease is thought to be a common source of the bacteria that causes pyelonephritis in cats.

Clinical signs of pyelonephritis can include increased urination, increased thirst, weight loss, and lethargy. There may also be low grade fever, pain in the kidneys, abdomen, or lumbar area when palpated, and even signs of cystitis. Many of these patients have an infection that has been ongoing for several weeks or longer and will often present for chronic renal failure.

Laboratory findings on a urinalysis can show bacteria, elevated protein, occult blood, and leukocyte (white blood cell) casts. If more than 75% of kidney function has been lost, the blood profile will include an increase in BUN, creatinine, and phosphorus, nonregenerative anemia, hypokalemia, and metabolic acidosis. An excretory urogram or ultrasound of the kidneys can be performed to confirm the diagnosis and assess damage done to the kidneys by the infection.

The cornerstone of treatment is identification of the bacteria causing the infection. Antibiotic therapy is prescribed for 4–6 weeks, based on

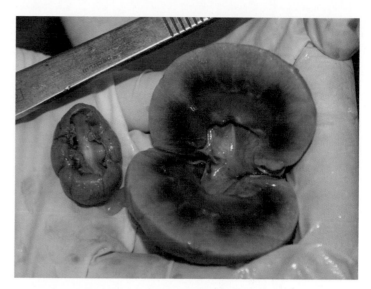

Figure 30-1 Pyelonephritis is characterized by a dilated renal pelvis. Both of these kidneys exhibit that characteristic. The small kidney was damaged severely and shrank. The large kidney sustained some damage but enlarged (hypertrophied) so it could do the work of both.

urine culture results. Some patients will require up to 12 weeks of therapy with a rotation of antibiotics based on bacterial culture and sensitivity findings. Urine cultures should be repeated approximately 1 week after the completion of antibiotics to confirm the infection has been cleared. If the culture is negative, it should be repeated 4–6 weeks later to verify that the infection has definitely cleared. Clients should be educated to return the cat for an examination anytime the cat is not acting well or is showing signs of cystitis (frequent urination, blood in the urine, or straining to urinate). If chronic renal insufficiency or failure has also occurred, long-term support for kidney function may be needed.

The prognosis is generally good if a diagnosis is made before extensive permanent damage occurs to the kidneys. Cats that are not treated early usually have some permanent kidney damage (see Figure 30-1), which will eventually lead to chronic renal failure; however, this may not occur for several years.

Polycystic Kidney Disease

Polycystic kidney disease (PKD) is an inherited disorder that occurs in man, cats, dogs, and mice. In cats it most commonly affects Persians and other long-haired cats. Studies in Persians have shown that the disorder is inherited as a dominant trait. PKD causes fluid-filled cysts to develop throughout the kidney, increasing in number and size over time (Fig. 30-2a). As the cysts grow, they compress and replace normal functioning kidney tissue with nonfunctional fluid-filled compartments, ultimately causing renal failure. Cysts can occur in one or both kidneys and may also develop in the liver. PKD can be present in kittens as well as older cats.

Clinical signs of a cat with severe PKD will be identical to those of a cat in chronic kidney failure. Enlargement of one or both kidneys may be palpated or seen on a radiograph. An ultrasound will reveal multiple fluid-filled cysts throughout the kidney (Fig. 30-2b).

Treatment is directed toward the resulting kidney failure that the cysts eventually cause. Secondary bacterial infections of the cysts are possible, requiring appropriate antibiotic therapy. There is not a treatment available to remove the cysts.

Cats affected with PKD will develop chronic kidney failure as adults. The average age of onset of kidney failure is 7 years, although in many cats it occurs at less than 3 years. The long-term prognosis depends on

(a)

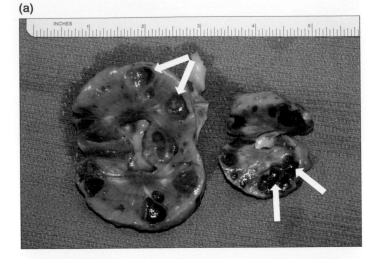

(b)

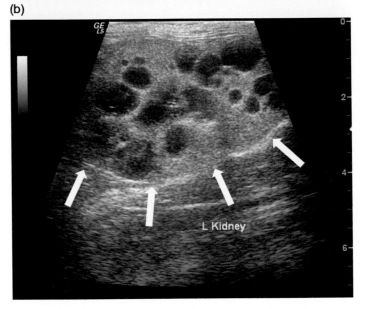

Figure 30-2 Polycystic kidney disease results in multiple cysts forming in the kidney tissue. (a) The arrows point to several cysts in both kidneys. As in Figure 30-1, the large kidney hypertrophied so it could do the work of both. (b) An ultrasound study of this polycystic kidney shows many cysts *(black areas)* of varying sizes. The arrows point to the renal capsule.

the age of the cat when clinical signs appear and the severity and progression of the resulting kidney failure. Some cats die within a few weeks of diagnosis, others can live comfortably for several years. Few cats with PKD live past 10 years of age.

Littermates and parents of affected cats should have periodic ultrasound screenings for PKD. Early detection allows early therapy to support kidney function.

Urolithiasis

Uroliths, also known as stones, are rocklike mineral structures that are formed in the urinary tract. The two most common types are struvite uroliths and calcium oxalate uroliths. Other types of uroliths that have been identified in cats include calcium phosphate and urate. Stones may also be of mixed composition, comprised of both struvite and calcium oxalate. Uroliths may occur singularly or as multiple stones. The size and shape of uroliths can also vary. Male and female cats are affected equally.

Clinical signs of a cat with bladder uroliths generally include hematuria (blood in the urine) and dysuria (straining to urinate). The irritated bladder can be painful. Hematuria occurs when the surface of the bladder wall bleeds from the irritation of the stones. Dysuria is caused by a stone partially or fully obstructing the passage of urine.

The specific cause of urolith formation is unknown. Diet may contribute in some cases. The urine commonly contains an increased concentration of materials that can produce crystals. For example, struvite crystals are composed of ammonium, magnesium, and phosphate. Cats that have crystals in their urine may not necessarily develop uroliths. Urine pH may also play a role in urolith formation. Struvite crystals dissolve readily in acidic urine, and form readily in alkaline urine. Uric acid crystals dissolve readily in alkaline urine but not in acid urine.

Diagnosis can be obtained with radiography or ultrasound (Fig. 30-3). Special procedure radiography may be ordered if stones are suspected but not visible on routine radiographs. Refer to Chapter 7. Palpation of uroliths within the bladder is not usually possible because the uroliths are typically relatively small. Imagine trying to locate a small pebble inside a water balloon. Every time the balloon is squeezed the pebble will quickly move way from your hand before you can grasp it.

There are several treatment options available. Cystotomy (surgical incision into the urinary bladder) can be performed to remove the uroliths if they are in the bladder. An alternative to surgery is using a therapeutic diet that will alter the pH of the urine, thereby dissolving the urolith. This treatment has been proven successful only with struvite uroliths. Not all cats will eat the special diet that must be fed exclusively for several months. Surgery is generally required for removal for removal of uroliths in the ureter or urethra (Fig. 30-3d).

If the chosen treatment is successful the prognosis is favorable. If the urolith is removed surgically or retrieved after passing out the urethra it should be sent to a commercial laboratory for analysis. To prevent recurrences a special diet or medications to adjust urine pH can be prescribed based on the urolith analysis.

Feline Idiopathic Cystitis

Cystitis is inflammation in the urinary bladder. A bacterial infection, a bladder stone, or bladder trauma can cause cystitis. However, cats have a specific form of cystitis that has eluded our understanding of its cause even after decades of research. It has been called by many terms: feline urologic syndrome, feline lower urinary tract disease (FLUTD), and interstitial cystitis. Currently the best term is feline idiopathic cystitis (FIC) because the cause is unknown.

Various causes have been proposed over the last 40 years including dry cat food, cat food with high ash (mineral) content, fish flavored cat food, high pH producing cat food, cat food with high magnesium content, and stress. None of these have been proven to be the cause, and it is possible that there are several factors that occur together to cause FIC.

FIC causes inflammation of the bladder wall, changes in urine pH, hematuria (blood in the urine), pollikuria (increased frequency of urination), and dysuria (difficulty urinating or straining to urinate). These clinical signs are common to all forms of cystitis because they represent the way the bladder responds to an insult of any type.

Diagnosis of FIC is based on the presence of two or more of the listed clinical signs and the ruling out of other causes of cystitis. The urinalysis of a cat with FIC may be normal, but it usually has abnormal changes in pH, blood content, and crystal content. Most affected cats have a high pH and struvite crystals; others have a low pH and calcium oxalate crystals. The consistent finding is the lack of bacteria on a urine culture.

There are two forms of FIC, the obstructive form and the nonobstructive form. The obstructive form results in formation of a mucous and crystal plug that obstructs the urethra (see below). The nonobstructive form causes the classic clinical signs of cystitis for several days and then spontaneously resolves.

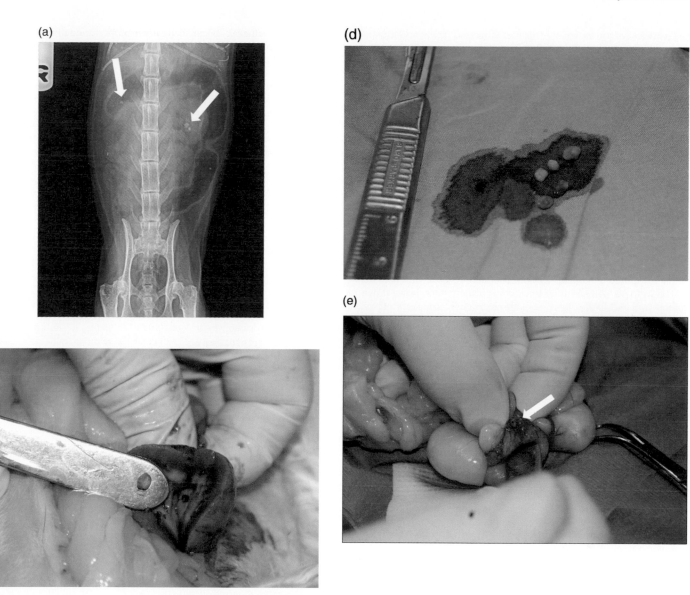

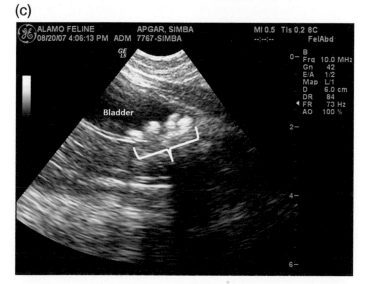

Figure 30-3 (a) This radiograph shows one small urolith in the pelvis of the right kidney and two medium-sized uroliths in the left kidney. The arrows point to the uroliths. (b) One of the uroliths in the left kidney is shown at necropsy. The kidney has been cut open. (c) Several uroliths are seen in this ultrasound study of the urinary bladder. They are within the bracket. (d) Five uroliths were removed from the bladder of the cat in figure c. (e) a 1-mm urolith is shown being removed from a ureter at surgery (arrow).

Treatment of the obstructive form is addressed herein and must occur promptly because urethral obstruction of any cause is life threatening. There have been many treatments used for the nonobstructive form, most of which have resulted in a cure. However, because this is a self-limiting disease, even no treatment, sometimes called tincture of time, will result in a cure. The use of anti-inflammatory or antispasmodic drugs is the most common approach.

Urethral Obstruction

Urethral obstruction is a serious emergency and requires immediate treatment. It can be fatal if urine flow is not restored within 24–48 hours. It is possible for a female cat to develop a urethral obstruction; however, it is much more common in males. In male cats even the smallest uroliths may be unable to pass because the male urethra tapers down to about 0.5 mm in diameter as it exits the body. Stones will travel down the urethra and become lodged, blocking the flow of urine out of the bladder (Fig. 30-4).

Uroliths are only one possible cause of urethral obstruction. Urethral plugs composed of a mucus-like material may also cause an obstruction.

The kidneys will continue to produce urine, which flows down the ureters into the bladder. Because of the obstruction, urine cannot pass out of the body, and the bladder will become excessively large and painful.

The most common clinical sign of a cat with a urethral obstruction is severe abdominal pain. Owners may report the cat making frequent trips to the litter box and unsuccessfully attempting to urinate. This is often misinterpreted as constipation. Physical examination will reveal a large firm bladder. Use caution when palpating or trying to express the bladder; the wall may be thin and fragile, and excessive force can cause it to rupture.

Diagnosis may be based on the obvious physical examination findings. Radiography or ultrasound can be used to confirm the diagnosis. Blood profiles should be ordered to determine if damage to the kidneys has occurred and to assess electrolyte status. Obstruction to urine flow will always result in elevated BUN and creatinine values that typically return to normal within 48–72 hours after relief of the obstruction.

Treatment includes relieving the obstruction. If the patient has multiple recurrences of urethral obstruction or if the veterinarian is unable to relieve an obstruction, a perineal urethrostomy may be recommended. Relieving urethral obstruction may be accomplished by using a technique to carefully flush the urethra and clear the obstruction. Once the obstruction is relieved an indwelling urinary catheter can be placed. The catheter must be placed carefully to prevent damage to the urethra. It can

be left in place for 1–2 days to allow for proper urine drainage from the bladder. During this time the cat may also need IV fluid therapy for rehydration and diuresis.

With proper treatment prognosis is favorable. Once the indwelling urinary catheter is removed the patient should be monitored closely for urine output because recurrence of a blockage within a few hours of catheter removal is possible. If the kidneys suffered damage treatment for kidney insufficiency may be required. The owner should monitor the cat's urine output closely and return for further treatment at the first signs of distress.

Bladder Atony

If the urethral obstruction is not relieved within 24 hours, the bladder may distend to the point that the muscles in the wall of the bladder become unable to contract. This is called bladder atony. This is a reversible condition as long as the bladder does not remain distended. Expression of the bladder several times per day, continued use of an indwelling catheter, or drugs that stimulate smooth muscle contraction, such as bethanechol, will usually reverse the condition in a few days. The cat is typically hospitalized until it can urinate freely on its own.

Perineal Urethrostomy

Perineal urethrostomy is a surgical procedure that removes the very narrow portion of the urethra in male cats. During the procedure, the penis is removed because this is the location of the smallest urethral diameter. The portion of the urethra with the larger diameter is then sutured to the skin, creating a new urethral opening and a urethra of consistently large diameter.

Postoperatively it is extremely important that an Elizabethan collar or other comfortable restraint device is used for about 48 hours so the cat cannot reach the surgery site to groom or clean. The urethra and skin are sutured with multiple tiny sutures. If the cat tries to clean the area too soon damage can occur to the surgery site, resulting in complications which are difficult to correct.

Suggested Readings

Colville J. 2008. The Urinary System. In T Colville, JM Bassert, eds., *Clinical Anatomy and Physiology for Veterinary Technicians*, 2nd ed. pp. 374–86. St. Louis: Mosby Inc.

Grace SF. 2011. Renal Failure, Acute. In GD Norsworthy, ed., *The Feline Patient*, 4th ed., pp. 452–54. Ames: Wiley-Blackwell.

Marshall R. 2011. Urethral Obstruction. In GD Norsworthy, ed., *The Feline Patient*, 4th ed., pp. 530–34. Ames: Wiley-Blackwell.

Norsworthy GD. 2011. Renal Failure, Chronic. In GD Norsworthy, ed., *The Feline Patient*, 4th ed., pp. 455–56. Ames: Wiley-Blackwell.

Norsworthy GD. 2011. Renal Insufficiency. In GD Norsworthy, ed., *The Feline Patient*, 4th ed., pp. 457–59. Ames: Wiley-Blackwell.

Norsworthy GD. 2011. Urolithiasis. In GD Norsworthy, ed., *The Feline Patient*, 4th ed., pp. 538–42. Ames: Wiley-Blackwell.

Weissova T, Norsworthy G. Feline Idiopathic Cystitis. In GD Norsworthy, ed., *The Feline Patient*, 4th ed., pp. 176–78. Ames: Wiley-Blackwell.

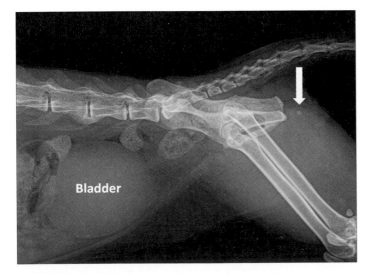

Figure 30-4 The arrow points to a urolith in the urethra. The resulting urethral obstruction resulted in a full urinary bladder.

Index

Abdomen
  physical exam of, 6, 26
  radiology of, 38–43
  ultrasound of, 43–6
Abortion, 21, 182, 194
Abscess, periapical, 147
ACE inhibitor *see* Angiotensin-converting
  enzyme (ACE) inhibitors
Acepromazine, 113, 124
Acetaminophen, toxicity, 210
Acetylcholine, 210
Acetylcholinesterase, 210
Achromotrichia, 27
Acidosis, 115, 127 *see also* Metabolic acidosis
  on blood chemistry, 92–3, 127
Acne, 167
Activated charcoal, 209–11
Acupuncture, 134, 140
Adenocarcinoma, cytology, 78
Adenosine triphosphate (ATP), 93
Adrenal gland
  location of, 40, 46
  on ultrasound, 46, 49
Age approximation, dental eruption times, 146
Agglutination, 101–2, 104
Aging changes, 26
Albumin
  in blood chemistry panel, 91, 92–3
  in conjugation of bilirubin, 182
Alcohol, for surgical scrub, 120
Aleurostrongylus Abstrusus, 201
Allergy, 164–6
Allergy testing, 164–5
Alopecia, 167–8, 197
Alopecia, psychogenic, 166
Alpha cells, function of, 178
Alpha-2 agonist
  blood pressure, 124
  and capillary refill time, 122
  contraindications, 124
  definition of, 124
  effects on heart function, 124
  and general anesthesia, 116
  and opiods for pain, 122
  and sedation, 123
Aluminum hydroxide, 214
Alveolar sac *see* Alveoli
Alveoli
  in capnography, 126
  damage to, 117
  function, 204
Amino acid
  in dilated cardiomyopathy, 161
  in red blood cell breakdown, 172
  in thyroid function, 178
Ammonia, conversion to urea, 92

Amylase, in blood chemistry, 94
Anal reflex, 15
Analgesia, 129–35
  definition of, 131
  multimodal, 131–2
Analgesic drugs, 132–4
Anaphylaxis, and Vitamin K administration,
  209
Ancylostoma tubaeforme, 201–2
Anemia
  evaluation by impedance counter, 87
  with hepatic lipidosis, 174
  with kidney diseases, 213–15
  on a manual blood smear, 89, 101
  and propofol use, 115
  types of, 91
  with parasite infestation, 199–202
  with toxicosis, 210
  with viral diseases, 183–4, 194
Anesthesia
  general, 113
  recovery, 136
  sedation, 113
Angiotensin-converting enzyme (ACE)
  inhibitors
  effects on anesthesia, 113
  heart disease, 159
Anisocoria, 5
Anisocytosis
  definition of, 102
  on hemogram, 91
  of platelets, 91
Anodontia *see* Missing teeth
Anorexia
  with abnormal blood values, 92–4
  with hepatic lipidosis, 173–5
  with inflammatory hepatitis, 175
  with lymphosarcoma, 79
  with parasite infestation, 199, 202
  with toxicosis, 208
Anterior chamber, 179, 187, 193
Anterior cruciate ligament *see* Cranial cruciate
  ligament rupture, physical therapy
Anticholinergic drug, 125
Anticoagulant
  rodenticides, 209
  sample handling, 82, 97
Anticonvulsant, permethrin toxicity, 210
Antifreeze, 209, 215
Antigen
  FeLV testing, 95, 189
  FIV testing, 95
  giardia testing, 203
  heartworm testing, 95, 207
Antiseptic, in surgical preperation, 120
Anxiolytics, 134

Aorta
  imaging, 37, 46, 157, 161
  position in the heart muscle, 165
Aortic thromboembolism *see*
  Thromboembolism
Apnea, monitoring, 136–7
Apomorphine, 211
Appetite stimulant, 174, 214
Arrector pili, 164
Arrhythmia
  during anesthesia, 124–6
  on ECG, 156
  and heart disease, 159–61
Arthritis *see* Osteoarthritis
Artifacts
  on blood smears, 74, 99–100
  radiology, 32–3; 41
Ascarids *see* Roundworms
Ascites, 159–60, 186
Aspiration
  of bladder, 67
  fine-needle, 70–71
  into lungs during anesthesia, 116, 119, 136
  ultrasound guided needle, 33, 36, 38
Aspirin, blood clots, 160
Aspirin toxicosis, 210
Assisted standing, 141, 143
Asthma, 204–5
Ataxia
  with ear mites, 195
  with FIV, 182
  with toxicosis, 208–10
Atenolol, 160
Atopic dermatitis *see* Atopy
Atopy, 164
Atrophy
  of iris, 26–7
  muscle, 138, 140, 152–3
  muscle, physical therapy for, 138,
    140, 142–3
Atropine
  for bradycardia, 125
  for SLUD treatment, 211
Aural hematoma, 205–6

Bain anesthesia system, 116
Balanced anesthesia, 124
Barium, 40–42
Barium series, 40
Basal cell tumor, 78
Base Narrow Canine Teet, 147
Basophil, 91, 106
Beetle, as intermediate host, 198–200
Benazepril, for kidney disease, 214
Benign characteristics, cytology, 78,
Benzodiazepines, 113

Nursing the Feline Patient, First Edition. Edited by Linda E. Schmeltzer and Gary D. Norsworthy.
© 2012 John Wiley & Sons, Inc. Published 2012 by John Wiley & Sons, Inc.